MW01291930

Turner Syndrome

Patricia Y. Fechner

Editor

Turner Syndrome

Pathophysiology, Diagnosis and Treatment

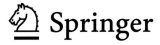 Springer

Editor
Patricia Y. Fechner
Division of Endocrinology
Seattle Children's Hospital
University of Washington
Seattle, WA
USA

ISBN 978-3-030-34148-0   ISBN 978-3-030-34150-3   (eBook)
https://doi.org/10.1007/978-3-030-34150-3

This Springer imprint is published by the registered company Springer Nature Switzerland AG
The registered company address is: Gewerbestrasse 11, 6330 Cham, Switzerland

To my parents, thank you for all of your love and support.

Preface

The purpose of this book is to provide a resource for providers who care for girls and women with Turner syndrome. Turner syndrome occurs in 1:1800–2000 females, yet many providers may not have a lot of experience caring for a female with Turner syndrome. Patients with Turner syndrome have many of the same health issues as other females, but some health issues are at a higher frequency that necessitates more frequent and earlier screening.

Many contributors to this work are experts in the care of females with Turner syndrome, while others are experts in their own field of medicine who can apply this expertise to the care of individuals with Turner syndrome. They all have worked on this project as a labor of love and for the benefit of the girl or woman with Turner syndrome. I wish to thank each of them for their significant contributions to this book.

The chapters in the book are organized by subspecialty and/or major health issue, with the goal to provide in-depth coverage of the health issues faced by those with Turner syndrome.

Seattle, WA, USA   Patricia Y. Fechner, MD

Contents

Contributors

Anna M. Acosta, MD Memorial Care and Miller Children's and Women's Hospital, Long Beach, CA, USA

Margaret P. Adam, MD Division of Genetic Medicine, Department of Pediatrics, University of Washington School of Medicine and Seattle Children's Hospital, Seattle, WA, USA

Philippe Backeljauw, MD The Cincinnati Center for Pediatric and Adult Turner Syndrome Care, Cincinnati Children's Hospital Medical Center, University of Cincinnati College of Medicine, Cincinnati, OH, USA

Lia Bernardi, MD, MSCI Division of Reproductive Endocrinology, Department of Obstetrics and Gynecology, Northwestern University Feinberg School of Medicine, Chicago, IL, USA

Carolina Di Blasi, MD Seattle Childrens Hospital, University of Washington, Seattle, WA, USA

Åsa Bonnard, MD, PhD Department of Clinical Science, Intervention and Technology, Division of Otorhinolaryngology, Karolinska Institutet, Stockholm, Sweden

Department of Otorhinolaryngology, Karolinska University Hospital, Stockholm, Sweden

Amanda Bradshaw, PA-C Gastroenterology, Seattle Children's Hospital, Seattle, WA, USA

Sarah Corathers, MD The Cincinnati Center for Pediatric and Adult Turner Syndrome Care, Cincinnati Children's Hospital Medical Center, University of Cincinnati College of Medicine, Cincinnati, OH, USA

Patricia Y. Fechner, MD Division of Endocrinology, Seattle Children's Hospital, University of Washington, Seattle, WA, USA

Courtney Finlayson, MD Division of Endocrinology, Department of Pediatrics, Ann & Robert H. Lurie Children's Hospital of Chicago, Northwestern University Feinberg School of Medicine, Chicago, IL, USA

Joseph T. Flynn, MD, MS University of Washington School of Medicine, Seattle, WA, USA

Division of Nephrology, Seattle Children's Hospital, Seattle, WA, USA

Aneta M. Gawlik, PhD Department of Pediatrics and Pediatric Endocrinology, School of Medicine in Katowice, Medical University of Silesia, Katowice, Poland

Claus H. Gravholt, MD, PhD Department of Endocrinology and Internal Medicine, Aarhus University Hospital, Aarhus, Denmark

Department of Molecular Medicine, Aarhus University Hospital, Aarhus, Denmark

Department of Endocrinology and Internal Medicine and Medical Research Laboratories, Aarhus University Hospital, Aarhus, Denmark

Reema Habiby, MD Division of Endocrinology, Department of Pediatrics, Ann & Robert H. Lurie Children's Hospital of Chicago, Northwestern University Feinberg School of Medicine, Chicago, IL, USA

Alessandra Haskin, BA Department of Dermatology, SUNY Health Science Center at Brooklyn, Brooklyn, NY, USA

Erin P. Herlihy, MD Department of Ophthalmology, University of Washington School of Medicine, Seattle, WA, USA

Division of Pediatric Ophthalmology, Seattle Children's Hospital, Seattle, WA, USA

Malou Hultcrantz, MD Department of Clinical Science, Intervention and Technology, Division of Otorhinolaryngology, Karolinska Institutet, Stockholm, Sweden

Department of Otorhinolaryngology, Karolinska University Hospital, Stockholm, Sweden

Darcy King, ARNP University of Washington, Seattle, WA, USA

Karen O. Klein, MD University of California, San Diego & Rady Children's Hospital, San Diego, CA, USA

Dale Lee, MD Pediatrics-Gastroenterology, Clinical Nutrition & Celiac Program, Seattle Children's Hospital, University of Washington, Seattle, WA, USA

Eve Lowenstein, MD, PhD Department of Dermatology, SUNY Health Science Center at Brooklyn, Brooklyn, NY, USA

Melanie A. Manning, MD Division of Medical Genetics, Department of Pediatrics, Stanford University School of Medicine and Lucile Salter Packard Children's Hospital, Stanford, CA, USA

Department of Pathology, Stanford University School of Medicine, Stanford, CA, USA

Nelly Mauras, MD Nemours Children's Health System, Jacksonville, FL, USA

Yosuke Miyashita, MD, MPH University of Pittsburgh School of Medicine, Pittsburgh, PA, USA

Angel Siu Ying Nip, MBChB University of Washington, Seattle, WA, USA

Charmian A. Quigley, MBBS Sydney Children's Hospital, Randwick, NSW, Australia

Alissa J. Roberts, MD Division of Endocrinology, Seattle Children's Hospital, University of Washington, Seattle, WA, USA

Robert L. Rosenfield, MD The University of Chicago Pritzker School of Medicine, Chicago, IL, USA

Jolene C. Rudell, MD, PhD Department of Ophthalmology, University of Washington School of Medicine, Seattle, WA, USA

Division of Pediatric Ophthalmology, Seattle Children's Hospital, Seattle, WA, USA

Richard J. Santen, MD University of Virginia, Charlottesville, VA, USA

Theo C. J. Sas, MD Albert Schweitzer Hospital Dordrecht and Sophia Children's Hospital Rotterdam, Rotterdam, The Netherlands

Michael Silberbach, MD Doernbecher Children's Hospital, Oregon Health & Sciences University, Portland, OR, USA

Suzanne E. Steinman, MD Department of Orthopedics and Sports Medicine, Seattle Children's Hospital, Seattle, WA, USA

Department of Orthopaedics and Sports Medicine, University of Washington, Seattle, WA, USA

Harlyn Susarla, DMD Seattle Childrens Hospital, University of Washington, Seattle, WA, USA

Mette H. Viuff, MD Department of Endocrinology and Medical Research Laboratories, Aarhus University Hospital, Aarhus, Denmark

Ghassan T. Wahbeh, MD Pediatrics-Gastroenterology, Inflammatory Bowel Disease Center, Seattle Children's Hospital, University of Washington, Seattle, WA, USA

Klane K. White, MD, MSc Department of Orthopedics and Sports Medicine, Seattle Children's Hospital, Seattle, WA, USA

Department of Orthopaedics and Sports Medicine, University of Washington, Seattle, WA, USA

Lauren White, ARNP Gastroenterology, Seattle Children's Hospital, Seattle, WA, USA

Luciana T. Young, MD Seattle Children's Hospital/University of Washington, Division of Cardiology, Seattle, WA, USA

Chapter 1
Description of Turner Syndrome

Alissa J. Roberts and Patricia Y. Fechner

Introduction

Turner syndrome was defined in 1938 by Dr. Henry Turner who described a constellation of findings in girls as "A Syndrome of Infantilism, Congenital Webbed
Neck and Cubitus Valgus." This same syndrome had been previously described by
Otto Ullrich in 1930, thus, in some countries the term Ullrich-Turner syndrome is
used. As knowledge and the field of genetics progressed, Turner syndrome was
further defined as phenotypic features consistent with Turner syndrome (which
could be as subtle as isolated short stature) in a female along with complete or
partial absence of a second sex chromosome on 20–30-cell karyotype, which could
include cell line mosaicism [1]. There have been many advances in the diagnosis
and management of females with Turner syndrome, and this chapter serves as an
introductory overview of the incidence, karyotype findings, and phenotype of
Turner syndrome, most of which will be described in further detail in appropriate
chapters following. For a summary of overall screening recommendations in
Turner syndrome, see Table 1.1, which incorporates 2017 clinical practice guidelines from the 2016 Cincinnati International Turner Syndrome Meeting [2].

A. J. Roberts (✉) · P. Y. Fechner
Division of Endocrinology, Seattle Children's Hospital,
University of Washington, Seattle, WA, USA
e-mail: Alissa.Roberts@seattlechildrens.org

© Springer Nature Switzerland AG 2020
P. Y. Fechner (ed.), *Turner Syndrome*,
https://doi.org/10.1007/978-3-030-34150-3_1

Table 1.1 Screening recommendations in Turner syndrome

Screening category	Screening	Frequency in childhood	Frequency in adulthood
Metabolic	BMI/weight	At diagnosis, at least annually	At least annually
	Lipid panel	Annually after age 10 years	Annually
	Liver function (AST, ALT, GGT, alkaline phosphatase)	Annually after age 10 year	Annually
	Hemoglobin A1c	Annually after age 10 years	Annually
Skeletal screening	Spine exam: scoliosis/kyphosis	Every 6 months if on growth hormone, annually if not on growth hormone, screen until growth complete	None
	Growth	Initiate growth hormone at age 5–6 years or when significant growth failure occurs	None
	Hip exam	In infancy	None
	Bone density (DEXA)	Baseline when completed puberty	Every 5 years
	25-Hydroxyvitamin D level	Start at age 9–11 years, then every 2–3 years	Every 3–5 years
	Orthodontic exam	Age 7, then as recommended by initial exam	As recommended by initial exam
Puberty and ovarian reserve	LH and FSH ±AMH and inhibin B	Age 11, then annually until initiate estrogen	As needed
Cardiovascular	Echocardiogram with cardiology evaluation	At diagnosis, every 3–5 years starting at age 12 years, cardiac MRI once	Every 5–10 years Cardiac MRI once
	Blood pressure	At diagnosis, at least annually	At least annually
Renal	Renal ultrasound	At diagnosis	None
Autoimmunity	Thyroid (TSH and free T4)	At diagnosis, annually	Annually
	Celiac screen (IgA level (once) and tissue transglutaminase IgA level)	Starting at age 2–3 years, every 2 years thereafter	Every 5 years
HEENT	Audiology screen	Age 9–12 months or at diagnosis whichever first, then every 3 years	Every 5 years
	Ophthalmological examination	Age 12–18 months or at diagnosis whichever first, then annually	Annually
Skin	Skin exam	At diagnosis, annually	Annually
Psychosocial	Neurocognitive evaluation	Preschool, school entry, transition to high school or higher education	As indicated

Table 1.1 (continued)

Screening category	Screening	Frequency in childhood	Frequency in adulthood
	Occupational, physical, and speech therapy evaluation	Preschool or school entry	
	Mental health screening	Annually after age 10	Annually
	Connect with social supports	At diagnosis, annually	Annually

Table 1.1 based on Gravholt et al. [2]

Incidence

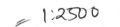

The true incidence of Turner syndrome is unknown, given that the presentation can be subtle and thus underdiagnosed, particularly in the mosaic forms. One large-scale study in Denmark, which looked at the incidence of chromosome abnormalities in almost 35,000 live births, found the incidence of Turner syndrome to be 1 per 1893 girls [3]. When looking at the presentation of phenotypic features in Turner syndrome, there is thought to be an ascertainment bias [4]. In other words, because the girls with milder phenotypes are less likely to be diagnosed with Turner syndrome, the distribution of features in those in whom the diagnosis is known tends to lean toward the more moderately or severely affected. The incidence of Turner syndrome and the number of afflicted females who have very few signs or symptoms is likely underrepresented in the medical literature.

As we move into a new era with the widely available cell-free fetal DNA prenatal testing, we will likely see an increase in prenatally diagnosed Turner syndrome and thus may have changes in the known incidence rate as well as a shift in the spectrum of phenotypes and karyotypes. Cell-free fetal DNA is placental DNA found in maternal blood, accessed by noninvasive venipuncture. This technology is becoming an increasingly popular routine screening test in the first trimester of pregnancy for aneuploidies—primarily trisomy 21 and 13 due to its noninvasive nature. However, with the information on these aneuploidies, the consumer also acquires information on the sex chromosomes of the fetus and sex chromosome differences such as 45,X. One systemic review determined the current sensitivity of cell-free fetal DNA for monosomy X is 94.1% and false positive is 0.53% [5]. Others though have found higher false positive rate. This demonstrates the limitations of this testing for diagnosis of monosomy X and that either invasive prenatal or postnatal karyotype is far superior. In addition, for any prenatal diagnosis of suspected monosomy X, a postnatal karyotype must be performed to confirm and establish a diagnosis of Turner syndrome. As this field rapidly evolves, we expect to see a growing body of literature on this topic.

Karyotype

The distribution in karyotypes in girls identified with Turner syndrome is approximately half 45,X, 35% mosaic, and the rest structural abnormalities in the X chromosome [6]. All these karyotypes have in common missing elements from the X chromosome. The X chromosome contains over 1000 genes (as compared to the Y chromosome which contains around 200 genes) [7]. In the case of the genetically typical female, 46,XX, in every cell, one of the X chromosomes is inactivated via lyonization. However, approximately 10–15% of the genes on the inactive X chromosomes escape inactivation and therefore remain active. Most of these genes are located on the tip of the short arm of the X chromosome in what is known as the pseudoautosomal region and have corresponding homologous genes on the Y chromosome. In the female with Turner syndrome, who lacks all or part of the inactive X chromosome, she also lacks those pseudoautosomal genes and genes that would continue to be expressed despite inactivation. Thus, she only has a "single dose" of these genes with the one X chromosome, and many of the phenotypic features present in Turner syndrome are from the haploinsufficiency or inadequate "dosing" of these genes.

45,X is the classic karyotype of Turner syndrome but can lead to a wide array of phenotypes, ranging from isolated short stature to multiple dysmorphic features and congenital heart disease. Specific phenotypic features of Turner syndrome are outlined in the next section. Mosaicism, where only some cell lines are 45,X, can also present in a variety of manners. Most common, 45,X/46,XX, is often the most subtle phenotype, and some, which are incidentally diagnosed, may not even warrant a clinical diagnosis of Turner syndrome. It must be cautioned that in mosaicism, karyotype distribution of cell lines cannot predict phenotype in that a lymphocyte karyotype may differ from the distribution of cell lines in other tissues [8].

Another mosaic form of Turner syndrome includes the presence of Y material, such as 45,X/46,XY, and conveys an increased risk of gonadoblastoma. This mosaic genotype can present with a variety of phenotypes, varying from typical appearing male with normal testes to a female with Turner syndrome. There may be some virilization of the patient with Turner syndrome with Y material, or there may not be any depending on the presence or absence of functional testicular tissue. The increased risk of gonadoblastoma in this population of females with Turner syndrome is notable and ranges from 12% to 60% risk depending on the cohort [9, 10]. Individuals with 45,X/46,XY karyotype who are phenotypically female have been found to have the highest risk of gonadoblastoma due to the intra-abdominal location of their gonads [11]. Standard of care remains prophylactic gonadectomy, though some controversies may exist if there is no evidence of gonadal failure (i.e., streak gonads) thus indicating some potential fertility [8]. However, there have been few reported cases in the literature of fertility with the 45,X/46,XY karyotype, and these had almost exclusively been in phenotypically male individuals (hence without intra-abdominal gonads) [12]. There is one case report of a successful pregnancy in a Turner syndrome 45,X/46,XY individual [13]. In most cases, the high risk of gonadoblastoma with intra-abdominal gonads outweighs any chance of fertility, especially if laboratory assessment is consistent with gonadal failure and dysplastic gonads, and gonadectomy should be strongly considered.

Another form of Turner syndrome involves structural abnormalities of the X chromosome. Potential abnormalities include ring X, Xq isochromosomes, and small deletions in the X chromosome (such as Xp-, deletions in the distal short arm). These patients have a variety of phenotypes that are often related to the specific X chromosome abnormality. For instance, those with a ring X chromosome tend to have a higher degree of cognitive and behavioral difficulties [14]. Though there are correlations between genotype and phenotype in these structural X abnormalities, in cases of mosaicism, presenting features have even more variation and are more difficult to predict from a karyotype.

Phenotype

The Turner syndrome phenotype consists of many possible features, including but not limited to short stature, primary ovarian failure, lymphatic obstruction, cardiac abnormalities, renal abnormalities, and skeletal abnormalities. In the sections below, we will outline the presentation of some of these phenotypic features as well as general management or screening. Most of these conditions will be explored and discussed in more detail in subsequent chapters. Therefore, the following serves as an overview.

Short Stature/Skeletal Manifestations

Short stature in Turner syndrome is universal and usually begins with in utero growth restriction. Typically, length will decline and fall off of the growth curve by the time girls are 1.5 years old. The etiology of short stature for females with Turner syndrome is haploinsufficiency of the SHOX gene, a gene located in the pseudoautosomal region of the X chromosome, encoding a transcription factor which regulates aspect of skeletal development and growth [15]. Of note, those who have mosaic forms of Turner syndrome do not lack as many copies of the SHOX gene, depending on the degree of mosaicism, and can have lesser degrees of short stature. In addition, females with mosaicism which includes Y material may have an even lesser degree of short stature because of the presence of Y material.

The other skeletal features of Turner syndrome are also related to SHOX haploinsufficiency and effects on the developing and maturing skeleton. Shortening of the 4th and 5th metacarpals can be seen. A widened carrying angle is often present. Body proportions are often abnormal with a greater upper to lower segment ratio (described as sitting height) than with an unaffected individual [16]. Furthermore, a Madelung deformity, dorsal subluxation of the distal ulna related to epiphyseal growth arrest of the distal radius, is a classic finding related to SHOX gene insuffi-ciency [17]. This finding does not often manifest until age 10–14 years.

Recombinant growth hormone therapy, via subcutaneous daily injections, is FDA approved for treatment of short stature in Turner syndrome. A large random-ized control trial demonstrated that early treatment with growth hormone, prior to the age of 4 years, improved height in girls with Turner syndrome over the course of the 2 year study. More importantly, the increase in height percentiles was present at a time when a decrease in height percentiles in females with Turner syndrome not receiving growth hormone at this young age occurred [18]. Long-term outcomes of very early treatment with growth hormone are still pending. Current recommenda-tions are to initiate growth hormone therapy at 4–6 years of age if there is evidence of growth failure to optimize height potential, decrease disadvantages that could be associated with severe short stature, and allow for more physiologic timing for induction of puberty [2].

Risk of rare side effects (all less than 0.5%) of growth hormone therapy in a child with Turner syndrome includes scoliosis, diabetes, cardiovascular events, intracra-nial hypertension, and slipped capital femoral epiphysis (SCFE). The use of growth hormone therapy has not been found to have any negative effect on aortic diameter [19] or middle ear disease and hearing loss [20] in this population. In addition to benefits pertaining to height, childhood growth hormone use in females with Turner syndrome has been found to favorably affect their lipid profile as adults [21]. Also, growth hormone seems to have a beneficial effect on diastolic blood pressure and normalization of upper to lower segment ratio (body proportions), even 5 years after discontinuing growth hormone therapy [22]. Unfortunately, no lasting positive effects on BMI have been observed [22]. Growth hormone use does not seem to impact bone mineral density [23]. Overall, the benefits of growth hormone seem to far outweigh any potential risk, and its use is now offered to families as standard of care in management of Turner syndrome.

Primary Ovarian Failure

Loss of oocytes in Turner syndrome begins mid-gestation, and females often have few viable oocytes at birth. This loss of oocytes is thought to be due to abnormal meiosis with the absence of a normal/complete second X chromosome [24]. However, despite this reduction in oocytes, up to 30% of women with Turner syn-drome will have spontaneous initiation of puberty (this is more likely with mosaic forms of Turner syndrome as compared to one cell line with monosomy X) [25]. About half of those with spontaneous puberty will also have spontaneous menarche. However, despite these encouraging statistics, over 90% of females with Turner syndrome will have premature ovarian failure, and a minority (up to 5.6% in a French cohort) achieve spontaneous pregnancies [26].

In most girls with Turner syndrome, pubertal induction is undertaken using exog-enous estradiol, typically in a transdermal form to avoid first-pass metabolism through the liver. Goals of estrogen therapy include development of secondary sexual characteristics at a time similar to peers and improved bone health, cardiovascular health, and potential benefits for neurocognitive development [27]. Typically, if there are no signs of spontaneous puberty by the age of 12 years with elevated gonadotropins, estradiol therapy is initiated [2]. This is done is a stepwise manner starting with very low doses increased over several years, to mimic physiologic puberty. Eventually, once breakthrough vaginal bleeding occurs or a certain estradiol dose is reached, cyclic progestin is added. It is a little less clear when to initiate exogenous estrogen in females with Turner syndrome who undergo spontaneous puberty but have biochemical evidence of gonadal failure. One study investigated the initiation of ultra-low-dose estrogen in young girls as early as age 5 years and identified some benefit to onset and tempo of puberty [28]. This is related to a premise that girls with Turner syndrome lack normal low levels of estradiol exposure in early childhood, which may impact several areas of physical and neurological development.

Pregnancy in Turner syndrome, as mentioned above, is rarely spontaneous and, if it is, is more likely in women with mosaic karyotypes. Assisted reproductive techniques are available, such oocyte cryopreservation and in vitro fertilization, if some follicles remain at the time of evaluation by a reproductive endocrinologist [29]. Becoming a receipient of oocyte donation is also an option. Importantly, pregnancy in a woman with Turner syndrome can be very risky in that the risk of aortic rupture may be up to 2% and should only be pursued if a thorough cardiovascular evaluation has been performed to assess the amount of risk [30]. The presence of congenital heart disease or a dilated aorta is considered a contraindication to pregnancy in Turner syndrome, and in these patients surrogacy or adoption may be proposed alternatives.

Congenital Heart Disease and Cardiovascular Concerns

The prevalence of cardiac malformations has been found to be around ¼ of live females with Turner syndrome, bicuspid aortic valve and aortic coarctation being the most common [31, 32]. In addition, those females that have a webbed neck and fetal lymphedema are at an increased risk for congenital heart disease [33, 34]. Most studies have found the incidence of bicuspid aortic valve to be 16% and aortic coarctation to be 11% [1].

Aortic dissection is one of the most fatal consequences of Turner syndrome and has been found to occur at an incidence of 36 per 100,000 Turner syndrome years, compared with an incidence of 6 per 100,000 in the general population [35]. In addition, it occurs at a young age with an average age of 35 years in females with Turner syndrome. Echocardiogram should be performed in all infants diagnosed with Turner syndrome and cardiac MRI in all older children, and adults in that MRI can detect cardiac abnormalities that may be missed by echocardiogram [36]. As mentioned above, the risk of aortic dissection is further increased during and following pregnancy, and careful counseling and consideration of any other risk factors must be considered in a female with Turner syndrome who desires a pregnancy.

In addition to structural abnormalities of the heart and vasculature, individuals with Turner syndrome are at risk for features of metabolic syndrome which impact cardiovascular health such as hypertension, dyslipidemia, and obesity. Hypertension has been found to occur in up to half of adolescents adults with Turner syndrome [37] and in even more adults. Hypertension is a risk factor for aortic dilatation and dissection [38] and should be managed aggressively in patients with Turner syndrome.

Mortality in females with Turner syndrome is increased threefold over the general population. Circulatory disease has been seen to be a major contributor to this, associated with 41% of excess mortality [39]. Other components of metabolic syndrome, obesity, impaired glucose metabolism, and dyslipidemia, occur at higher rates in females with Turner syndrome and thus appropriate screening, nutritional and lifestyle counseling, and medical management when indicated are key components of care of these individuals to mitigate this risk [40].

Lymphatic Obstruction

Aberrant development of the fetal lymphatic system in Turner syndrome often results in fetal lymphedema and cystic hygromas that lead to peripheral lymphedema and neck webbing in the infant. Initial peripheral lymphedema is temporary and often resolves spontaneously but may recur at any time throughout the life of a female with Turner syndrome. Neck webbing is a stable feature and is often a cardinal sign in diagnosing Turner syndrome and has been associated with increased risk of congenital heart anomalies.

Renal

Structural kidney abnormalities can occur in approximately 30–40% of individuals with Turner syndrome [41], most commonly collecting system abnormalities and horseshoe kidneys. A postnatal renal ultrasound should be done at the time of diagnosis of Turner syndrome to evaluate for urologic abnormalities. It has been found that structural abnormalities of the kidney occur more frequently in non-mosaic monosomy X karyotypes, while collecting system defects occur more frequently in mosaic or structural X karyotypes [41].

Autoimmunity

As with many other chromosomal abnormalities, individuals with Turner syndrome have a higher risk of autoimmune conditions. Most commonly, females with Turner syndrome develop Hashimoto's thyroiditis and primary hypothyroidism, and in a study of children with Turner syndrome, hypothyroidism occurred in 24% [42]. Graves' disease is a risk as well, occurring in 2.5% [42]. Thus, annual thyroid function tests are essential. Celiac disease is the next most common autoimmune disorder in this population, after thyroid disease, occurring in up to 6% of females [43]. The majority of cases are subclinical, so serological screening every 2–5 years after age 2 years is recommended [2, 44]. Other autoimmune conditions such as type 1 diabetes [45] have been reported to occur at higher rates in Turner syndrome and should be considered if symptoms arise.

Psychological/Cognitive

In general, females with Turner syndrome have normal intelligence. However, they often have impairments in certain domains of learning related to nonverbal skills such as visual-spatial abilities, mathematics, and executive function [46]. They can also have some difficulty with social skills and maturity as well as anxiety [47]. To address these, all females with Turner syndrome should have formal psycho-educational evaluation to assess for learning disabilities and allow for early interventions. In addition, continued psychological support with both individual counseling as well as support group involvement should be encouraged [1].

Support groups and resources for females with Turner syndrome exist such as the Turner Syndrome Society (www.turnersyndrome.org), which offers national conferences, various events, and many electronic resources. The Turner Syndrome Foundation (www.turnersyndromefoundation.org) also offers many electronic resources and information on research opportunities.

Cancer Risk

Women with Turner syndrome have recently been identified as having an increased risk for various malignancies in several national cohort studies [48–51]. This is thought to be related to the X chromosome abnormality as well as potentially related to hormone differences with lack of innate estrogen and chronic estrogen replacement that are observed in this population. Additionally, the use growth hormone in this population has been considered as an important risk factor, but there have been no studies that have demonstrated this [51]. In addition, data from three growth hormone registries does not support an increase in risk of neoplasia in females with Turner syndrome treated with growth hormone therapy [52–54].

In a Swedish study including 1409 women with Turner syndrome [48], it was found that the overall risk of cancer was 1.34 for women with Turner syndrome and risk was increased only for solid tumors, specifically melanoma and central nervous system tumors. There was no increase in hematological malignancies in this group. Another cohort study in Great Britain of 3435 women with Turner syndrome [49] found that these women had in increased risk of meningioma and childhood brain tumors, and possibly bladder cancer, melanoma, and corpus uteri cancer, but a decreased risk of breast cancer. Additionally, those with Y chromosome material had a higher risk of gonadoblastoma (cumulative risk of 7.9% by age 25 years). In a Danish cohort of 597 women [50], an increased overall relative risk of cancer of 1.1 was observed with a particular increase in colon cancer. However, this increased colon cancer risk has not been observed in the larger aforementioned cohort studies. A retrospective study done in Italy evaluated 87 women with Turner syndrome and found 17 neoplasms in 14 of the patients: 6 skin neoplasia, 3 central nervous system tumors, 3 gonadal neoplasia, 2 breast tumors, 1 hepatocarcinoma, 1 carcinoma of the pancreas, and 1 follicular thyroid cancer [51]. A high incidence of adenomyoma gallbladder (15.3%) was also found in this group. Case reports of patients with Turner syndrome and central nervous system malignancies such as meningioma, medulloblastoma, and cerebellar astrocytoma have been published to further support the increased incidence of brain tumors in this population [55, 56].

The causes and contributing factors to this observed increased cancer risk need to be further elucidated. At this point, there is a need for general counseling of patients and families around these potential increased cancer risks and a heightened clinical suspicion if concerning symptoms for malignancy arise.

References

1. Bondy CA, Turner Syndrome Study G. Care of girls and women with Turner syndrome: a guideline of the Turner Syndrome Study Group. J Clin Endocrinol Metab. 2007;92(1):10–25.
2. Gravholt CH, Andersen NH, Conway GS, et al. Clinical practice guidelines for the care of girls and women with Turner syndrome: proceedings from the 2016 Cincinnati International Turner Syndrome Meeting. Eur J Endocrinol. 2017;177(3):G1–G70.
3. Nielsen J, Wohlert M. Chromosome abnormalities found among 34,910 newborn children: results from a 13-year incidence study in Arhus, Denmark. Hum Genet. 1991;87(1):81–3.
4. Gunther DF, Eugster E, Zagar AJ, Bryant CG, Davenport ML, Quigley CA. Ascertainment bias in Turner syndrome: new insights from girls who were diagnosed incidentally in prenatal life. Pediatrics. 2004;114(3):640–4.
5. Kagan KO, Hoopmann M, Singer S, Schaeferhoff K, Dufke A, Mau-Holzmann UA. Discordance between ultrasound and cell free DNA screening for monosomy X. Arch Gynecol Obstet. 2016;294(2):219–24.
6. Savendahl L, Davenport ML. Delayed diagnoses of Turner's syndrome: proposed guidelines for change. J Pediatr. 2000;137(4):455–9.
7. Spatz A, Borg C, Feunteun J. X-chromosome genetics and human cancer. Nat Rev Cancer. 2004;4(8):617–29.
8. Davenport ML. Approach to the patient with Turner syndrome. J Clin Endocrinol Metab. 2010;95(4):1487–95.
9. Matsumoto F, Shimada K, Ida S. Tumors of bilateral streak gonads in patients with disorders of sex development containing y chromosome material. Clin Pediatr Endocrinol. 2014;23(3):93–7.
10. Tam YH, Wong YS, Pang KK, et al. Tumor risk of children with 45,X/46,XY gonadal dysgenesis in relation to their clinical presentations: Further insights into the gonadal management. J Pediatr Surg. 2016;51(9):1462–6.

11. Coyle D, Kutasy B, Han Suyin K, et al. Gonadoblastoma in patients with 45,X/46,XY mosaicism: a 16-year experience. J Pediatr Urol. 2016;12(5):283.e1–7.
12. Flannigan RK, Chow V, Ma S, Yuzpe A. 45,X/46,XY mixed gonadal dysgenesis: a case of successful sperm extraction. Can Urol Assoc J. 2014;8(1–2):E108–10.
13. Landin-Wilhelmsen K, Bryman I, Hanson C, Hanson L. Spontaneous pregnancies in a Turner syndrome woman with Y-chromosome mosaicism. J Assist Reprod Genet. 2004;21(6):229–30.
14. Kuntsi J, Skuse D, Elgar K, Morris E, Turner C. Ring-X chromosomes: their cognitive and behavioural phenotype. Ann Hum Genet. 2000;64(Pt 4):295–305.
15. Fukami M, Seki A, Ogata T. SHOX haploinsufficiency as a cause of syndromic and nonsyndromic short stature. Mol Syndromol. 2016;7(1):3–11.
16. Malaquias AC, Scalco RC, Fontenele EG, et al. The sitting height/height ratio for age in healthy and short individuals and its potential role in selecting short children for SHOX analysis. Horm Res Paediatr. 2013;80(6):449–56.
17. Huguet S, Leheup B, Aslan M, et al. Radiological and clinical analysis of Madelung's deformity in children. Orthop Traumatol Surg Res. 2014;100(6 Suppl):S349–52.
18. Davenport ML, Crowe BJ, Travers SH, et al. Growth hormone treatment of early growth failure in toddlers with Turner syndrome: a randomized, controlled, multicenter trial. J Clin Endocrinol Metab. 2007;92(9):3406–16.
19. Bondy CA, Van PL, Bakalov VK, Ho VB. Growth hormone treatment and aortic dimensions in Turner syndrome. J Clin Endocrinol Metab. 2006;91(5):1785–8.
20. Davenport ML, Roush J, Liu C, et al. Growth hormone treatment does not affect incidences of middle ear disease or hearing loss in infants and toddlers with Turner syndrome. Horm Res Paediatr. 2010;74(1):23–32.
21. Irzyniec TJ, Jez W. The influence of hormonal replacement and growth hormone treatment on the lipids in Turner syndrome. Gynecol Endocrinol. 2014;30(3):250–3.
22. Bannink EM, van der Palen RL, Mulder PG, de Muinck Keizer-Schrama SM. Long-term follow-up of GH-treated girls with Turner syndrome: BMI, blood pressure, body proportions. Horm Res. 2009;71(6):336–42.
23. Bakalov VK, Van PL, Baron J, Reynolds JC, Bondy CA. Growth hormone therapy and bone mineral density in Turner syndrome. J Clin Endocrinol Metab. 2004;89(10):4886–9.
24. Hovatta O. Ovarian function and in vitro fertilization (IVF) in Turner syndrome. Pediatr Endocrinol Rev. 2012;9(Suppl 2):713–7.
25. Pasquino AM, Passeri F, Pucarelli I, Segni M, Municchi G. Spontaneous pubertal development in Turner's syndrome. Italian Study Group for Turner's Syndrome. J Clin Endocrinol Metab. 1997;82(6):1810–3.
26. Bernard V, Donadille B, Zenaty D, et al. Spontaneous fertility and pregnancy outcomes amongst 480 women with Turner syndrome. Hum Reprod. 2016;31(4):782–8.
27. Ross JL, Roeltgen D, Feuillan P, Kushner H, Cutler GB Jr. Effects of estrogen on nonverbal processing speed and motor function in girls with Turner's syndrome. J Clin Endocrinol Metab. 1998;83(9):3198–204.
28. Quigley CA, Wan X, Garg S, Kowal K, Cutler GB Jr, Ross JL. Effects of low-dose estrogen replacement during childhood on pubertal development and gonadotropin concentrations in patients with Turner syndrome: results of a randomized, double-blind, placebo-controlled clinical trial. J Clin Endocrinol Metab. 2014;99(9):E1754–64.
29. Oktay K, Bedoschi G, Berkowitz K, et al. Fertility preservation in women with Turner syndrome: a comprehensive review and practical guidelines. J Pediatr Adolesc Gynecol. 2015;29(5):409–16.
30. Practice Committee of American Society For Reproductive M. Increased maternal cardiovascular mortality associated with pregnancy in women with Turner syndrome. Fertil Steril. 2012;97(2):282–4.
31. Mazzanti L, Cacciari E. Congenital heart disease in patients with Turner's syndrome. Italian Study Group for Turner Syndrome (ISGTS). J Pediatr. 1998;133(5):688–92.
32. Gotzsche CO, Krag-Olsen B, Nielsen J, Sorensen KE, Kristensen BO. Prevalence of cardiovascular malformations and association with karyotypes in Turner's syndrome. Arch Dis Child. 1994;71(5):433–6.

33. Berdahl LD, Wenstrom KD, Hanson JW. Web neck anomaly and its association with congenital heart disease. Am J Med Genet. 1995;56(3):304–7.
34. Loscalzo ML, Van PL, Ho VB, et al. Association between fetal lymphedema and congenital cardiovascular defects in Turner syndrome. Pediatrics. 2005;115(3):732–5.
35. Gravholt CH, Landin-Wilhelmsen K, Stochholm K, et al. Clinical and epidemiological description of aortic dissection in Turner's syndrome. Cardiol Young. 2006;16(5):430–6.
36. Bondy CA. Aortic dissection in Turner syndrome. Curr Opin Cardiol. 2008;23(6):519–26.
37. Los E, Quezada E, Chen Z, Lapidus J, Silberbach M. Pilot study of blood pressure in girls with Turner syndrome: an awareness gap, clinical associations, and new hypotheses. Hypertension. 2016;68:133.
38. Elsheikh M, Casadei B, Conway GS, Wass JA. Hypertension is a major risk factor for aortic root dilatation in women with Turner's syndrome. Clin Endocrinol. 2001;54(1):69–73.
39. Schoemaker MJ, Swerdlow AJ, Higgins CD, Wright AF, Jacobs PA, United Kingdom Clinical Cytogenetics G. Mortality in women with turner syndrome in Great Britain: a national cohort study. J Clin Endocrinol Metab. 2008;93(12):4735–42.
40. Mavinkurve M, O'Gorman CS. Cardiometabolic and vascular risks in young and adolescent girls with Turner syndrome. BBA Clin. 2015;3:304–9.
41. Bilge I, Kayserili H, Emre S, et al. Frequency of renal malformations in Turner syndrome: analysis of 82 Turkish children. Pediatr Nephrol. 2000;14(12):1111–4.
42. Livadas S, Xekouki P, Fouka F, et al. Prevalence of thyroid dysfunction in Turner's syndrome: a long-term follow-up study and brief literature review. Thyroid. 2005;15(9):1061–6.
43. Bonamico M, Pasquino AM, Mariani P, et al. Prevalence and clinical picture of celiac disease in Turner syndrome. J Clin Endocrinol Metab. 2002;87(12):5495–8.
44. Hill ID, Dirks MH, Liptak GS, et al. Guideline for the diagnosis and treatment of celiac disease in children: recommendations of the North American Society for Pediatric Gastroenterology, Hepatology and Nutrition. J Pediatr Gastroenterol Nutr. 2005;40(1):1–19.
45. Jorgensen KT, Rostgaard K, Bache I, et al. Autoimmune diseases in women with Turner's syndrome. Arthritis Rheum. 2010;62(3):658–66.
46. Ross J, Zinn A, McCauley E. Neurodevelopmental and psychosocial aspects of Turner syndrome. Ment Retard Dev Disabil Res Rev. 2000;6(2):135–41.
47. McCauley E, Feuillan P, Kushner H, Ross JL. Psychosocial development in adolescents with Turner syndrome. J Dev Behav Pediatr. 2001;22(6):360–5.
48. Ji J, Zoller B, Sundquist J, Sundquist K. Risk of solid tumors and hematological malignancy in persons with Turner and Klinefelter syndromes: a national cohort study. Int J Cancer. 2016;139(4):754–8.
49. Schoemaker MJ, Swerdlow AJ, Higgins CD, Wright AF, Jacobs PA, Group UKCC. Cancer incidence in women with Turner syndrome in Great Britain: a national cohort study. Lancet Oncol. 2008;9(3):239–46.
50. Hasle H, Olsen JH, Nielsen J, Hansen J, Friedrich U, Tommerup N. Occurrence of cancer in women with Turner syndrome. Br J Cancer. 1996;73(9):1156–9.
51. Larizza D, Albanesi M, De Silvestri A, et al. Neoplasia in Turner syndrome. The importance of clinical and screening practices during follow-up. Eur J Med Genet. 2016;59(5):269–73.
52. Bell J, Parker KI, Swinford RD, Hoffman AR, Maneatis T, Lippe B. Long-term safety of recombinant human growth hormone in children. J Clin Endocrinol Metab. 2010;95(2):167–77.
53. Bolar K, Hoffman AR, Maneatis T, Lippe B. Long-term safety of recombinant human growth hormonein Turner syndrome. J Clin Endocrinol Metab. 2008;93(1):344–51.
54. Child CJ, Zimmermann AG, Chrousos GP, et al. Safety outcomes during pediatric GH therapy: final results from the prospective GeNeSIS observational program. J Clin Endocrinol Metab. 2019;104(2):379–89.
55. Pier DB, Nunes FP, Plotkin SR, et al. Turner syndrome and meningioma: support for a possible increased risk of neoplasia in Turner syndrome. Eur J Med Genet. 2014;57(6):269–74.
56. Alexiou GA, Varela M, Dimitriadis E, et al. Brain tumors in Turner syndrome. Eur J Med Genet. 2014;57(6):312–3.

Chapter 2
The Genetics of Turner Syndrome

Margaret P. Adam and Melanie A. Manning

Introduction

On the surface the genetics of Turner syndrome (TS) would appear straightforward, as many affected females have 45,X. This chapter reviews the structure and function of the sex chromosomes and the multitude of chromosomal differences that can be seen in females with TS, including sex chromosome mosaicism. This chapter also explores the unique features of the X chromosome, including X-chromosome inactivation, and evidence for and against the existence of imprinted genes on the X chromosome. In order to fully understand the clinical features seen in individuals with TS, mechanisms leading to structural rearrangements of the sex chromosomes are discussed, as is an overview of important genes that reside on the X chromosome. Finally, this chapter summarizes the recommended genetic testing when Turner syndrome is suspected in both a prenatal and a postnatal setting and recurrence risks when a family has had one girl with Turner syndrome.

M. P. Adam (✉)
Division of Genetic Medicine, Department of Pediatrics, University of Washington School of Medicine and Seattle Children's Hospital, Seattle, WA, USA
e-mail: margaret.adam@seattlechildrens.org

M. A. Manning
Division of Medical Genetics, Department of Pediatrics, Stanford University School of Medicine and Lucile Salter Packard Children's Hospital, Stanford, CA, USA

Department of Pathology, Stanford University School of Medicine, Stanford, CA, USA

© Springer Nature Switzerland AG 2020
P. Y. Fechner (ed.), *Turner Syndrome*,
https://doi.org/10.1007/978-3-030-34150-3_2

Structure and Function of Sex Chromosomes

In humans, normal internal and external sexual differentiation relies on the presence and composition of the sex chromosomes (see Chap. 1). Most phenotypic females have two X chromosomes (Fig. 2.1), while most phenotypic males have one X chromosome and one Y chromosome. Females with Turner syndrome typically have only one X chromosome (45,X; Fig. 2.2). The Y chromosome contains genes that are important in initiating a complex molecular signaling pathway that induces the bipotential gonad to differentiate into a functioning testis between 6 and 10 weeks of gestation [28]. Therefore, sex determination in humans is dependent upon the presence (male) or absence (female) of a functional Y chromosome in the bi-potential gonadal tissue and not on the number of X chromosomes. However, while only one X chromosome is needed for differentiation of the bi-potential gonad into an ovary in the absence of functional Y chromosomal material, two X chromosomes are required for ovarian maintenance over time; thus women with 45,X without detectable mosaicism for a 46,XX cell line typically have ovarian dysgenesis [44, 59].

One of the best recognized master regulators of male differentiation is the transcription factor encoded by *SRY* (sex-determining region Y), located on the short arm at Yp11.2 [60]. The long arm of the Y chromosome contains several families of genes which allow normal spermatogenesis to occur [32]. At the very end of each arm of the Y chromosome is an area that contains housekeeping genes that are

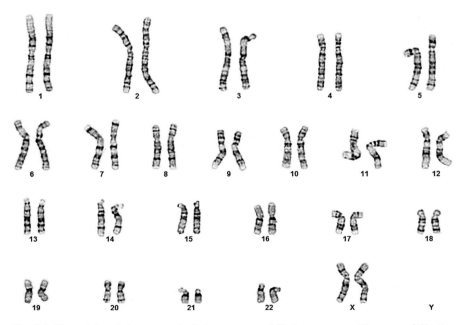

Fig. 2.1 Normal female karyotype depicting two normal X chromosomes. (Courtesy of Charles D. Bangs and Athena M. Cherry, Stanford University, Stanford, CA)

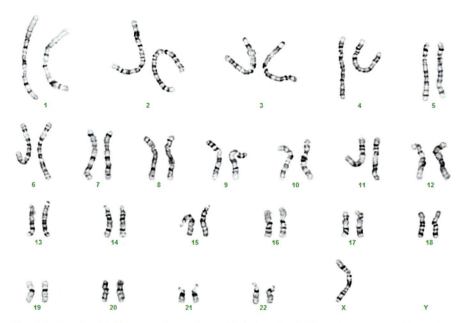

Fig. 2.2 Female with Turner syndrome due to 45,X. Note the single X chromosome with no other sex chromosome present. (Courtesy of Charles D. Bangs and Athena M. Cherry, Stanford University, Stanford, CA)

expressed in multiple organ systems. These areas, called the pseudoautosomal regions (PARs) [8], pair with homologous regions on the ends of the X chromosome and recombine during meiosis, meaning that these genes are represented in a diploid state (i.e., two alleles) in both males and females [48]. The majority of genes in the PAR region escape X-inactivation, such that in females (similar to males) both alleles are expressed [15]. PAR1, located at the terminus of Xp/Yp, is approximately 2.7 Megabases (Mb) in size and contains 25 known genes (16 of which code for proteins); PAR2, located at the terminal end of Xq/Yq, is 0.33 Mb in size and contains five known genes (three of which are known to escape X-inactivation) [5, 14, 50].

X-Inactivation

In order to maintain balanced gene expression levels between the sexes, the X chromosome undergoes regulation that ensures dosage compensation. One of the mechanisms responsible for this is X-chromosome inactivation (XCI) in females [15]. While the Y chromosome houses very few genes that are important for functions other than internal/external genital development and fertility in males, the X chromosome contains hundreds of genes that are important for normal cognitive development (see section "X-Linked Disorders") [15, 70].

Most genes located in the PAR regions of the X chromosome and approximately 15% of genes located elsewhere on the X chromosome escape X-inactivation [15, 48]. Furthermore, the specific genes that are inactivated and the extent to which they are inactivated may differ depending on the tissue type and the developmental stage, adding yet another layer of complexity to this process. Since all of the genes in PAR1 escape X-inactivation, haploinsufficiency for any dosage-sensitive genes in this area could be responsible for the clinical features seen in individuals with Turner syndrome [5]. It is also hypothesized that since males do not have features of Turner syndrome, a majority of the phenotype (excepting the female-specific findings such as ovarian dysgenesis) is due to loss of biallelic expression for genes in the PAR regions that escape XCI [15]. However, the most likely determinant of the severity of the features seen in any given individual with Turner syndrome is the degree of mosaicism for a normal (either 46,XX or 46,XY) cell line in various tissues.

Between 70% and 99% of non-mosaic 45,X human embryos do not survive to term. Studies using human stem cells have suggested that the genes that are present in the PAR regions and those that escape X-inactivation are important in early development and placental function [25, 64]. Furthermore, there may be more variability in the expression of X-linked genes in the early embryo prior to the development of the gonads [15].

The process of X-inactivation in human females is not completely understood but is facilitated by a gene on Xq13.2 termed *XIST* (X-inactivation-specific transcript). *XIST* in humans does not appear to be imprinted, but rather is expressed between the 4- and 8-cell stage in both males and females [46, 65]. Despite the presence of *XIST* mRNA (messenger RNA) at this early stage, both X chromosomes appear to remain active in the trophectoderm and the inner cell mass of the embryo, suggesting that in humans the actual process of XCI occurs in the 10–20 cell epiblast, just after the blastocyst stage [15, 36]. The *XIST* gene product is a noncoding RNA which is thought to coat the inactive X chromosome, leading to chromatin modification and gene repression [45]. In general, XCI is stochastic (i.e., random) with all daughter cells maintaining the same inactive X chromosome as the original parent cell. This means that patches of somatic tissues that arose from one progenitor cell all express genes from either the paternally derived or the maternally derived X chromosome. During the process of gametogenesis, however, the inactive X chromosome is reactivated, which may be the reason that functional germ cells are not made in individuals who have only one X chromosome (see section "Genes on the X Chromosome that Contribute to the Features of Turner Syndrome").

There are several exceptions to the stochastic inactivation of the X chromosome. For example, if a deletion on one X chromosome includes the entire *XIST* gene, this deleted X chromosome will not be able to undergo XCI, leaving the normal X chromosome to be inactive in all cells. However, large X chromosome deletions in which *XIST* is retained are frequently preferentially inactivated to allow expression of the normal X chromosome in most, if not all, cells. When a woman has an X chromosome-autosome translocation, the normal (nontranslocated) X chromosome is typically preferentially inactivated to allow normal gene dosage expression for the autosomal material translocated onto the X chromosome and to avoid overexpression of X-linked genes that are translocated onto the autosome [54].

Imprinted Genes on the X Chromosome

Imprinting is a process by which a gene or group of genes is differentially expressed depending on whether the allele is on the maternally or paternally derived chromosome. In other words, both alleles at a locus are not equally expressed; instead one allele is expressed and the other allele silenced, depending on the parent of origin of the allele.

Turner syndrome (TS) is not truly considered an imprinting disorder, but in any given individual with 45,X, the single X chromosome can be inherited either from the egg (maternal) or the sperm (paternal) [68]. It is estimated that the single X chromosome is inherited from the mother in approximately 80% of females with TS and from the father in the remaining 20% [23]. While substantial evidence points to the existence of imprinted genes on the X chromosome in mice [47], there have not been any definitively identified genes on the human X chromosome that have been shown to be imprinted.

The possibility that the human X chromosome harbors imprinted genes has been studied by evaluating clinical and learning differences between individuals with TS who have a paternally derived X chromosome (X_p) and those who have a maternally derived X chromosome (X_m). Early studies found a better response to growth hormone therapy and a lower probability of having sensorineural hearing loss in females with TS who inherited X_m [22]. Another study identified kidney malformations only in females with TS who had inherited X_m and a higher likelihood of ocular anomalies in those who had inherited X_p [52]. In this study, parent of origin of the X chromosome also appeared to play a role in body mass index and lipid profiles but not in response to growth hormone therapy [52].

Later studies found no significant differences between individuals with 45,X due to X_p and X_m when comparing audiologic, cardiovascular, lymphatic, skeletal, ocular, or renal anomalies. Similarly, no significant differences were seen between girls and women with $45,X_p$ and $45,X_m$ when comparing body mass index, height, or response to growth hormone therapy [7, 29]. Instead both studies found a selective maternal effect on final height in females with TS that was not associated with the parent of origin of the X chromosome. Further studies have also failed to identify any differences in response to growth hormone therapy between females with TS who inherited X_m and those who inherited X_p [16, 37]. Therefore, growth may be impacted by imprinting on autosomal genes but is not likely to be due to imprinted genes on the X chromosome itself.

Psychosocial and cognitive abilities have also been heavily studied with the aim of determining whether these abilities could be impacted by imprinted genes on the X chromosome. It is well known that individuals with TS have a relatively specific neurocognitive profile which includes difficulties with motor abilities, attentional processes, visuospatial perception, and memory with strengths in verbal intelligence quotient (IQ) [9, 41, 49]. Furthermore, individuals with TS frequently have a discrepancy between verbal IQ (VIQ) and performance IQ (PIQ), with PIQ most often being lower than VIQ [43]. An initial study suggested a relationship between the neurocognitive profile and the parent of origin of the X chromosome in Turner syndrome, with females who had $45,X_m$ having significantly lower VIQ scores and worse performance on measures of social cognition and adjustment compared to those with $45,X_p$ [61]. However, a more recent study suggested the opposite, that females with $45,X_p$ performed worse on scales that assess verbal skills compared with those with $45,X_m$ [39].

Studies of the anatomic differences between brain structures in women with $45,X_m$ and $45,X_p$ have also been inconclusive. While some studies suggest that women with X_p have a larger volume of white matter in the temporal lobes bilaterally and in the gray matter in the caudate nuclei and women with $45,X_m$ have increased gray matter in the left superior temporal gyrus, other studies did not find a significant difference in the size of different structures in the brain in women with TS based on parent of origin of the X chromosome [21, 27, 68].

Another argument for the existence of imprinted genes on the X chromosome is the observation that both females with TS and males (who by default inherited their only X chromosome from their mother) have an increased risk of being diagnosed with an autism spectrum disorder (ASD) compared to normal females [12]. This has led to a hypothesis that the paternally derived X chromosome might play a protective role against sociocognitive disorders [9]. While this seems like a logical hypothesis, it is now clear that ASD is a heterogeneous disorder with a variety of identifiable genetic causes in a minority of cases [53]. Individuals with many genetic conditions, including fragile X syndrome, have autistic features as one facet of their condition. Given the large number of genes on the X chromosome that are important for normal neurocognitive development ([70]; see section on "X-Linked Disorders"), it is more likely that the increased risk of "autism" is due to the fact that both females with TS and males who have only one X chromosome, such that a mutation in an important neurodevelopmental gene on the X chromosome and not the parent of origin of the X chromosome itself is the determinant of this finding. Since both females with TS and males do not have a second X chromosome to compensate for haploinsufficiency of an X-linked gene or genes that contribute to normal neurologic and cognitive development, both groups are at increased risk of having X-linked conditions that lead to intellectual disability and/or autistic features.

Most of the studies comparing physical and learning profiles in women with $45,X_m$ and $45,X_p$ are fraught with small sample sizes, typically evaluating less than 100 affected individuals, with the exception of Devernay et al. [16], in which 180 individuals were included. Furthermore, while statistically significant differences can be found in some studies, this does not always translate into clinically significant differences [34]. Altogether, the overlap in features between females with $45,X_m$ and $45,X_p$ is much greater than the overlap in features between all individuals with $45,X$ (regardless of parent of origin of the X chromosome) and those with 46,XX or 46,XY.

One hallmark of imprinted loci on autosomes is the existence of differentially methylated regions (DMRs) that control the epigenetic modification required for parent of origin-specific gene expression. Molecular genetic techniques have been developed to identify such regions, with the goal of defining which regions of the genome are likely to be subjected to imprinting effects [57]. Perhaps the most compelling evidence against the existence of imprinted genes on the human X chromosome is the failure to identify any DMRs on the X chromosome using these assays [58].

Genes on the X Chromosome that Contribute to the Features of Turner Syndrome

The majority of genes that are responsible for the phenotypic features of TS have not been identified, although it is hypothesized that genes in the PAR regions or those that escape XCI are the most likely candidates [15, 71]. However, it is also possible that some of the phenotypic features of TS may be secondary to lymphedema, such as widely spaced nipples, low-set ears, and neck webbing, as these features can also be seen in other conditions, such as Noonan spectrum disorders, in which lymphatic malformations are common [71].

By studying the phenotypes of females who have partial X chromosome deletions, it may be possible to ascertain which genes lead to which components of the phenotype. Initial studies suggested that short stature, ovarian failure, and highly arched palate mapped to the Xp11.2-p22.1 locus [71] and that the neurocognitive phenotype mapped to an area just distal to this, at Xp22.3 [72]. One attractive gene in the Xp22.3 region which may be responsible for a portion of the neurocognitive phenotype is *NLGN4X*, heterozygous (or hemizygous) mutation of which has also been identified to lead to an increased susceptibility to autism [35].

SHOX (short stature homeobox), also located on Xp22.33, is one of the only genes that has unambiguously been associated with short stature and may also be responsible for various skeletal manifestations of TS [19]. Heterozygous (or hemizygous) mutation or small deletion of *SHOX* in individuals with a normal sex chromosome complement causes nonsyndromic (isolated) short stature and Leri-Weill dyschondrosteosis. Biallelic mutations or deletions cause Langer mesomelic dysplasia. *SHOX* is expressed in early embryogenesis in the developing bone and in the prepubertal growth plate chondrocytes during prepubescence [5]. Females who have biallelic preservation of this gene (i.e., those with solely an Xq deletion) typically do not have short stature.

The genes responsible for ovarian function have been mapped to the ends of both Xp and Xq, and in general, the more X chromosome material that is missing, the higher the chance of premature ovarian failure [55]. In fact, reactivation of the inactive X chromosome and an increase in the biallelic expression of X-linked genes are needed for normal ovarian function, which explains why individuals who have a preponderance of 45,X cells in their gonads have ovarian dysgenesis [15]. However, in addition to genes on the X chromosome itself, a number of autosomal genes are also needed for normal ovarian development. Autosomal genes may play a role in the increased expression of X-linked genes during gametogenesis. For example *PRDM14* located on 8q13.3 is a transcription factor that acts in the primordial germ cells to modify epigenetic markers and aid in the reactivation of the inactive X chromosome [15, 45].

The gene *BMP15*, which encodes an oocyte-specific growth factor, is located on Xp11.22 and is important in facilitating normal folliculogenesis and in stimulating granulosa cell growth. Heterozygous mutation of this gene leads to premature ovarian failure and/or ovarian dysgenesis in those with a normal 46,XX karyotype, and therefore absence of one copy of this gene in women with 45,X may predispose to the ovarian phenotype seen in Turner syndrome [17].

How Structural Rearrangements Occur

During meiosis each chromosome pairs with its homologue and crossing-over between the two homologues occurs. A ring X chromosome results from two breaks in the same X chromosome; one break occurs at each end of the chromosome with fusion of the broken end of the short arm with the broken end of the long arm (Fig. 2.3). This may or may not result in a net gain or loss of coding genetic material at one or both of the ends of the ring chromosome. Ring chromosomes are also mitotically unstable, typically leading to mosaic cell lines which lack the ring and/ or which have more than one ring chromosome. The clinical significance of a ring X chromosome depends on the degree of mosaicism for the cell lines without the ring and cell lines with duplicate rings, the presence of *XIST* on the ring chromosome, and the overall genomic content of the ring.

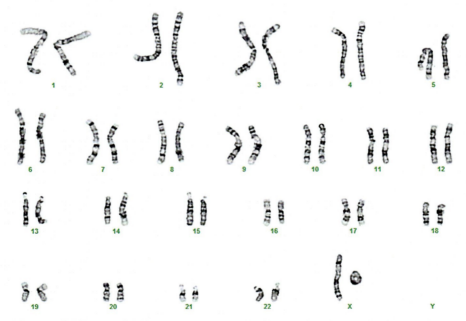

Fig. 2.3 Female with a 46,X,r(X) karyotype. Note the presence of one normal X chromosome and a ring X chromosome in which there is net loss of genetic material. (Courtesy of Charles D. Bangs and Athena M. Cherry, Stanford University, Stanford, CA)

Smaller deletions and duplications of genetic material may result from non-allelic homologous recombination (NAHR), in which highly similar genomic sequences erroneously pair during meiosis with a resulting cross-over event, leading to one daughter cell having a tandem duplication of the DNA segment between the non-allelic sequences and the other daughter cell harboring a deletion of this same segment. NAHR most often leads to small deletions and duplications of genetic material which are not appreciable by high-resolution karyotype, but instead require chromosomal microarray or targeted fluorescence in situ hybridization (FISH) techniques for detection.

In males, the X and Y chromosomes act as homologous pairs. Errors in pairing and in crossing-over can lead to structural chromosome abnormalities. A cross-over between palindrome arms of the Y chromosome can lead to an isodicentric Y chromosome (two centromeres are present with either two mirror image long arm segments at each end and fused mirror image short arms between the two centromeres or vice versa) or to a Y isochromosome (a chromosome with one centromere in which the arms of the chromosomes are mirror images of each other) [4]. Structurally abnormal Y chromosomes, particularly those with two centromeres, are likely to be lost during the process of mitosis, leading to mosaicism for a 45,X cell line.

No environmental factors have unequivocally been associated with an increased risk of structural chromosome abnormalities in the offspring of exposed individuals. Mutagens (agents or exposures that work in a stochastic manner to cause adverse consequences, typically at the DNA level) have the potential to induce chromosome breaks, translocations, deletions, and point mutations. However, studies of the offspring of individuals who were exposed to the atomic bomb blasts or survivors of childhood cancer (who have undergone combination chemotherapy and radiation therapy) have not shown a detectable increase in external anomalies, although large-scale chromosome studies on these offspring to detect balanced chromosomal translocations have not been done [1]. Whether the grandchildren of those who underwent the initial exposure will demonstrate an increased rate of aneuploidy due to a parent with an asymptomatic balanced translocation has yet to be studied.

X-Linked Disorders

Over 10% of genes on the X chromosome (more than 100 protein coding genes alone) have been identified that, when mutated in hemizygous (i.e., only one X) males, cause intellectual disability [15, 70]. In heterozygous 46,XX females, features may or may not be present, owing to X-chromosome inactivation (XCI). Some 46,XX females who have a pathogenic variant (i.e., mutation) in one gene on one of their X chromosomes have features that are the same as affected males, owing to unfavorable XCI of the X chromosome that contains the normally functioning gene. Conversely, skewing of XCI in favor of the X chromosome that expresses the normal allele may lead to minimal or no features at all in such women. Therefore, the terms "X-linked recessive" and "X-linked dominant" are no longer preferred in clinical practice to refer to genes on the X chromosome that can lead to disease, as "X-linked recessive" genes can lead to variable features of the condition in 46,XX females, depending on XCI. For example, 46,XX women who are heterozygous for a pathogenic variant in *DMD*, which leads to Duchenne and Becker muscular dystrophy in males, typically do not have classic features of DMD, but they are at risk for the development of adult-onset dilated cardiomyopathy, which requires screening [3].

Females with Turner syndrome due to 45,X who have a pathogenic variant in an X-linked gene would be expected to have classic features of the X-linked condition, similar to males who are also hemizygous. While a phenotypic female who expresses classic features of an X-linked condition could potentially have Turner syndrome, other causes (i.e., a 46,XX female with skewed XCI or a 46,XY phenotypic female with complete androgen insensitivity syndrome) are also possible. Performing a karyotype would distinguish between these possibilities.

Genetic Testing

Prenatal Testing

The term Turner syndrome (TS) is used to describe phenotypic females who have characteristic physical features and complete or partial absence of the second sex chromosome, with or without cell line mosaicism. Within the definition of Turner syndrome, the following are specifically excluded: (1) those with a 45,X cell line (i.e., mosaicism) but without clinical features of TS; (2) phenotypic males, regardless of karyotype; (3) small terminal deletions of Xp that do not include Xp22.3, which may lead only to short stature; and (4) deletions of Xq distal to Xq24 for which the diagnosis of premature ovarian failure is more appropriate [6].

A diagnosis of TS may be suspected on prenatal ultrasound, particularly when a thickened nuchal translucency is identified through first trimester screening or if a cystic hygroma develops. A fetus with Turner syndrome may also have other ultrasound anomalies, such as left-sided congenital heart defects and renal anomalies, although none of these findings is specific to the diagnosis of TS. A sex chromosome anomaly, such as 45,X/46,XY, may also be suspected if the fetus is found to have the appearance of ambiguous genitalia on prenatal ultrasound [2]. However, if there is a low level of mosaicism for the 45,X cell line in combination with a normal cell line (i.e., 46,XX), there may be no suggestive prenatal ultrasound findings [30]. In fact, for most prenatal incidentally diagnosed (i.e., fetal karyotype completed because of maternal age) fetuses with a 45,X/46,XY chromosome complement, the outcome is a normal phenotypic male who would not be considered to have Turner syndrome [66].

In 2011, noninvasive prenatal screening (NIPS) was introduced as a new method to evaluate pregnancies for fetal aneuploidy. As this screening test relies on obtaining a maternal blood sample as opposed to a placental or an amniotic fluid sample, it carries no risk of fetal mortality; therefore, it has been rapidly implemented into clinical practice. This method relies on sampling extracellular fetal DNA that can be extracted from maternal plasma during the pregnancy. NIPS can be done as early as 9 weeks of gestation up until term and has a high specificity and sensitivity for both trisomy 21 and trisomy 18, but lower sensitivity and specificity for the detection of sex chromosome aneuploidy [10]. In fact, a recent study of 216 pregnant women who underwent NIPS followed by further prenatal cytogenetic or chromosomal microarray studies found that for monosomy X the positive predictive value was only 23%, meaning that NIPS currently has a high false-positive rate for TS [42]. This may be related in part to the low prevalence of a fetus with 45,X in an unselected population of pregnant women. If monosomy X is suggested by NIPS, a diagnostic study, such as amniocentesis or postnatal karyotype, is recommended to confirm the result. It is unknown if NIPS is accurate for the detection of Turner syndrome due to a structural rearrangement or deletion of a portion of one X chromosome, as it is designed specifically to screen for aneuploidy (i.e., loss or gain of an entire chromosome).

Invasive prenatal diagnosis for chromosome anomalies includes chorionic villus sampling (CVS), performed between 10 and 12 weeks of gestation, and amniocentesis, most typically performed after 16 weeks of gestation until 23 weeks of gestation (amniocentesis can be performed at later gestational ages but leads to an increasing risk of preterm birth). CVS relies on the collection of placental tissue, which has a fetal component; there is a risk of both confined placental mosaicism (i.e., when a mosaic chromosome abnormality is found only in placental tissue and not in the fetus) and maternal cell contamination (when a portion or all of the cells cultured for the study are of maternal and not fetal origin). When a diagnosis of mosaic Turner syndrome is detected through CVS, a confirmatory study, which may include amniocentesis or postnatal testing, is required to determine if the abnormal cell line is present in the fetus, as placental tissues are better able to tolerate chromosome abnormalities than is the fetus. Because amniocentesis does not carry a risk of confined placental mosaicism or maternal cell contamination, the finding of a mosaic sex aneuploidy does not typically prompt a second prenatal sample, but postnatal confirmation is recommended [69].

When multiple fetal anomalies are found on prenatal ultrasound or after birth, a chromosomal microarray (CMA; typically obtained through amniocentesis if it is pursued prenatally) may be performed as a first-line test instead of a karyotype. This study will reveal monosomy X in addition to loss of a portion of one X chromosome. It is estimated that CMA is able to detect mosaicism to a level of about 10–15% [56], but it is not able to determine the structure of an abnormal X chromosome (i.e., if it is in a ring configuration). One advantage of CMA is that it can determine the exact gene content of a deletion or duplication of genetic material, such as whether *XIST* is present on a structurally abnormal X chromosome.

Postnatal Testing

When TS is suspected postnatally, a chromosome analysis from peripheral blood is typically performed. Evaluation of a buccal smear for Barr bodies (X chromatin bodies) should not be done as a diagnostic test, as such testing has low sensitivity and specificity for TS, may lead to a false-negative result in individuals who have mosaicism for 45,X/46,XX, and will not detect Y chromosome material, if it is present [18]. Similarly, in the absence of cognitive impairment, chromosomal microarray is not recommended as a first-line test for an individual suspected of having TS because of its limited ability to detect low levels of mosaicism [69]. Of individuals with TS who undergo a peripheral blood karyotype, approximately 45% will be found to have non-mosaic 45,X; the remainder of affected individuals have a variety of structural chromosome abnormalities or mosaicism for a 45,X cell line and another cell line (see Table 2.1) [69].

Because the presence of Y chromosomal material in an individual with a 45,X cell line increases the risk of the development of gonadoblastoma [11, 63], clinicians and patients are frequently concerned about whether genetic testing can rule out the presence of Y chromosomal material. Using standard cytogenetic techniques, between 6% and 11% of individuals with TS have been identified to have mosaicism for a cell line that contains either a normal or an abnormal Y chromosome [69]. Unfortunately, no test can absolutely guarantee that there is no mosaicism for a second cell line in individuals with 45,X. Furthermore, the question of whether mosaicism exists in the cells in a gonad or streak gonad would require evaluation of the tissue itself, which is impractical. Therefore, the American College of Medical Genetics and Genomics (ACMG) has developed laboratory guidelines for the diagnosis of Turner syndrome [69]; these guidelines were reaffirmed in 2014 by the ACMG Laboratory Quality Assurance Committee.

Methods to detect occult mosaicism for Y chromosomal material have included the use of molecular genetic techniques (polymerase chain reaction [PCR] and/or Southern blot) or interphase fluorescence in situ hybridization (FISH) with a Y centromere probe [13, 67]. Unfortunately PCR for the detection of Y chromosomal material has a high false-positive rate [67], and the ACMG recommends that confirmation of a positive result be performed through FISH analysis [69].

The current laboratory standard for the evaluation of an individual suspected of having a sex chromosome abnormality is a standard 20-cell karyotype done on a peripheral blood sample. If mosaicism for a sex chromosome abnormality is found

Table 2.1 Karyotypes in individuals with Turner syndrome

Karyotype	Percentage (%) of individuals with TS
45,X	45
46,X,i(X)(q10) with or without 45,X	15–18
46,X,+mar or + r with or without 45,X	7–16
45,X/46,XX or 45,X/47,XXX	7–16
46,X,del(Xp) with or without 45,X	2–5
46,XY or 46,X,del(Y) or 46,X,r(Y) with 45,X	6–11
Others	2–8

From Wolff et al. [69]
mar marker chromosome, *r* ring chromosome

in the first 20 cells, the analysis is complete. However, if only one cell with a sex chromosome gain, loss, or rearrangement is identified in the first 20 metaphases analyzed, then a minimum of 10 additional metaphase cells should be evaluated. If a full 30-cell analysis demonstrates a non-mosaic 45,X karyotype, interphase FISH analysis on a minimum of 200 cells using X and Y centromere probes to evaluate for a low level of mosaicism for a second cell line is recommended. In the event that an affected female has evidence of virilization, such as clitoromegaly or posterior fusion of the labia majora, yet the chromosome analysis and FISH studies do not reveal a second cell line, then evaluation of a second tissue, such as skin fibroblasts, should be considered. Similarly, in a female with features of TS in whom cytogenetic studies have identified only 46,XX cells, evaluation of a second tissue can be pursued if the clinical suspicion for a diagnosis of TS remains high. However, it should also be noted that women normally undergo an age-related loss of the X chromosome [51] and, therefore, some women without TS may be found to have a low level of mosaicism for 45,X (typically <10%) on a standard peripheral blood cytogenetic analysis [69].

When a ring X chromosome is identified either in a mosaic or non-mosaic form, the outcome is quite variable. Further microarray studies can determine if *XIST* is present on the ring, in which case it may be selectively inactivated, particularly if the ring is missing a significant amount of X chromosomal material. In general, individuals with a ring X chromosome have a high risk of cognitive impairment along with other features of TS, particularly if *XIST* is absent on the ring chromosome [31, 38]; however, exceptions to this general rule exist. Cognitive impairment may also be a feature when individuals have an X chromosome-autosome translocation, because the X chromosome involved in the translocation most often remains active with selective inactivation of the normal X chromosome.

Recurrence Risks

Unaffected Parents

Turner syndrome due to 45,X is typically a sporadic condition unrelated to parental age. Approximately 70–80% of cases are due to a nondisjunction event involving the paternal X chromosome (leading to $45,X_m$) [23, 40]. When a couple has a daughter with 45,X, the risk of recurrence in a subsequent pregnancy is very low, with the highest reported rate being 1.4% [33]. The increased risk of recurrence compared to the background risk in the population has been postulated to be related to an increased risk of nondisjunction in certain families. The causes of an increased risk of nondisjunction in some families are unknown, although mechanisms that impact DNA methylation status, such as genetic polymorphisms in *MTHFR* which encodes the enzyme methylenetetrahydrofolate reductase, have been implicated in some studies [26]. Similarly, it is postulated that individuals who have detectable mosaicism for 45,X/46,XX or 45,X/46,XY likely had a normal sex chromosome complement at conception but subsequently underwent somatic loss of one sex chromosome during later embryonic or fetal development. Therefore, the recurrence risk for an unaffected couple to have another affected pregnancy is low.

The recurrence risk for a couple who has a daughter with one normal X chromosome and a second, structurally abnormal X chromosome depends on the chromosomal complement of the mother. If the mother does not have any evidence of an X chromosome abnormality on peripheral blood cytogenetic studies, then the recurrence risk is low. Paternal testing for an X chromosome abnormality is typically not required in a father who has undergone normal growth and development.

Affected Mother

Most women with TS due to 45,X are infertile due to ovarian dysgenesis [59]. However, women with detectable mosaicism for a 46,XX cell line (or rarely those who have 45,X without a detectable 46,XX cell line) may undergo spontaneous puberty and menarche, although they appear to have an increased risk for premature ovarian failure. In this population, there also appears to be an increased risk of spontaneous miscarriage, although the possibility of a secondary cause, such as uterine or other Mullerian anomalies or maternal factors, may contribute to this increased rate [20, 24]. There is also an increased risk above the general population risk of having a child with 45,X, other chromosome abnormalities, or birth defects [62]. The overall risk to any given affected mother is unknown and it should be noted that most reports of offspring with chromosome anomalies or birth defects are derived from case reports or small case series, meaning that the literature may be biased and not representative of the true risk. In any event, high-resolution ultrasound is recommended and prenatal diagnosis for chromosome abnormalities (see section "Genetic Testing") is available.

Women who themselves have a structural X chromosome abnormality (including ring X) in which the Xq13-q26 region is preserved may also have preserved fertility [62]. Depending on the amount of X chromosome material that is missing, affected women may also be at increased risk for premature ovarian failure [20]. In those who are able to conceive with their own ovum, theoretically half of the female conceptuses will inherit the structurally abnormal X and the other half will inherit the normal X. The risk of having a liveborn female with the structurally abnormal maternal X, however, may be less than 50%. For example, a woman with a ring X chromosome will inevitably also have mosaicism for a 45,X cell line. If a female fetus inherits the maternal ring X chromosome, the fetus also will ultimately have mosaicism for a 45,X cell line. The fetus may have an increased risk of spontaneously aborting, depending on the degree of mosaicism for a 45,X cell line. Liveborn female offspring with mosaicism for a ring X chromosome born to women who also have mosaicism for a ring chromosome have been reported [20]. Unfortunately empiric recurrence risks are not available due to the very small number of families in which fertility is preserved and pregnancy outcome is known and may be falsely elevated due to publication bias [20].

A male fetus who inherits the structurally abnormal maternal X chromosome may not be viable, leading to an increased rate of miscarriage in women with a structurally abnormal X chromosome, or may have congenital anomalies and/or cognitive impairment, depending on the specific X chromosome abnormality present in the mother. Preconception genetic counseling to address these issues for the specific X chromosome abnormality in any given family is recommended.

Father with a Structurally Abnormal Y Chromosome

In individuals who have mosaicism for a 45,X cell line and a second cell line that contains a structurally abnormal Y chromosome (i.e., an isodicentric Y that retains *SRY* and genes important for male fertility), it is possible that this structurally abnormal Y chromosome was inherited from an asymptomatic father. Paternal peripheral blood chromosome analysis is recommended. If the father of the affected child is not found to harbor the abnormal Y chromosome in his blood, recurrence risks are low. A father who has this Y chromosome rearrangement would have a 100% chance of passing it onto each son and will not pass it on to any daughter. Structurally abnormal Y chromosomes in which *SRY* is nonfunctional are unlikely to be inherited from an asymptomatic father. Similarly, Y chromosome abnormalities in which important genes for male fertility are missing are unlikely to be inherited from a father without the use of assisted reproductive technology. Prenatal diagnosis for Y chromosome abnormalities is also available.

Commentary

While it is clear that the chromosomal nature of Turner syndrome has been extensively researched, there is still much that could be learned about the pathogenesis of the clinical features seen in Turner syndrome. For example, most of the genes that lead to the features of TS have not been identified. Determining which genes predispose to the congenital malformations (i.e., the specific constellation of congenital heart defects seen in TS, the renal anomalies, etc.) could be invaluable to our overall understanding of the etiology of these types of malformations, both as isolated birth defects and as parts of other multiple malformation syndromes. This may lead to the identification of new developmental pathways, perturbations of which could lead to these features in isolation. Similarly, further dissection of the causes of the specific neurocognitive and social difficulties in girls with TS will improve our understanding of the complexities of the brain and could potentially lead to improved treatments, including targeted pharmacologic therapies, to aid affected individuals. Clearly, we have only scratched the surface in our understanding of the complexities of the X chromosome and the various genes it houses.

References

1. Adam MP. The all-or-none hypothesis revisited. Birth Defects Res A ClinMolTeratol. 2012;94:664–9. https://doi.org/10.1002/bdra.23029.
2. Adam MP, Fechner P, Ramsdell LA, Badaru A, Grady RE, Pagon RA, et al. Ambiguous genitalia: what prenatal genetic testing is practical? Am J Med Genet Part A. 2012;158A:1337–43. https://doi.org/10.1002/ajmg.a.35338.
3. American Academy of Pediatrics Section on Cardiology and Cardiac Surgery. Cardiovascular health supervision for individuals affected by Duchenne or Becker muscular dystrophy. Pediatrics. 2005;116:1569–73.
4. Bellott DW, Hughes JF, Skaletsky H, Brown LG, Pyntikova T, Cho TJ, et al. Mammalian Y chromosomes retain widely expressed dosage-sensitive regulators. Nature. 2014;508:494–9. https://doi.org/10.1038/nature13206.
5. Blaschke RJ, Rappold G. The pseudoautosomal regions, *SHOX*, and disease. CurrOpin Genet Dev. 2006;16:233–9.
6. Bondy CA, The Turner Syndrome Consensus Study Group. Care of girls and women with Turner syndrome: a guideline of the Turner Syndrome Study Group. J ClinEndocrinolMetab. 2007;92:10–25.
7. Bondy CA, Matura LA, Wooten N, Troendle J, Zinn AR, Bakalov VK, et al. The physical phenotype of girls and women with Turner syndrome is not X-imprinted. Hum Genet. 2007;121:469–74.
8. Burgoyne PS. Genetic homology and crossing over in the X and Y chromosomes of mammals. Hum Genet. 1982;61:85–90.
9. Burnett AC, Reutens D, Wood AG. Social cognition in Turner's syndrome. J ClinNeurosci. 2010;17:283–6. https://doi.org/10.1016/j.jocn.2009.09.006.
10. Committee Opinion No. 640. Cell-free DNA screening for fetal aneuploidy. American College of Obstetrics and Gynecologists. Obstet Gynecol. 2015;126:e31–7. https://doi.org/10.1097/AOG.0000000000001051.
11. Cools M, Drop SL, Wolffenbuttel KP, Oosterhuis JW, Looijenga LH. Germ cell tumors in the intersex gonad: old paths, new directions, moving frontiers. Endocr Rev. 2006;27:468–84.
12. Creswell CS, Skuse DH. Autism in association with Turner syndrome: genetic implications for male vulnerability to pervasive developmental disorders. Neurocase. 1999;5:511–8.
13. Da Silva-Grecco RL, Trovo-Marqui AB, de Sousa TA, Da Croce L, Balarin MA. Identification of Y-chromosome sequences in Turner syndrome. Indian J Pediatr. 2016;83:405–9. https://doi.org/10.1007/s12098-015-1929-6.
14. De Bonis ML, Cerase A, Matarazzo MR, Ferraro M, Strazzullo M, Hansen RS, et al. Maintenance of X- and Y-inactivation of the pseudoautosomal (PAR2) gene *SPRY3* is independent from DNA methylation and associated to multiple layers of epigenetic modifications. Hum Mol Genet. 2006;15:1123–32.
15. Deng X, Berletch JB, Nguyen DK, Disteche CM. X chromosome regulation: diverse patterns in development, tissues and disease. Nat Rev Genet. 2014;15:367–78. https://doi.org/10.1038/nrg3687.
16. Devernay M, Bolca D, Kerdjana L, Aboura A, Gerard B, Tabet AC, et al. Parental origin of the X chromosome does not influence growth hormone treatment effect in Turner syndrome. J ClinEndocrinolMetab. 2012;97:E1241–8. https://doi.org/10.1210/jc.2011-3488.
17. Di Pasqualie E, Beck-Peccoz P, Persani L. Hypergonadotropic ovarian failure associated with an inherited mutation of human bone morphogenic protein-15 (BMP15) gene. Am J Hum Genet. 2004;75:106–11. https://doi.org/10.1086/422103.
18. Frias JL, Davenport ML, Committee on Genetics and Section on Endocrinology. Health supervision for children with Turner syndrome. Pediatrics. 2003;111:692–702.
19. Fukami M, Naiki Y, Muroya K, Hamajima T, Soneda S, Horikawa R, et al. Rare pseudoautosomal copy-number variations involving *SHOX* and/or its flanking regions in individuals with and without short stature. J Hum Genet. 2015;60:553–6. https://doi.org/10.1038/jhg.2015.53.

20. Gardner RJM, Sutherland GR. Chromosome abnormalities and genetic counseling. 3rd ed. New York: Oxford University Press; 2004.
21. Good CD, Lawrence K, Thomas NS, Price CJ, Ashburner J, Friston KJ, et al. Dosage-sensitive X-linked locus influences the development of amygdala and orbitofrontal cortex, and fear recognition in humans. Brain. 2003;126:2431–46.
22. Hamelin CE, Anglin G, Quigley CA, Deal CL. Genomic imprinting in Turner syndrome: effects on response to growth hormone and on risk of sensorineural hearing loss. J ClinEndocrinolMetab. 2006;91:3002–10.
23. Hassold T, Benham F, Leppert M. Cytogenetic and molecular analysis of sex-chromosome monosomy. Am J Hum Genet. 1988;42:534–41.
24. Homer L, Le Martelot MT, Morel F, Amice V, Kerlan V, Collet M, et al. 45,X/46,XX mosaicism below 30% of aneuploidy: clinical implications in adult women from a reproductive medicine unit. Eur J Endocrinol. 2010;162:617–23. https://doi.org/10.1530/EJE-09-0750.
25. Hook EB, Warburton D. Turner syndrome revisited: review of new data supports the hypothesis that all viable 45,X cases are cryptic mosaics with a rescue cell line, implying an origin by mitotic loss. Hum Genet. 2014;133:417–24. https://doi.org/10.1007/s00439-014-1420-x.
26. Ismail MF, Zarouk WA, Ruby MO, Mahmoud WM, Gad RS. Methylenetetrahydrofolate reductase gene polymorphisms in Egyptian Turner Syndrome patients. Acta Biochim Pol. 2015;62:529–32. https://doi.org/10.18388/abp.2015_974.
27. Kesler SR, Blasey CM, Brown WE, Yankowitz J, Zeng SM, Bender BG, et al. Effects of X-monosomy and X-linked imprinting on superior temporal gyrus morphology in Turner syndrome. Biol Psychiatry. 2003;54:636–46.
28. Knarston I, Ayers K, Sinclair A. Molecular mechanisms associated with 46,XX disorders of sex development. Clin Sci (London). 2016;130:421–32. https://doi.org/10.1042/CS20150579.
29. Ko JM, Kim J-M, Kim GH, Lee BH, Yoo HW. Influence of parental origin of the X chromosome on physical phenotypes and GH responsiveness of patients with Turner syndrome. Clin Endocrinol. 2010;73:66–71. https://doi.org/10.1111/j.1365-2265.2010.03782.x.
30. Koeberl DD, McGillivary B, Sybert VP. Prenatal diagnosis of 45,X/46,XX mosaicism and 45,X: implications for postnatal outcome. Am J Hum Genet. 1995;57(3):661–6.
31. Kubota T, Wakui K, Nakamura T, Ohashi H, Watanabe Y, Yoshino M, et al. The proportion of cells with functional X disomy is associated with the severity of mental retardation in mosaic ring X Turner syndrome females. Cytogenet Genome Res. 2002;99:276–84.
32. Lahn BT, Page DC. Functional coherence of the human Y chromosome. Science. 1997;278:675–80.
33. Larizza D, Danesino C, Maraschio P, Caramagna C, Klersy C, Calcaterra V. Familial occurrence of Turner syndrome: casual event or increased risk? J Pediatr Endocrinol Metab. 2011;24:223–5.
34. Lawrence K, Kuntsi J, Coleman M, Campbell R, Skuse D. Face and emotion recognition deficits in Turner syndrome: a possible role for X-linked genes in amygdala development. Neuropsychology. 2003;17:39–49.
35. Lawson-Yuen A, Saldivar JS, Sommer S, Picker J. Familial deletion within NLGN4 associated with autism and Tourette syndrome. Eur J Hum Genet. 2008;16:614–8. https://doi.org/10.1038/sj.ejhg.5202006.
36. Lee JT, Bartolomei MS. X-inactivation, imprinting, and long noncoding RNAs in health and disease. Cell. 2013;152:1308–23. https://doi.org/10.1016/j.cell.2013.02.016.
37. Lee HJ, Jung HW, Lee GM, Kim HY, Kim JH, Lee SH, et al. No influence of parental origin of intact X chromosome and/or Y chromosome sequences on three-year height response to growth hormone therapy in Turner syndrome. Ann Pediatr Endocrinol Metabol. 2014;19:127–34. https://doi.org/10.6065/apem.2014.19.3.127.
38. Leppig KA, Sybert VP, Ross JL, Cunniff C, Trejo T, Raskind WH, et al. Phenotype and X inactivation in 45,X/46,X,r(X) cases. Am J Med Genet A. 2004;128A:276–84.
39. Loesch DZ, Bui QM, Kelso W, Huggins RM, Slater H, Warne G, et al. Effect of Turner's syndrome and X-linked imprinting on cognitive status: analysis based on pedigree data. Brain and Development. 2005;27:494–503.

40. Mathur A, Stekol L, Schatz D, MacLaren NK, Scott ML, Lippe B. The parental origin of the single X chromosome in Turner syndrome: lack of correlation with parental age or clinical phenotype. Am J Hum Genet. 1991;48:682–6.
41. McCauley E, Kay T, Ito J, Treder R. The Turner syndrome: cognitive deficits, affective discrimination, and behavior problems. Child Dev. 1987;58:464–73.
42. Meck JM, Kramer Dugan E, Matyakhina L, Aviram A, Trunca C, Pineda-Alvarez D, et al. Noninvasive prenatal screening for aneuploidy: positive predictive values based on cytogenetic findings. Am J Obstet Gynecol. 2015;213:214.e1–5. https://doi.org/10.1016/j.ajog.2015.04.001.
43. Mullaney R, Murphy D. Turner syndrome: neuroimaging findings: structural and functional. Dev Disabil Res Rev. 2009;15:279–83. https://doi.org/10.1002/ddrr.87.
44. Ogata T, Muroya K, Matsuo N, Shinohara O, Yorifuji T, Nishi Y, et al. Turner syndrome and Xp deletions: clinical and molecular studies in 47 patients. J Clin Endocrinol Metab. 2001;86:5498–508.
45. Ohhata T, Wutz A. Reactivation of the inactive X chromosome in development and reprogramming. Cell Mol Life Sci. 2013;70:2443–61. https://doi.org/10.1007/s00018-012-1174-3.
46. Okamoto I, Patrat C, Thépot D, Peynot N, Fauque P, Daniel N, et al. Eutherian mammals use diverse strategies to initiate X-chromosome inactivation during development. Nature. 2011;472:370–4. https://doi.org/10.1002/gcc.20890.
47. Raefski AS, O'Neill MJ. Identification of a cluster of X-linked imprinted genes in mice. Nat Genet. 2005;37:620–4.
48. Raudsepp T, Chowdhary P. The Eutherian pseudoautosomal region. Cytogenet Genome Res. 2015;147:81–94. https://doi.org/10.1159/000443157.
49. Ross JL, Zinn AR, McCauley E. Neurodevelopmental and psychosocial aspects of Turner syndrome. Ment Retard Dev Disabil Res Rev. 2000;6:135–41.
50. Ross MT, Grafham DV, Coffey AJ, Scherer S, McLay K, Muzny D, et al. The DNA sequence of the human X chromosome. Nature. 2005;434:325–37.
51. Russell LM, Strike P, Browne CE, Jacobs PA. X chromosome loss and ageing. Cytogenet Genome Res. 2007;116:181–5.
52. Sagi L, Zuckerman-Levin N, Gawlik A, Ghizzoni L, Buyukgebiz A, Rakover Y, et al. Clinical significance of the parental origin of the X chromosome in Turner syndrome. J Clin Endocrinol Metab. 2007;92:846–52.
53. Schaefer GB, Mendelsohn NJ, Professional Practice and Guidelines Committee. Clinical genetics evaluation in identifying the etiology of autism spectrum disorders: 2013 guideline revisions. Genet Med. 2013;15:399–407. https://doi.org/10.1038/gim.2013.32.
54. Schinzel A. Catalogue of unbalanced chromosome aberrations in man. 2nd ed. Berlin: De Gruyter; 2001.
55. Schlessinger D, Herrera L, Crisponi L, Mumm S, Percesepe A, Pellegrini M, et al. Genes and translocations involved in POF. Am J Med Genet. 2002;111:328–33.
56. Scott SA, Cohen N, Brandt T, Toruner G, Desnick RJ, Edelmann L. Detection of low-level mosaicism and placental mosaicism by oligonucleotide array comparative genomic hybridization. Genet Med. 2010;12:85–92. https://doi.org/10.1097/GIM.0b013e3181cc75d0.
57. Sharp AJ, Migliavaccal E, Durprel Y, Stathaki E, Sailani MR, Baumer A, et al. Methylation profiling in individuals with uniparental disomy identifies novel differentially methylated regions on chromosome 15. Genome Res. 2010;20:1271–8. https://doi.org/10.1101/gr.108597.110.
58. Sharp AJ, Stathaki E, Migliavacca E, Brahmachary M, Montgomery SB, Dupre Y, et al. DNA methylation profiles of human active and inactive X chromosomes. Genome Res. 2011;21:1592–600. https://doi.org/10.1101/gr.112680.110.
59. Simpson JL, Rajkovic A. Ovarian differentiation and gonadal failure. Am J Hum Genet. 1999;89:186–200.
60. Sinclair AH, Berta P, Palmer MS, Hawkins R, Griffiths BL, Smith M, et al. A gene from the human sex-determining region encodes a protein with homology to a conserved DNA-binding motif. Nature. 1990;346:240–5.

61. Skuse DH, James RS, Bishop DV, Coppin B, Dalton P, Aamodt-Leeper G, et al. Evidence from Turner's syndrome of an imprinted X-linked locus affecting cognitive function. Nature. 1997;387:705–8.
62. Tarani L, Lampariello S, Raguso G, Colloridi F, Pucarelli I, Pasquino AM, et al. Pregnancy in patients with Turner's syndrome: six new cases and review of the literature. Gynecol Endocrinol. 1998;12:83–7.
63. Tsuchiya K, Reijo R, Page DC, Disteche CM. Gonadoblastoma: molecular definition of the susceptibility region on the Y chromosome. Am J Hum Genet. 1995;57:1400–7.
64. Urbach A, Benvenisty N. Studying early lethality of 45,XO (Turner's syndrome) embryos using human embryonic stem cells. PLoS One. 2009;4:e4175. https://doi.org/10.1371/journal.pone.0004175.
65. van den Berg IM, Laven JS, Stevens M, Jonkers I, Galjaard RJ, Gribnau J, et al. X chromosome inactivation is initiated in human preimplantation embryos. Am J Hum Genet. 2009;84:771–9. https://doi.org/10.1016/j.ajhg.2009.05.003.
66. Wheeler M, Peakman D, Robinson A, Henry G. 45,X/46,XY mosaicism: contrast of prenatal and postnatal diagnosis. Am J Med Genet. 1988;29:565–71.
67. Wiktor AE, Van Dyke DL. Detection of low level sex chromosome mosaicism in Ullrich-Turner syndrome patients. Am J Med Genet. 2005;138A:249–61.
68. Wilkins JF, Ubeda F. Diseases associated with genomic imprinting. Prog Mol Biol Transl Sci. 2011;101:401–45. https://doi.org/10.1016/j.cub.2011.02.027.
69. Wolff DJ, Van Dyke DL, Powell CM, Working Group of the ACMG Laboratory Quality Assurance Committee. Laboratory guideline for Turner syndrome. Genet Med. 2010;12:52–5. https://doi.org/10.1097/GIM.0b013e3181c684b2.
70. Zechner U, Wilda M, Kehrer-Sawatzki H, Vogel W, Fundele R, Hameister H. A high density of X-linked genes for general cognitive ability: a run-away process shaping human evolution? Trends Genet. 2001;17:679–701.
71. Zinn AR, Tonk VS, Chen Z, Flejter WL, Gardner HA, Guerra R, et al. Evidence for a Turner syndrome locus or loci at Xp11.2-p22.1. Am J Hum Genet. 1998;63:1757–66.
72. Zinn AR, Roeltgen D, Stefanatos G, Ramos P, Elder FF, Kushner H, et al. A Turner syndrome neurocognitive phenotype maps to Xp22.3. Behav Brain Funct. 2007;3:24. https://doi.org/10.1186/1744-9081-3-24.

Chapter 3
Pattern and Etiology of Growth Disturbance in Turner Syndrome and Outcomes of Growth-Promoting Treatments

Charmian A. Quigley

Spontaneous Growth Pattern in Childhood and Adolescence, and Adult Height of Untreated Women

Growth Pattern and Height During Infancy, Childhood, Adolescence, and Adulthood

In 1932 Dr. Henry Turner, an Oklahoma obstetrician and gynecologist, evaluated his first patient with the condition that subsequently came to bear his name, and in 1938 he published his seminal paper reporting the clinical features of seven patients between the ages of 15 and 23 years who had been referred to him for "dwarfism" and lack of secondary sexual development [1]. Although Dr. Turner was the first to synthesize the clinical features into a recognizable pattern, medical historians have deduced that anatomist Giovanni Morgagni may have described the first case of the condition in 1768, when he reported autopsy findings of a woman with short stature and gonadal dysgenesis [2]. Furthermore, 8 years before Turner's publication German physician Dr. Otto Ullrich had reported a patient with classical features of Turner syndrome (TS) and made the prescient speculation that the physical anomalies might be due to generalized dilatation of the lymphatics [3]. Thus the condition is commonly known as Ullrich-Turner syndrome (UTS) in Europe. Studies in the 1970s and 1980s focused on describing the phenotype of women with TS, and in 1985 Lyon and colleagues compiled the data from five patient cohorts and published the first comprehensive TS growth chart [4–8], reporting that average adult height (AH) of untreated women with TS was around 143 ± 7 cm, about 20 cm shorter than the mean height of women without TS. However, in "tall" regions such as the Netherlands and Scandinavia, mean heights are up to 5 cm greater both for women in the general population and for women with TS (Table 3.1; Fig. 3.1). Because the

C. A. Quigley (✉)
Sydney Children's Hospital, Randwick, NSW, Australia

© Springer Nature Switzerland AG 2020
P. Y. Fechner (ed.), *Turner Syndrome*,
https://doi.org/10.1007/978-3-030-34150-3_3

Table 3.1 Summary of Turner syndrome growth charts

Country/Region	Number subjects	Data type	Age, yr	Estrogen age, yr (n)[a]	Adult height mean±SD, cm	Age at AH, yr (n)	Reference	Year published
Argentina	254	Cross	0–22	14.0±1.2 (90)	137.9±5.7	18.1 (110)	Garcia-Rudaz et al. [9]	1995
Austria	141	Mixed	0–18	None	Median, 143.8	≥18 (18)	Haeusler et al. [10]	1992
Belgium	100	Mixed	0–22	15.0±1.2 [11.3–18.0] (83[b])	143.4±5.6	≥16 (34)	Massa et al. [11]	1990
Canada	116	Mixed	0–20	17.0 (38)	142.0±7.6	17[c] (28)	Park et al. [12]	1983
Denmark	78	Long	6.5–17.5	17.0±2.0; Baseline, ≥13.2 (71)	146.8±5.8	≥21 (76)	Naeraa and Nielsen [13]	1990
Denmark Netherlands Sweden	108 372 118 Total: 598	Long	0–20+	17.7 [14.8–20.1] (n/p)[d] 15.1 [12.8–19.9] (n/p)[d] Insufficient data	146.9±7.8	19–45 (50)	Rongen-Westerlaken et al. [14]	1997
Egypt	93	Cross	0.5–24	n/p	~144[e]	n/p	El-Bassyouni et al. [15]	2012
England Finland France Germany	93 55 60 251 Total: 459	Mixed	1–20+	Baseline, ≥19 (29)[f]	143.2±4.5[g] 142.9±7.3[h]	19–24 (29)[g] ≥19 (138)[h]	Lyon et al. [4]	1985
France	167	Mixed	0–22	n/p	142.1±5.6	22 (106)	Sempe et al. [16]	1996
Japan	704	Mixed	0–20	None	139.5±4.0[i]	≥18 (23)	Suwa [17]	1992
Japan	1447/118[j]	Mixed	0.75–23.25	None[k]	141.3±5.6	≥20 (26)	Isojima et al. [18, 19]	2009/2010
Israel	47	Long	0.25–3.0	n/a	n/a	n/a	Even et al. [20]	2000
Italy	772	Mixed	0–20+	Baseline, ≥13 (225)	142.5±7.0	20.7[l] (105)	Bernasconi et al. [21]	1994
USA	112	Long	0–8	n/a	n/a	n/a	Davenport et al. [22]	2002

Abbreviations: (*n*) number of subjects, *n/a* not applicable (children in these 2 series were up to age 8 only), *n/p* not provided, *cross* cross-sectional, *long* longitudinal, *mixed* mixed cross-sectional and longitudinal data - in most cases of "mixed" data the majority of data points are cross-sectional, *none* no subjects received estrogen

[a]Mean (± SD), median [range] or baseline age at which estrogen replacement was initiated; (*n*) = number of subjects who received estrogen

[b]*n* = 83 with "induced puberty", calculated by deducting 17 subjects with spontaneous puberty from the total 100 subjects

[c]In this study "maturity" was defined as bone age equivalent to 17 years

[d]Median age [10–90 percentile]; n/p = no data are provided for numbers of patients who received estrogen but it appears this was all or most

[e]Mean height estimated from graph, actual value and subject number not provided

[f]Estrogen data were provided for English cohort only, all other series had received "no hormone treatment"

[g]AH and age data provided separately for English cohort

[h]Values for AH and age for pooled Finnish, French and German cohorts

[i]Calculated as weighted average of mean values for 18 subjects with, and 5 subjects without, spontaneous menarche

[j]Two consecutive studies comprising an initial sample and a validation sample

[k]Reports do not specify whether or not estrogen was given, but subjects with signs of puberty were specifically excluded

[l]Median age

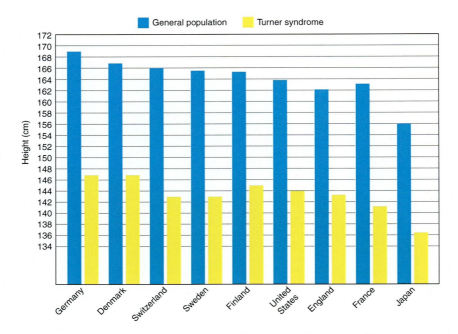

Fig. 3.1 Heights of non-GH-treated women with Turner syndrome (yellow bars) compared to heights of women in the general population (blue bars) in various countries. On average, women with Turner syndrome are about 20 cm shorter than their countrywomen. (Reproduced with permission from *Turner Syndrome: A Comprehensive Guide*, copyright Office of Lilly CME)

initial studies of stature in TS were derived from clinic populations, they may reflect a degree of ascertainment bias toward shorter subjects. In addition, a number of studies, including an analysis of over 7200 patients enrolled in a large international observational database, have demonstrated secular trends toward greater height (and other features) of girls and women with TS, similar to those observed in the general population [18, 21, 23]. Nevertheless, it remains clear that short stature is a consistent feature of untreated patients with TS.

The natural history of growth in TS was extensively examined in the 1970s–1990s in a series of European and North American studies [4–8, 11–14, 16, 21, 24–35] and can be summarized as a pattern of inexorable growth failure over the 20+-year period from birth to maturity. The growth disturbance is already established by the second trimester of fetal development [33], resulting in mild intrauterine growth restriction, with average birth weight about 300–400 grams and length approximately 1–2 cm (0.5–1.0 standard deviation [SD]) below normative means, depending on population and gestational age [12–14, 20–22, 24, 25, 35]. Linear growth is slow during infancy and childhood [20–22, 36] and there is absence of the typical robust pubertal growth spurt (Fig. 3.2) [4, 5, 13, 24–26].

The early comprehensive height surveys led to development of various country-specific TS growth curves in the 1980s and 1990s (Table 3.1; Fig. 3.2b).[1] However,

---

[1] For detailed review and analysis of various international Turner syndrome growth charts, see reference [37].

these percentile charts are comprised mainly of cross-sectional rather than longitudinal data and therefore serve primarily to allow assessment of an individual's position relative to other patients with TS at a given age, but do not provide the optimal template for tracking the growth patterns of individual patients over time. Because these TS-specific percentiles tended to parallel the general population growth curves in the first few years of life (Fig. 3.2b), possibly due to their construction mainly from smoothed cross-sectional data [4, 21], the growth failure that occurs during infancy was not initially appreciated. Subsequently, longitudinal data from Sweden [35, 36], Israel [20], the USA [22], and Japan [19] elucidated the marked growth failure evident in the first 2–3 years of life, revealing persistently below-average height velocity (HV)[2] for age, or declining height SDS, resulting in

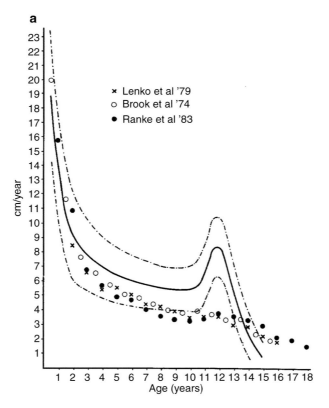

Fig. 3.2 (**a**) Mean height velocities of girls with Turner syndrome from 3 independent cohorts (•, °, ×) compared to height velocities of British girls in the general population published by Tanner et al. (1966 Arch Dis Child, 41:613) (curves). (Reprinted with permission from Springer Nature Publishing. *European Journal of Pediatrics.* Ranke et al. [5]). (**b**) Growth curves (5th - 95th percentiles) for girls ages 2–19 years: Turner syndrome, lower curves, purple lines; U.S. general population, upper curves, red lines. Reproduced with permission from the Office of Lilly CME, based on data from Lyon et al. [4]

---

[2] *Height velocity* is alternatively referred to in some publications as *growth velocity*. However, as *growth* can refer to any measurable parameter, such as head circumference, weight, body mass index, etc., the more specific term *height velocity* (HV) is used in this chapter.

Fig. 3.2 (continued)

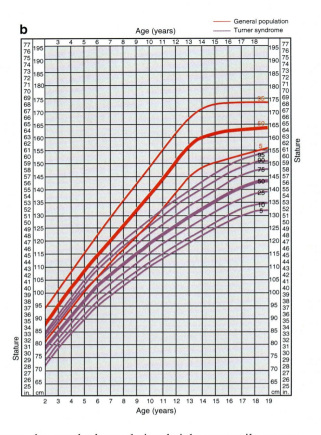

a downward trajectory across the standard population height percentile curves. Davenport and colleagues [22] demonstrated progressive declines in mean length/ height SDS over the first 8 years of life, from mean length SDS of around −0.7 at birth to a nadir of −2.3 SDS by 4 years. Height SDS decreased most rapidly in the first 18 months of life, such that 95% of girls with TS had height below the 50th percentile of the standard (non-TS) growth curve by 1.5 years of age; by school entry at around 4–6 years of age the mean height deficit relative to peers was ~10 cm. The early growth failure was observed regardless of karyotype in the Swedish, Israeli, and US cohorts [20, 22, 35, 36]. It should be noted, however, that all of these studies report data for girls enrolled in clinical studies on the basis of postnatal diagnosis and therefore may suffer from ascertainment bias toward more severely affected cases. Highlighting this point, a study of 88 subjects, of whom 16 (18%) were diagnosed with TS for reasons other than clinical suspicion (e.g., prenatal karyotype performed for advanced maternal age), found that length/height at around 2 years of age was about 0.6 SDS greater for girls diagnosed incidentally than for those diagnosed on clinical grounds [38]. Nevertheless, the conclusions regarding growth deficits in TS remain valid for the majority of patients.

Three studies have analyzed linear growth in girls with TS according to the infancy-childhood-puberty (ICP) model of Karlberg [39]. This mathematical model describes normal growth in terms of three distinct, additive, but partially superimposable phases reflecting different hormonal influences on growth: the infancy phase, representing the transition from intrauterine to extrauterine life, is notable for the precipitous deceleration in HV in the first 2 years of life, with less marked slowing thereafter (Fig. 3.2a); the childhood phase, which begins at around 0.5–1.0 year of age in typical girls and overlaps the infancy phase, is initiated by a minor increase in growth rate (the infancy-childhood spurt) due to the onset of GH-dependent growth; and the puberty phase, the timing of which varies widely, is marked by the dramatic sex steroid-fueled pubertal growth spurt. The growth pattern of TS is disturbed, with subnormal growth rate during the infancy phase [22] followed by delayed transition to the childhood phase by about 0.3–0.4 years [20, 22, 35] suggesting late onset of predominantly GH-dependent growth, resulting in reduced height gain between 0.5 and 3.0 years of age [22, 35]. Even and colleagues [20] pointed out that about half of the 3 standard deviations of the overall height deficit of TS has already occurred before birth, and the majority of the total AH deficit has occurred by age 3 years. Consequently, efforts to restore height to within the normal range with growth-promoting therapies will likely be only partially effective.

During middle and late childhood (around ages 5–12 years) height continues to drift further below the standard percentile curves (Fig. 3.2b) [35], as girls with TS do not undergo the slight mid-childhood (preadolescent) increase in growth rate that occurs around age 8–10 years in typical girls under the influence of a subtle prepubertal rise in estrogen secretion [40]. Thereafter, the absence of the marked estrogen-mediated growth spurt of puberty further exacerbates the height deficit from peers, although a few studies have reported a minor increase in growth rate (or a slowing of the rate of decline) around the late-childhood, early-teen years [10–12]. Nevertheless, by age 14–15 years average height is ~4 SD (>20 cm) below the population mean [4, 21, 25, 36]. After their peers have attained AH in the mid-teen years, untreated girls with TS, whose epiphyses remain open due to absence of the maturational effects of high estrogen concentrations, may continue to grow very slowly until their early 20s, eventually resulting in slight catch up back toward the lower end of the population height curve (Fig. 3.2b).

Despite their extended growth period the mean AH of cohorts of women with TS is around 143–146 cm [range 132–155 cm], which is ~20 cm (~3 SD) below the mean height of women in the general female population in the same country [4, 18, 24, 28, 31, 41] (Fig. 3.1). Women with TS are also ~20 cm shorter than their midparental (genetic target) heights [5, 14], however, there remains a strong correlation between subject height and genetic target height [11, 21, 27, 34], indicating that a significant component of linear growth is modulated by non-X chromosomal genes. The genetic influences on height are further complicated by the finding that height SDS in TS correlates with mother's height, but not with father's height, irrespective of subject age or the parental origin of the retained X chromosome (i.e., whether the single intact X chromosome was inherited from the father or mother) [42–44]. This finding suggests potential genomic imprinting effects, with differential height influence of genes inherited from maternal vs. paternal autosomes.

Prediction of Mature Height

The ability to predict the growth pattern and height of an individual girl with TS represents a potentially important factor for decision-making regarding the use of growth-promoting therapies. In practice, the typical approach for prediction of untreated AH is the projected AH method [4] or modifications thereof [45, 46]. This method assumes that an untreated girl will continue to grow along the same percentile channel as her height at presentation, when plotted on a TS-specific height chart. For example, a 9 year-old girl with TS who presents to the clinic with height of 112 cm (~25th percentile on the TS curve) would be predicted to attain AH of ~140 cm if untreated (~25th percentile for age 19). However, this height projection method provides only a rough estimate, tends to overpredict AH [46], and cannot be considered accurate on an individual patient basis [41]. This issue is illustrated by data from a Canadian study, in which the subjects' actual heights at maturity were compared with the baseline predictions of their untreated AH [47]. At completion of growth subjects in the control group, who received no GH treatment, were up to 1.1 SD shorter or taller than the AH projected at study entry, equivalent to an "error" of up to 7 cm either side of the estimate (i.e., up to 14 cm for an individual patient).[3] Although detailed mathematical prediction models may provide greater accuracy by including factors such as bone age or bone age SDS (methods are compared in ref. [46]), these models are not helpful in girls under the age of about 9 years and may be impractical for use in the clinical setting.

Body Proportions and Skeletal Anomalies

In addition to overall short stature, individuals with TS tend to have disproportionate growth, with greater disturbance in the longitudinal axis (e.g., height) than in the horizontal axis (e.g., pelvic or shoulder width). These growth variations result in a "stocky" appearance, with a relatively large trunk, and broad shoulders and pelvis compared to height, accompanied by increased ratio of sitting height to leg length [48–51]. The proximal leg segment (femur) is relatively shorter than the lower leg segment (tibia/fibula) [48]; hands and feet are also relatively large compared with height [48–51] (Fig. 3.3). Findings such as short neck, cubitus valgus, genu valgum, short fourth/fifth metacarpals, and, occasionally, Madelung deformity of the wrist result from developmental variations of individual bones [52]. It has been suggested that infants with TS are at increased risk of congenital hip dysplasia [53, 54]. However, objective evidence supporting this suggestion is lacking (discussed in Chap. 14). Scoliosis risk is increased in TS, with 41% prevalence in non-GH-treated girls in one cross-sectional study [55], compared with ~2% of girls in the general

---

[3] According to the 2000 data from the US National Center for Health Statistics, 1 SD for height at age 20 years is ~6.5 cm [www.cdc.gov].

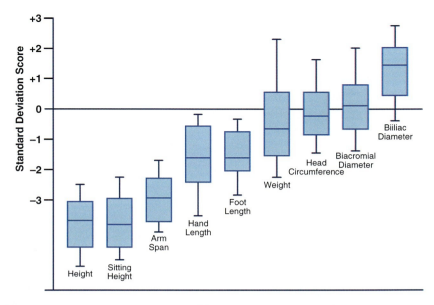

Fig. 3.3 Body proportions of women with Turner syndrome. Box-and-whiskers plots display the range (whiskers), 25th and 75th percentiles (lower and upper boundaries of the box), and median/50th percentile (central horizontal line in each box) of the data distribution for each parameter. Reproduced with permission based on data from Gravholt CH [49]

population [56, 57]; in addition, kyphosis and/or vertebral wedging also appear to be more common in TS than in the general population [56, 57].

Skeletal maturation in TS is typically delayed and shows a unique pattern with greatest delay in the short bones (e.g., phalanges), least delay in the long bones (e.g., radius and ulna), and intermediate delay in the carpal bones [58].

Etiology of the Growth Disturbance

The 7 young women described in Turner's initial 1938 report were all referred to him because of lack of pubertal development and marked short stature [1]. Assuming that the clinical features resulted from pituitary dysfunction, Dr Turner treated his patients with various pituitary extracts, without significant clinical benefit. Subsequently, a number of studies suggested deficits in GH secretion in TS [59–63], whereas other researchers hypothesized that GH secretion was essentially normal after accounting for sex steroid deficiency and relative overweight [64, 65].

More than half a century after Turner's initial clinical description, genetic studies mapping the critical deletion interval for short stature in the pseudoautosomal regions of the X and Y chromosomes [66–71] led eventually to the identification of the *short stature homeobox*-containing *(SHOX)* gene by two independent research groups [72, 73].

Although SHOX deficiency is now considered to play a preeminent role in the etiology of the growth disturbance of TS, the pathogenesis appears to be multifactorial, with disturbances of GH/IGF-I physiology, estrogen secretion, and growth plate responsiveness likely contributing to deficient genetic/hormonal interactions with SHOX-dependent factors at critical periods of growth [74]. Brief summaries of key contributors to the growth disturbances of TS are provided in the following sections.

SHOX Deficiency

Because they lack all or part of the second sex chromosome, individuals with TS have only a single copy of the *SHOX* gene typically located on the distal short arm of each of the two the X chromosomes in 46,XX individuals at Xp22.33 [66–81], and also on the distal Y chromosome at Yp11.3 in 46,XY individuals (Fig. 3.4). Unlike most genes on the X chromosome, which undergo X inactivation to maintain dosage equivalence between male and female, the pseudoautosomal location of *SHOX* means that

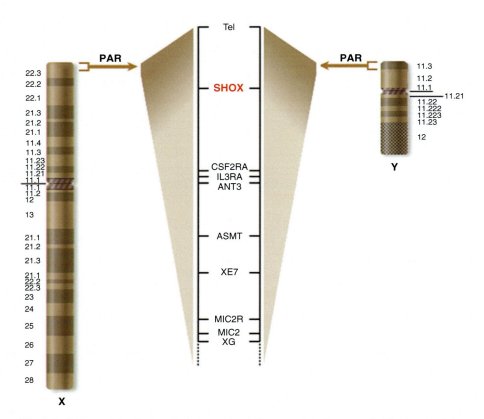

Fig. 3.4 Cartoon of the *SHOX* (*short stature homeobox*-containing) gene at the distal ends of the pseudoautosomal regions of the X and Y chromosomes. (Reproduced with permission from *Turner Syndrome: A Comprehensive Guide*, copyright Office of Lilly CME)

the gene does not undergo inactivation of the second copy in typical 46,XX individuals and functions essentially as an autosomal gene [82]. Two intact copies of the gene are required for normal growth, and the homeodomain transcription factor encoded by the *SHOX* gene is expressed during prenatal and postnatal development of the long bones (radius, ulna, tibia, and distal femur) and the first and second pharyngeal arches [81, 83]. Notably, as early as the 1970s, Brook and colleagues suggested that the growth failure in TS was likely associated with the "abnormally coarse trabecular structure of the bones" due to the "missing chromosomal material" [25]. Subsequently, Hochberg proposed that the unique profile of disordered bone maturation in TS suggests an insult to chondroplasia [58] and this hypothesis is consistent with the demonstrated role for SHOX as a regulator of apoptosis in hypertrophic chondrocytes during growth plate fusion [82, 84–86]. Thus, the skeletal dysplasia of TS is believed to result primarily from insufficient transactivation of SHOX-dependent target genes (such as *NPPB*, encoding brain natriuretic peptide [87]) involved in the regulation of chondrocyte proliferation and differentiation in the growth plate [81, 82], but the exact pathophysiological and cellular mechanisms by which SHOX deficiency results in short stature remain to be determined.

Isolated deletions and mutations of the S*HOX* gene are also found in some individuals with the skeletal dysplasia referred to as Léri-Weill dyschondrosteosis (or syndrome) and in a subset of individuals with so-called "idiopathic" short stature (i.e., short stature without skeletal dysplasia or other dysmorphic features) [81]. Patients who have small X-chromosomal deletions including *SHOX* and genes distal to it typically have short stature and other skeletal anomalies but do not have the broad multisystem phenotypic and functional anomalies seen in TS [88]. The milder growth deficit observed in patients with Léri-Weill syndrome and apparent "idiopathic" short stature suggests that haploinsufficiency of additional genes on the short arm of the X-chromosome contributes to the more severe growth and skeletal deficits seen in TS; other fundamental genetic factors such as aneuploidy/chromosomal imbalance may also play roles in the spectrum of phenotypic and functional anomalies [70, 89, 90].

Alterations of GH and IGF-I Physiology

Variations in GH physiology in TS have been reported since the 1980s, including reduced responses to classical provocative stimuli, diminished spontaneous pulsatile GH secretion, and suboptimal response to GH-releasing hormone [59–65, 91–93]. Although some studies tended to explain the apparent GH "insufficiency" on the basis of sex-steroid deficiency or relative overweight [62, 65], it seems plausible that in fact there may be a degree of functional or secondary GH inadequacy in some individuals with TS contributing to their growth disturbance; such functional deficits might be at least partially remediable by treating the confounding factor(s), such as adiposity or estrogen deficiency. In addition to modestly inadequate GH secretion, individuals with TS may have a degree of GH resistance or reduced GH "bioactivity" [94, 95] possibly associated with a combination of factors including increased concentrations of GH binding protein [96] and/or reduced GH receptor expression and signaling as a consequence of estrogen deficiency [97]. GH resistance, if present, seems unlikely to be due to variations in the GH receptor (GHR), as the distribution of GHR isoforms (full-length, major allele vs. exon 3-deleted, minor allele) associated with variations in GH sensitivity is similar in TS to the general population distribution [98, 99]. In conjunction with mild GH resistance, there is evidence of altered IGF-I physiology in TS [100], with low-normal total serum IGF-I; increased proteolysis of IGFBP-3, which may be responsive to estrogen replacement [101]; reduced free IGF-I [101–103]; and resistance to IGF-I [94, 101].

Estrogen Deficiency

Ovarian failure due to gonadal dysgenesis, a cardinal feature of TS, begins in midgestation with accelerated apoptosis of germ cells [104] resulting in prenatal degeneration of the ovary and deficiency of endogenous estrogen secretion. However, estrogen deficiency seems unlikely to contribute to the prenatal growth deficit of TS, given the very high intrauterine estrogen environment of all fetuses as a result of maternal estrogen production. Furthermore, an animal model of profound estrogen deficiency - the estrogen receptor (ER)-null mouse - does not have a growth-retarded phenotype [105]. In contrast, there is good evidence of a role for estrogen deficiency in the postnatal growth failure of TS. Estrogens impact growth at a number of levels, by increasing GH secretion and modulating GH action, and as the principal effectors of epiphyseal maturation and fusion [74, 75, 97, 106].

The fact that typical female infants are smaller than male infants at birth, yet show more rapid growth and skeletal maturation during the first few years of life, is believed to be due to the greater estrogen secretion of female vs. male children during the prepubertal years [40, 107]. However, the most dramatic effects of estrogens on growth in both male and female children are the stimulation of the pubertal growth spurt and the mediation of epiphyseal maturation and fusion through the mechanism of growth plate senescence [108, 109]. In vivo human evidence of this latter role is seen in the prolonged period of linear growth and absence of epiphyseal maturation of rare individuals with mutations in the genes encoding ERα or the estrogen-producing enzyme, aromatase [110–113]. Ross, Cutler, and colleagues hypothesized that the role of estrogens in growth was biphasic, and their exploratory work conducted in the 1980s demonstrated a dose-dependent pattern of response to estrogen: very low doses (markedly lower than conventionally used to induce pubertal feminization) stimulated linear growth whereas higher doses did not [114].

Girls with TS lack both the GH-modulatory effects and the local epiphyseal effects of endogenous estrogens, likely contributing to their subnormal growth rates, reduced sensitivity to GH and delayed skeletal maturation during early and mid-childhood, as well as the absence of the pubertal growth spurt and the prolonged period of slow growth into the late teenage years and early 20s [4, 5, 24] (Fig. 3.2b).

Growth-Promoting Therapies

Because significant short stature is an almost universal clinical feature of untreated adult women with TS [53, 115] and can present substantial physical and social challenges, various therapeutic approaches to increase height have been tested in anecdotal studies and clinical trials since the 1930s, beginning with GH treatment by Dr. Henry Turner himself [1]. His treatment attempts were unsuccessful, likely due to a combination of factors including the use of bovine GH (the only form available at the time) administered in subtherapeutic doses to teenage girls with limited growth potential.

Goals of Growth-Promoting Therapies

The initial goals of growth-promoting therapies for girls with TS are to maintain the child's height potential within the normal range relative to her peers, or to correct growth failure that has already occurred at the time of presentation by increasing HV to stimulate catch-up growth. Depending on age at presentation, these strategies should allow puberty to begin at a physiological age and facilitate attainment of adult height within the lower part of the reference range for the general female population. These goals are based on the assumption that height within or close to the normal range will help to minimize stigmatization, juvenilization, physical restrictions, and their associated psychological impacts.

To provide realistic expectations for the child and family it is important that clinicians discuss the likely height outcomes without or with pharmacologic intervention, based on certain patient and family factors such as age, bone age, height and pubertal status at presentation, maternal height, midparental height, and difference between the child's height and her midparental height (i.e., height deficit relative to genetic target height). Prediction of mature height, either without or with growth-promoting treatment, is an inexact art; families should be made aware that the common projection method for untreated AH [4] (i.e., carrying height forward along the same TS percentile as found at presentation) may have a substantial margin for error in some girls, of up to 7 cm higher or lower than the AH estimate [47]. Mathematical prediction models [45, 46, 116] can increase the accuracy of predictions, but may be impractical for clinical use.

Growth Hormone (GH)

The cornerstone of growth-promoting therapy is recombinant human growth hormone (GH), which increases HV during childhood, stimulates catch-up growth (i.e., crossing upward over percentiles) and for most patients results in modest increases in adult stature, compared with expected height if untreated [117, 118].

History of GH Treatment in TS

More than 40 years after Turner's initial unsuccessful trial of bovine GH, a small placebo-controlled study of pituitary-derived human GH in TS was initiated in 1984, but was aborted the next year when pituitary GH was withdrawn from all human use. Nevertheless, this trial formally demonstrated the proof of concept that GH could significantly increase HV in TS [119]. Subsequently, once recombinant GH became available for GH-deficient children in the mid-1980s, numerous small-group studies and large clinical trials of GH effectiveness in TS, most of which lacked concurrent untreated controls [117, 118, 120], were initiated in Europe, North America, and Australia [121–123]. Early results demonstrating improvements in HV fueled enthusiasm for GH treatment, and its use became common in TS even before formal licensing was obtained for this condition. In the 20 years following its approval for TS in the 1990s, dozens of papers reported results of GH treatment using a variety of regimens, either alone or in varying combinations with sex steroids or with anabolic steroids such as oxandrolone. Notwithstanding the limitations, a large body of evidence combining clinical trial outcomes and historical data led to the approval of recombinant GH for TS in most of Europe in 1993, in the USA in 1996 and in Japan in 1999.

Randomized Controlled Trials with Parallel Placebo or Nontreatment Control Groups

Despite the plethora of studies of GH treatment in TS, a 2007 Cochrane Center review [117] identified only four trials (from almost 50 papers reviewed) in which GH treatment was compared in a randomized, design with a concurrent (parallel) nontreatment or placebo control group for at least 1 year [47, 121, 124, 125]; two further studies fulfilling these criteria were published in the following decade [126, 127]. Of these six randomized, controlled trials (RCTs), one study was excluded from the Cochrane analysis because no outcome data were published [125], and only two have followed non-GH-treated subjects to (near) adult height ([N]AH) or final height[4] [47, 127] (Table 3.2). Apart from this handful of RCTs, most other studies have compared outcomes for a selected (nonrandomized) GH treatment group with either a matched historical control group (i.e., an untreated group selected from clinic records and not followed in parallel with treated subjects) or with mature heights expected for the study participants if they had remained untreated (projected or predicted AH). Many additional studies have examined other aspects of growth-promoting treatment, including dose-response to GH

---

[4] In this review the terms adult height (AH) and near-adult height (NAH) or final height (FH) refer to the most mature heights of study subjects, typically obtained after demonstration of minimal remaining growth potential (e.g., HV < 2.0 cm/year or bone age > 14 years). It is expected that most women will gain an additional ~1–2 cm after attainment of this milestone.

Table 3.2 Randomized, controlled trials with at least 1 year period of parallel untreated or placebo-treated control

Initial Report	Rosenfeld 1989	Quigley 2002	Stephure 2005	Davenport 2007	Ross 2011
Follow-up Report	Rosenfeld 1998	–	–	Quigley 2020	Quigley 2014
Control type	Untreated	Placebo, double-blind	Untreated	Untreated	Placebo, double-blind
Duration of control	1 year	18 months	To completion (AH)	2 years	To completion (AH)
Number control	18	41	43	45	39[a]
Number GH-treated	17	38[b]	61	43 (→66)[c]	52[a]
Baseline age (yr)	4.7–12.4	≥5.0, ≤12.0	7.0–13.0	0.75–4.0	5.0–12.5
Baseline height SDS, control	n/a	−2.9±0.9 (US[d])	−0.1±0.8 (TS[d])	−1.6±1.1 (US[d])	−2.8±0.8[e]
Baseline height SDS, GH-treated	−0.2±0.9 (TS[d])	−2.9±0.9 (US[d])	−0.2±0.9 (TS[d])	−1.4±1.1 (US[d])	−2.6±0.9[e]
GH dose mg/kg/week	0.375	0.36	0.30	0.35	0.30
GH injections per week	3 → 7	3 → 6	6	7	3
Duration GH (yr)	7.6±2.2	5.5±1.6	5.7±1.6	10.7±2.5	7.1±2.5[e]
Age at estrogen start (yr)	15	13.5[f]	13	12.2	>12[f]
Age at (N)AH	18.0±2.2	16.7±1.5	16.0±0.8	15.0±0.8	17.0±1.0[e]
AH SDS[g], control	n/a	n/a	−0.3±0.8 (TS[d])	n/a	−3.1±0.8 (US[d])[e]
AH SDS[g], GH-treated	n/a	−1.9±1.0 (US[d])	0.7±0.9 (TS[d])	−1.5±1.1 (US[d])	−2.2±1.1 (US[d])[e]
AH (cm), control	144.2±6.0 (historical)	n/a	141.0±5.4	n/a	142.5±5.2[e]
AH (cm), GH-treated	150.4±5.5	150.4±6.0	147.5±6.1	151.2±7.1	148.6±6.9[e]
AH criteria	Bone age >14 HV <2.5 cm/yr	Bone age≥14	Bone age ≥14 HV<2.0 cm/yr	Bone age ≥14.5 HV ≤2.0 cm/yr	HV <1.5 cm/yr
GH effect (cm or SDS)[g]	7.4 cm vs. historical control	1.3±0.6 (TS[d]) vs. baseline	7.2 cm vs. untreated control	1.6±0.6 (US[d]) vs. untreated control[h]	0.8±0.1 SDS (US[h]) vs. placebo[i]

Studies are presented by year of initial publication. Data are mean±SD. *AH* refers to study-defined age at assessment of adult height, *HV* height velocity, *n/a* not available

[a] Adult height population

[b] Subjects who received GH alone (0.36 mg/kg/week) without early low-dose estrogen from age 8; data not shown for 0.27 mg/kg/week groups

[c] 43 subjects received GH during initial 2-year controlled phase; 66 subjects received GH during extension phase to AH, including subjects who transitioned from control group to GH after 2-year randomized phase

[d] TS = SDS calculated using Turner syndrome height data; US = SDS calculated using US general population height data

[e] Study comprised 4 treatment groups: 2 GH groups (with or without childhood low-dose estrogen [LDE]) and 2 placebo-control groups (with or without childhood LDE). Values represent weighted averages for pooled GH or placebo groups (+/- LDE).

[f] Age at start of pubertal estrogen replacement for subjects in "GH alone" groups (i.e., those who did not receive childhood low-dose estrogen for growth stimulation)

[g] GH effect at endpoint was calculated in each study using ANCOVA with baseline age and baseline height SDS as covariates (additional covariates in some studies); using US general female population standards (Centers for Disease Control) 1 SD is equivalent to ~6.5 cm at age ≥16 yr

[h] Between-group difference at end of 2-year control period

[i] GH treatment effect at AH was calculated by ANCOVA for pooled groups of GH-treated subjects (with or without childhood low-dose estrogen) vs. pooled groups of placebo-treated subjects (with or without childhood low-dose estrogen)

and effects of supplemental treatments such as low-dose estrogen or anabolic steroids (e.g., oxandrolone), summarized later in the chapter.

Characteristics and Limitations of Studies

The RCTs designed in the 1980s typically enrolled girls from the ages of about 5 to 12 years. The "Toddler Turner" study, initiated in the late 1990s, specifically targeted a much younger population (9 months to 4 years) with the aim to prevent growth failure in preschool girls. GH regimens in the initial clinical trials were modeled on the pituitary-derived (cadaveric) GH regimens used in the 1980s, with total weekly dosage of approximately 0.30 mg/kg divided into three doses given on alternate days; in later studies the dosage was increased to 0.375 mg/kg/week divided into six or seven doses (dosage equivalent to ~54 µg/kg/day). A crucial factor contributing to variation between studies was the estrogen replacement regimen (timing of onset, formulation, and pattern of escalation) considered particularly relevant because of the dose-response effects of estrogen with respect to growth stimulation vs. skeletal maturation (see earlier section on "Estrogen Deficiency"). Another fundamental study design difference is the definition of the clinical endpoint, typically referred to as "adult" or "final" height[4], in terms of chronological age, bone age, and/or HV, all of which may substantially impact the comparability of treatment group and individual subject results.

An important limitation of many published reports is the lack of detail regarding statistical methodology. For example, *a priori* analysis for definition of sample size and power was provided in the published report for only one of the six RCTs [127], although power analyses were provided in the protocols for three of the remaining five studies [47, 124, 126] [unpublished data, Quigley]. The following sections focus on published data from the five RCTs that followed an untreated or placebo-treated control group for at least 1 year, generally reporting mean data unless stated otherwise (Table 3.2); supportive data from the numerous studies evaluating treatment effect by comparison with historical control data or the patient's own predicted/projected height without treatment are provided in a later section.

Short-Term Growth Response (Height Velocity, Height SDS)

One of the key goals of GH treatment in TS is to maintain height within, or restore height to, the normal range during childhood. Therefore, early response such as height increase over the first year or so of treatment, is an important aspect of GH efficacy. Furthermore, first-year response (i.e., increase in HV vs. pretreatment HV– GH "responsiveness") is one of the most powerful predictors of long-term outcome [116, 128]. HV in healthy children varies with age, from an average of around 8 cm/year at age 3 to a nadir of <6 cm/year at age 9 [129]. Therefore, because of the difficulty of comparing HV values across varying ages of study participants, some studies present standardized data, such as change in HV SDS or height SDS (HtSDS), the latter being the more robust measure.

In the large US placebo-controlled trial of 224 girls (Table 3.2, Quigley 2002) [124], mean pretreatment HV was 3.9 cm/year at the average age of 9.7 years, compared with 50th percentile HV for typical North American girls of around 6.0 cm/year at this age [129]. Mean HV after 6 months on study remained around 4 cm/year for the placebo group, but increased markedly to 7–8 cm/year for the GH-treated groups. In a smaller US study that maintained an untreated control group for the first

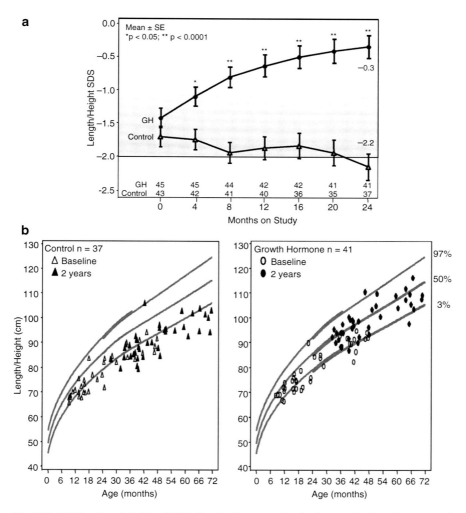

Fig. 3.5 (**a**) Mean length/height SDS during the 2-year, randomized, controlled "Toddler Turner" study for the nontreatment control group (open symbols) and the GH treatment group (filled symbols). Between-group difference at 2-year endpoint was 1.6 ± 0.6 SDS ($P < 0.0001$) by ANCOVA. (Reprinted with the permission of the Endocrine Society from Davenport et al. [126]. (**b**) Baseline (*open symbols*) and 2-year (*filled symbols*) length/height measurements (cm) for the nontreatment control group (*left*) and the GH treatment group (*right*), relative to the third, 50th, and 97th percentiles for the US female reference population from birth to 6 years. (Reprinted with the permission of the Endocrine Society, from Davenport et al. [126])

year, the mean HV of the controls was 3.8 cm/year vs. 6.6 cm/year for the GH-treated group after one year on study (Table 3.2, Roselfeld 1989) [121]. The National Institutes of Health (NIH) placebo-controlled study reported short-term results as changes in height SDS rather than HV. After one year the GH-treated group had 0.3 SDS (~1.7 cm) greater height increase than the placebo group (Table 3.2, Ross 2011) [127]. In the "Toddler Turner" study of preschool girls, whose average baseline age was 2 years, first-year HV was 8.0 cm/year for untreated controls vs. 11.7 cm/year for GH-treated girls and the height SDS difference between the GH-treated and control groups was significant as early as 4 months on study. Over the 2-year study period height SDS of the control group declined by mean 0.5 SDS, whereas that of the GH-treated group increased by 1.1 SDS, resulting in a between-group difference of 1.6 SDS by analysis of covariance (ANCOVA) at the end of the controlled period (Table 3.2, Davenport 2007) [126] (Fig. 3.5). Despite their divergent designs, these four controlled studies demonstrated a consistent, robust initial GH treatment effect vs. non-GH-treated control. Both the Cochrane Center review and the more recent meta-analysis concluded that across studies, GH-treated girls grew approximately 3 cm/year faster than untreated girls after 1 year [117, 118].

The initial catch-up growth afforded by the early increase in HV or HtSDS and restoration of height within the normal range may be particularly important to affected girls and their families: first, by helping to promptly reduce the height gap between the girl and her peers and, second, by facilitating physiological timing of puberty. However, as in all GH-treated conditions, the initial brisk response is not maintained and HV wanes over time, though it remains consistently greater than the untreated growth rate [117, 124, 130, 131].

Long-Term Outcomes (Height in cm, Height SDS, Percentage of Subjects who Attain AH Within Normal Range)

Attainment of AH within the normal range for the general female population represents the usual long-term goal of GH treatment in TS. Because of varying height standards across different reference populations, as well as different ages at assessment of (N)AH, the most common approach to assess mature height uses population-specific AH SDS (i.e., SDS calculated using data for adult women in the reference non-TS population). Unlike height SDS based on TS data, general population standards have the advantage of providing direct comparison with the young woman's peer group – the people with whom she will interact on a daily basis. For individual patients measured height in cm is more easily understood and for clinical trials the proportion of study patients who achieve heights within the population normal range (typically defined as above −2.0 SDS) is a useful efficacy parameter.

Only two studies, one Canadian and one US, have reported data for both GH-treated and non-GH-treated groups followed in parallel to AH, although the results cannot be easily compared between studies due to substantial differences in study design [47, 127]. In the Canadian nontreatment-controlled trial (Table 3.2, Stephure 2005), the treated group ($n = 61$) received a GH dosage of 0.3 mg/kg/week in six divided doses, while the non-GH-treated control group ($n = 43$)

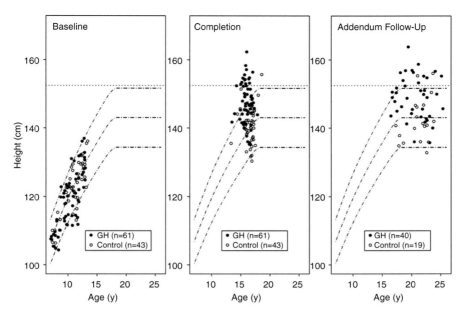

Fig. 3.6 Height data from individual subjects in the Canadian randomized, controlled trial of GH treatment to adult height, plotted against 10th, 50th, and 90th percentile curves for Turner syndrome: baseline (left), protocol completion (center), and addendum follow-up, at least 1 year after protocol completion (right); open symbols, non-GH-treated control; filled symbols, GH-treated subjects. (Reprinted with permission of the Endocrine Society, from Stephure [47])

received no injections: both groups underwent induction of puberty at age 13 using escalating doses of ethinyl estradiol (EE2) with addition of medroxyprogesterone acetate from age 15 [47]. After 5.7 years on study at average ages of 16.0 (GH) and 16.5 (Control) years, the mean NAH of the GH-treated group was 147.5 ± 6.1 cm vs. 141.0 ± 5.4 cm for the untreated control group, representing a difference of 7.2 cm by ANCOVA (Fig. 3.6).

In the US placebo-controlled study (Table 3.2, Ross 2011) 149 girls were randomized to four groups: GH (0.3 mg/kg/week in three divided doses) plus childhood low-dose estrogen from age 5–12; GH alone (plus oral placebo in place of estrogen from age 5-12); estrogen alone (plus placebo injection); and double placebo (placebo injection plus oral placebo) [127]. The prepubertal ultra-low-dose estrogen regimen is detailed on page 64; all groups underwent pubertal induction from age 12. After an average of 7.2 years on study at an average age of 17.0 years, the mean AH SDS values were (from shortest to tallest): −3.4 ± 0.7 (estrogen alone), −2.8 ± 0.9 (double placebo), −2.3 ± 1.1 (GH alone), and −2.1 ± 1.0 (GH + estrogen). By ANCOVA the mean height gain from GH treatment vs. placebo injection was 0.77 SDS, equivalent to ~5.0 cm. Notably, the group that received supplemental low-dose EE2 (for growth enhancement rather than pubertal induction) from age 5-12 years in addition to GH had the tallest AH, suggesting a modest synergistic effect between childhood estrogen (at the ultra-low doses used in this regimen) and GH. The authors pointed out that the somewhat lower magnitude of the height gain in this study than that reported in some other studies likely resulted from a number of factors, including use of a GH dosage and injection frequency considered suboptimal by current standards. Despite limitations, the data from these two stringent RCTs appear broadly representative of the average results across a wide variety of studies. This conclusion is supported by a 2018 meta-analysis of nine studies, which reported a mean FH gain from GH alone of approximately 7.2 cm (95% CI, 5.3–9.2 cm) [118], similar to the 6 cm mean estimate of GH effect provided by the Cochrane review a decade earlier [117].

In both the Canadian and the US RCTs there was wide variation in the mature heights of individual GH-treated subjects, from ~136 to 166 cm in the Canadian study and ~137 to 163 cm in the US study.[5] These broad height ranges are reflected by the proportions of subjects who attained AH within the general population normal range (i.e., above −2.0 SDS or ~150 cm). For the Canadian study about 50% of GH-treated subjects vs. ~16% of untreated controls had AH in the normal range[6] [47]; in the US study ~40% of GH-treated patients vs. 4% of placebo recipients attained normal AH [127].

In the remaining three RCTs that included parallel control groups for initial periods of 1–2 years, the untreated subjects transitioned onto active treatment after their control periods and were followed thereafter to AH [124, 132, 133]. As shown in Table 3.2, mean AH outcomes are somewhat greater than those of the GH-treated groups in the aforementioned Canadian and US RCTs, with average final heights above 150 cm for GH-treated groups overall.

In summary, the RCT data conclusively demonstrate the efficacy of GH in terms of both short-term and long-term height outcomes. First-year HV increases on average by about 3 cm/year vs. pretreatment HV, and long-term height gain vs. expected AH if untreated is about 5–8 cm over 5 or more years of treatment; that is, about 1 cm of height gain per year of GH treatment. Because height gains accumulate slowly, families should be counseled to have realistic expectations of treatment outcomes and should be advised of the importance of adherence to treatment, to prevent catch-down growth and loss of height potential if treatment is discontinued prematurely.

Studies without Parallel Control Groups (Historical Control, Predicted/Projected Height Comparison, Dose-Response)

In addition to the handful of RCTs detailed in the preceding sections, many studies have examined short- and long-term outcomes of GH treatment in TS using matched historical control groups [134, 135] or comparison with baseline predicted/projected AH [133, 136, 137]. Other studies have focused on exploratory aspects of treatment such as dose-response [137–139], combination with other growth-

---

[5] Calculated by conversion of height SDS to centimeters using height data from US Centers from Disease Control for age 20 years [www.cdc.gov]

[6] Calculated by analysis of Ref. [47], Fig. 2.

promoting agents [124, 140–142], young age at initiation of GH treatment [126, 143, 144], variation in timing of estrogen replacement [124, 134, 145–147], and comparison with other (non-TS) SHOX-deficient patients [148]. Initial treatment responses are comparable to those reported in the RCTs, with brisk increases in HV and height SDS in the first year or two of treatment and slower incremental gains thereafter. Similarly, long-term outcomes are consistent with those seen in the RCTs, with overall height gains attributed to GH of around 1.0 SD, equivalent to 6–7 cm depending on age, height standards used, and statistical methods [133, 134, 136, 149]. Notable exceptions are a French study and a Dutch study using escalating GH doses (45 vs. 67.5 vs. 90 µg/kg/day, equivalent to 0.32-0.63 mg/kg/week) starting at young ages, that demonstrated mean AH values well within the normal range (155.3 cm in the French study [137], 157.6–163.6 cm for different groups in the Dutch study [139]) and dramatic mean height gains of 15–17 cm versus baseline projected AH (i.e., height extrapolated from the baseline percentile using TS standards). The wide variability in reported or apparent efficacy has fueled efforts to identify factors associated with greater height gain from baseline and greater attained (measured) height, as described in the next section.

Observational Studies, Height Prediction Models, and Factors Influencing Response to GH Treatment

Because of the potential lack of generalizability of data obtained under the stringent conditions of RCTs, various groups have followed large numbers of patients with TS (and other conditions) in company and country-specific databases [128, 130, 150–153]. Well-designed observational studies can provide results that are highly consistent with RCT data on the same topic [154], and the volume of data allows robust assessment of both safety and efficacy outcomes under more naturalistic settings than those imposed by RCTs. Furthermore, these long-term observational databases provide the opportunity to develop mathematical models to predict response to treatment under "real-world" conditions [116, 128, 155–157].

Results from large observational studies generally support the efficacy findings from the RCTs of GH treatment in TS. A 1998 analysis of ~2500 patients followed in the US National Cooperative Growth Study reported mean height gain of 0.8 ± 0.7 SDS (US standard) after a mean of 3.2 years of GH treatment starting at an average age of 10 years [130]. Height gain was similar in an international cohort of ~140 patients treated for mean 4.5 years, averaging 0.9 SDS [158] based on Swiss general population height standards [159]. A German observational study of ~190 young women with TS at median age ~19 years reported median AH of ~152 cm, a 6 cm gain over baseline projected AH [136]. In a national registry of 675 French patients mean AH for subgroups analyzed by type of puberty ranged from 148.0 cm (spontaneous puberty) to 150.5 cm (induced puberty) after an average of 5 years' GH treatment starting at an average age of 11–12 years [151].

Although the average AH values for groups of patients are quite similar across many RCTs and observational studies – in the vicinity of 148–152 cm – the values for individual patients show a typical degree of variance, with one SD from the mean being about 6.5 cm, as it is for mature height in women in the general population. Thus the range of AH values across many studies and thousands of GH-treated patients is around 136–164 cm, with most subjects' final height values clustered round the mean of an essentially Gaussian (normal) distribution. Means and ranges of AH values are up to 5 cm greater for subjects from countries that have particularly tall populations such as the Netherlands [139].

Given the broad variation in potential outcome, substantial effort has been expended to define pretreatment and treatment-related variables associated with *greater AH* or greater *height gain from baseline* to AH. It might seem logical that greater height gain from baseline would lead directly to taller AH, but this is not the case. Children who are shorter at baseline have a "greater distance to travel" to attain a given adult height (e.g., the lower limit of the female population range, around 150 cm). Conversely, for a given height gain (e.g., 5 cm) the child who is taller at baseline will be a taller adult, assuming age at AH is held constant (e.g., 18 years). Not surprisingly, children with taller parents (i.e., greater MPH) are likely to be taller at baseline, given the correlation between subject height and parental height, which is retained in TS [42, 43]. Thus, two of the key factors associated with taller AH are taller baseline height and taller MPH (which, due to their correlation, are not independent variables).

Factors influencing adult height after GH treatment can be grouped as either intrinsic factors that are not modifiable or extrinsic factors that can be changed. Intrinsic factors include genetic influences such as parents' heights, discussed above, and growth-related genetic variants such as GH receptor isoforms, *SOCS2* polymorphism, or other single nucleotide polymorphisms [98, 160, 161]. Although these features cannot be manipulated, they may provide helpful information for setting realistic family expectations of treatment outcome, particularly if further research into genetic polymorphisms uncovers stronger links to GH responsiveness [160]. Certain factors are to some extent modifiable, such as age at diagnosis, which may be improved by greater vigilance for clinical features linked to TS (see Chap. 1); earlier diagnosis in turn provides the opportunity for earlier initiation of treatment and a longer period of treatment before puberty (either spontaneous or induced).

The other readily modifiable aspect of treatment is the GH regimen (e.g., dose, timing and duration of treatment). Although it might be assumed that a greater GH dose would be associated with greater treatment effect, the dose-response relationship is nonlinear, and the overarching goal is to use the lowest effective dose. Initial responsiveness to GH is highly predictive of subsequent response [126, 155, 158], leading to the proposal for individualized GH dosing strategies, rather than standard weight or body surface area-based dosing. These personalized algorithms are based on various factors including pretreatment auxologic and/or genetic variables and early treatment response variables such as the patient's initial change in HV or HtSDS with the goal of optimizing outcomes while using the lowest effective dose to maintain IGF-I in the normal range, and to minimize risk and cost [162].

The data from various subgroups of a 2350-subject cohort followed in one of the longest-standing GH observational studies have been used to develop mathematical models to predict outcomes such as prepubertal growth response [163], pubertal growth response [164], height gain during long-term GH treatment, and measured AH [116, 155]. The variables contributing the greatest influence to models of *mature height (AH or NAH)* were (in order of importance) taller height at GH start, greater first-year response to treatment, taller midparental height, older age at onset of puberty, younger age at GH start, and greater GH dose. These findings are supported by data from independent cohorts [126, 139, 155]. The *height gain* from start of treatment to AH was predicted by the same factors as those in the primary model, with the exception that younger age at GH start had the highest rank in the regression model, and height at GH start was a negative predictor (meaning the shorter the starting height, the greater the height gain). This study and others have placed particular emphasis on the importance of maximizing height gain prior to puberty, for example, by ensuring a longer period of GH treatment before induction of puberty [137, 139, 150, 155–157, 165, 166], in view of the maturational effects of high estrogen concentrations on the epiphyses. Ranke and colleagues, among others, have pointed out that GH appears to be more cost-effective when given during pre-puberty, in part due to the fact that older children are heavier, thereby increasing the total GH dose when prescribed based on body weight [163, 164].

Thus, current TS treatment guidelines suggest aiming for a period of at least 4 years of GH treatment before onset/induction of puberty [167]. However, the potential benefit of low-dose estrogen as adjunctive therapy for growth enhancement, as distinct from the issue of pubertal replacement, is a separate topic discussed below. Additional factors associated with *height gain from baseline* in some studies include difference between baseline height SDS and MPH SDS (i.e., greater height gain if the child is relatively short for her parental heights), taller maternal height (associated with greater response in a young cohort who started treatment before age 4 [144]), and weight SDS. The following sections review two key factors – age at GH initiation and GH regimen.

Age at GH Initiation

No specific age for initiation of GH treatment can be recommended, but various lines of evidence indicate that earlier treatment start [47, 116, 124, 136, 157], including at least 4 years of GH prior to puberty [131, 143, 144, 150], is associated with taller AH. The mean adult heights of cohorts of women with TS after completion of GH treatment during RCTs that began in the 1980s and 1990s were typically around -2 SD (i.e., at the lower end of the general population height range; Table 3.2). This outcome infers that about half of GH-treated women remained short despite many years of GH treatment, leading our group and others to examine the issue of age at GH initiation. We questioned whether early treatment of very young girls with TS might maintain the child's height percentile relative to non-TS peers and prevent the growth failure that would otherwise occur, thereby protecting the individual's genetic height potential. Importantly, the majority of height deficit of individuals with TS has occurred before the age of 3 years [20], so there is already a substantial gap to be bridged for most girls before they enter preschool. The Toddler Turner study clearly demonstrated that established growth failure could be halted, heights deficits repaired, and further growth failure prevented, by initiation of GH treatment at the average age of 2 years [126]. Supportive evidence for early GH initiation comes from matched or historically-controlled studies [143, 144] and from large cohorts followed in national or company-sponsored registries. Younger age at start of GH treatment is a highly significant predictor of treatment outcome when age is included as a continuous variable in regression and prediction models [47, 116, 151, 155–158, 168]. From the patient's perspective, early treatment may allow girls with TS to experience childhood without the challenges of significant short stature, and, by maintaining height within the normal range, can provide the opportunity for affected girls to undergo a normally timed puberty.

A 10-year follow-up study of the Toddler Turner cohort evaluated changes in height SDS, pubertal onset, and NAH in the two original treatment groups followed in a long-term extension [132]. Whereas only one of the two groups received GH during the 2-year controlled phase of the study (average ages 2-4 years), almost all girls in both groups received GH in the long-term extension from around age 8–16. Consistent with the mathematical models developed from the large observational studies, the most important factor in determining NAH in the Toddler long-term cohort was height SDS at start of treatment (i.e., the taller the girl was at start of treatment, relative to population standards for age, the taller she was at NAH). Because growth failure is progressive with increasing age in untreated girls, taller height SDS at GH start correlates moderately with younger age at start. In the Canadian study to AH detailed in the preceding section on RCTs (Table 3.2, Stephure 2005) the effect of baseline age was assessed by ANCOVA [47]. For each year of earlier GH initiation a mean incremental gain of 0.22 SDS (~1.5 cm) greater AH was demonstrated, although there was substantial interindividual variation.

In summary, relatively early GH initiation around 4–6 years of age should result in normalization of growth during childhood, maintenance of height potential and age-appropriate feminization (either spontaneous or induced), such that the goals for both physiological timing of puberty and optimal adult stature can be achieved. Contrary to previous published guidelines [53], current evidence suggests that treatment should be initiated promptly, without waiting to confirm the expected postnatal growth failure (i.e., by observing untreated growth for 6–12 months). Furthermore, early treatment is particularly relevant if the child already is short, has documented growth failure (e.g., HV < 50th percentile in the absence of other treatable cause of poor growth such as hypothyroidism or celiac disease), or has a strong likelihood of significantly short stature (e.g., short parents or short predicted AH). Nevertheless, GH treatment initiated in later childhood or even the early teen years (e.g., in girls whose diagnosis is delayed) may result in acceptable AH, as long as baseline bone age is no greater than ~12 years [169]. However, this outcome may be at the expense of delaying puberty to allow additional time for growth to occur. Therefore, the girl and her family will need to weigh the relative importance of height versus feminization. Depending on individual goals, GH treatment may be continued until the patient is satisfied with her height or until little growth potential remains (approximately bone age ≥ 14 years, representing ~98% of mature height, and/or HV <2 cm/year). Even after discontinuation of GH treatment most young women will gain an additional 1 or 2 cm in height.

GH Dose and Frequency of Administration

There are slight regional variations in GH regimens in terms of maximum approved dosage, basis for calculation (bodyweight vs. body surface area), and whether based on daily or weekly dosage (the latter inherited from the era of pituitary-derived GH). Approximate standard dosage ranges are as follows: Australia, 4.5–9.5 mg/m^2/week (equivalent to ~0.16–0.34 mg/kg/week or 23–49 µg/kg/day); Europe, 45–50 µg/kg/day; Japan, up to 0.35 mg/kg/week (~50 µg/kg/day), and North America, 0.350–0.375 mg/kg/week (50–54 µg/kg/day), typically administered in divided doses by subcutaneous injection in the evening 6–7 days/week.[7] Despite evidence of GH dose-response for randomized cohorts of patients in clinical trials, potential safety concerns and financial cost of increased total GH exposure have to be weighed when judging the benefit/risk/cost balance of higher GH dosages. Therefore, dosage should be individualized for age, pubertal status, and height potential, considering factors such as baseline predicted AH and parental heights. Given the clear evidence that a dose of 45–50 µg/kg/day can normalize height for most girls during early childhood [126, 144] and normalize adult stature for many [47, 124, 133, 137, 139, 149], and that substantially higher doses produce relatively small incremental height gains [139], there does not appear to be a rationale for starting GH at higher doses, particularly in view of potential increase in risk of dose-related adverse events. However, if treatment cannot be initiated at a relatively young, prepubertal age, a higher starting dose (up to 68 µg/kg/day) may be warranted in girls who have limited growth potential (e.g., delayed diagnosis, already pubertal, short parents). Similarly, if early response is inadequate or wanes dramatically (in the absence of poor treatment adherence or remediable growth-impairing process), dosage escalation may be considered, particularly if this would allow puberty to begin at an age similar to peers [137–139, 170]; however, dose-response effect may not be maintained to AH [139].

A question that has not been addressed in girls with TS is whether proactively increasing the GH dosage during the time for puberty, in conjunction with appropriate estrogen replacement, may stimulate a more robust pubertal growth spurt. However, this strategy has not proven helpful in children with GH deficiency [171]. Body surface area-based GH dosing, particularly in children whose GH treatment is initiated before 8 years of age, may result in more physiological IGF-I concentrations, reduced cumulative GH dose, cost of treatment, and potential risk, without reducing effectiveness [172]. Another approach that warrants investigation is IGF-I-based dosing, which has been used successfully in children with GH deficiency and idiopathic short stature but not yet tested in girls with TS. Titrating GH dose based on measured IGF-I concentrations has the advantage of using lower total GH dosages while maintaining the growth response, potentially enhancing both cost-effectiveness and safety [173, 174].

---

[7] Some clinicians choose to prescribe GH injections on 6 rather than 7 days per week to give the child one injection-free night per week.

GH is more effective when given daily rather than three days per week [175–177] and there is no evidence of incremental benefit of twice-daily GH injection [178]. There have been no published studies of treatment with long-acting GH in patients with TS. However, a study was initiated in 2017 in China using weekly subcutaneous injections of pegylated GH at two different dosages [www.clinicaltrials.gov; NCT03189160].

Individual Patient Outcomes

Extrapolating from study group data to individual patient outcomes suggests that, depending on age and starting height, catch-up growth should result in height within the lower end of the age-appropriate female reference range within the first 1–2 years of treatment. If treatment continues uninterrupted and HV is maintained around the reference population mean for chronological age during childhood, followed by adequate pubertal growth, then a resonable outcome of 5–8 cm height increment can be expected. For most patients these responses should allow attainment of AH within the lower part of the normal range, between the fifth and 50th percentiles on the standard height curve. Comparison of individual growth responses against general population ranges for HV and height SDS may be unreliable during the pubertal age range, because girls with TS lack the pubertal growth spurt resulting from the synergistic actions of endogenous GH and estrogen that occurs in girls with healthy ovaries. During this period girls with TS may lose ground when height SDS is calculated according to general standards, but height SDS should still continue to increase in GH-treated girls compared with untreated TS standards. However, interruption or discontinuation of GH treatment before completion of growth will likely result in growth deceleration ("catchdown"), with decline across the percentile channels and loss of height potential.

Height gains accumulate slowly over a long duration of treatment in girls with TS [133, 136, 145], perhaps as a consequence of their SHOX-related skeletal dysplasia, so patience and persistence are required. However, for certain patients with intrinsically low GH responsiveness the pursuit of "normal" stature may be an unattainable goal. In such cases it may be helpful for families to be made aware of this potential outcome sooner rather than later to avoid the futility, expense, and unnecessary risk of prolonged pharmacologic interventions.

Effects of GH Treatment on Psychosocial, Neurocognitive and Quality of Life Outcomes

Studies of the effects of GH and other growth-promoting treatments on quality of life, neurocognitive and psychosocial outcomes in patients with TS are challenging to analyze, and detailed review is beyond the scope of this chapter. There is wide variation in instruments used, populations studied, presence or absence of concomitant therapies such as estrogen or oxandrolone, timing of assessment (during vs. after growth-promoting treatment), use of different comparator groups (TS control vs. non-TS control vs. population reference values), and evaluation by patient vs. parent report [179–187]. In addition, published studies typically lack stringent statistical methods, such as *a priori* power analysis to define patient numbers or effect sizes needed to detect significant differences, or statistical adjustments to account for multiple comparisons across the wide variety of measures used. Bearing in mind such limitations, a systematic review of 13 studies in TS found a general trend toward reduced quality of life, but suggested that inconclusive results may reflect inadequate understanding of life factors most important to patients with TS [188]. Nevertheless, there appears to be no detrimental effect of growth-promoting therapies on psychosocial adjustment in women with TS relative to general population standards [153, 186].

Monitoring and Safety of GH Treatment

Efficacy Monitoring

The suggested approach to monitoring GH efficacy is to assess growth response approximately every 4 months during the first year of treatment and every 6 months thereafter, preferably with height measured around the same time of day, by the same person, using the same stadiometer, although this may be impractical in some settings. Because of the importance of initial response in predicting long-term outcome, the first-year HV should be compared with pretreatment HV based on height obtained at least 6 months prior to start of GH [117, 124, 130, 131, 189]. Plotting the data on general population height charts (and HV charts, where available) allows the clinician and family to readily assess the child's position relative to her peers, with whom she interacts on a daily basis, rather than to other girls with TS, whom she will likely see only on rare occasions such as clinic days. Failure to achieve catch-up growth (HV above the mean for chronological age [189] or increase in height SDS above baseline [163]) by the end of the first treatment year should prompt evaluation for adherence/compliance problems, errors in GH dosing or administration, and additional growth-impairing conditions such as hypothyroidism or celiac disease. However, comparison with general population growth standards during the time for puberty may be less helpful, as girls with TS typically lag behind their peers during this period due to absence of the estrogen-mediated pubertal growth spurt. This is one situation in which use of TS-specific height curves may provide reassurance, by demonstrating continued improvements in comparison with historical data for TS.

The initial brisk response to GH wanes after the first 6–12 months in all GH-treated conditions, and dosage escalation regimens have been used to address this known issue [131, 137, 138, 170]. However, as long as treatment is continued and overall growth rate remains around the 50th percentile for age, the initial height gains should be maintained. GH treatment may be discontinued once the patient and her family feel she has reached a satisfactory height, or linear growth is essentially complete (e.g., HV <2.0 cm/year or bone age ≥ 14 years, at which time 98% of mature height has been attained in most girls). There is no rationale for continuing GH treatment through the transition period and into adulthood in patients with TS.

Safety Overview

Clinical trials of GH treatment in TS have raised no serious or unexpected safety concerns. Published reports have provided reassurance with respect to blood pressure and risk factors for cardiovascular disease, heart morphology, aortic diameter and distensibility [190–193]; carbohydrate and lipid metabolism [191, 194–196]; body composition [191, 195]; bone mineralization [197]; body proportions [190]; and occurrence of otitis media and hearing loss [198, 199]. However, clinical trials do not have adequate patient numbers to detect rare events, are generally of inadequate duration to detect events with long latency periods, and are not designed with statistical power to evaluate safety endpoints. Large observational studies that follow substantial numbers of patients [200–203] can provide more robust assessment of the longer-term safety of GH. By comparing outcomes across groups of patients with various underlying diagnoses, these studies can help address the differences between effects of the drug and effects of the primary condition itself.

Data from two observational cohorts indicate increased risks of reversible intracranial hypertension, slipped capital femoral epiphysis, and possibly pancreatitis during GH treatment in girls with TS compared with children who have idiopathic GH deficiency or idiopathic short stature [201, 204]. Greater rates of onset or progression of scoliosis in girls with TS than in children with other growth disorders [200], may result from the underlying skeletal dysplasia of TS exacerbated by rapid catch-up growth stimulated by GH [204].

Specific monitoring for potential adverse outcomes during GH treatment in patients with TS is needed for two reasons: first, girls with TS have increased underlying risks for certain comorbid conditions (e.g., diabetes, dyslipidemia, hypertension, aortopathy, scoliosis, slipped capital femoral epiphysis, excessive cutaneous nevi, intracranial hypertension) that potentially could be aggravated by GH treatment; second, GH doses used in TS are supraphysiologic, thereby potentially increasing the risk for possible treatment-related hazards. The general guidelines for monitoring of lipids, cardiovascular status, otitis media and hearing deficits, scoliosis, slipped capital femoral epiphysis [56, 57, 167, 204, 205], and cutaneous nevi [206, 207] as proposed in current TS guidelines are likely adequate whether or not the child receives GH [167]. Adequate patient numbers to detect rare long-term outcomes require continued surveillance in large observational studies, particularly in adulthood, for an extended period after completion of treatment.

Mortality and Cardiovascular Disorders

Women with TS have increased risks of many comorbidities and of premature death [208, 209], but available data do not allow elucidation of relative risk of death *in adulthood* following GH treatment *in childhood*. A British cohort study of almost

3500 women with TS diagnosed between 1959 and 2002 found a threefold increase in standardized mortality ratio associated with increased risk of death from cardiovascular disorders, particularly aortic aneurysm [209]. However, the study did not collect information regarding GH exposure. In addition, a study of 5220 patients with TS followed in a company-sponsored GH observational study reported four deaths from aortic aneurysm and one from aortic dissection in patients aged 14–16 years [152]. In contrast, another observational study of ~950 GH-treated girls with TS reported two deaths (neither one from cardiovascular disease) vs. four expected deaths in ~7000 person-years of follow-up, for a standardized mortality ratio of 0.51 [210]. Although girls and women with TS have intrinsic increases in risks of various cardiovascular disorders, the available data do not suggest an effect of long-term GH treatment on the risks of hypertension, left ventricular hypertrophy, aortic dilatation, or aortic stiffness [190, 192, 193, 211–214]. Nevertheless, the baseline risk of cardiovascular mortality clearly warrants careful long-term surveillance, irrespective of GH treatment. Cardiovascular issues are discussed further in Chap. 6.

Neoplasia

There have been occasional case reports of neoplasia in both untreated and GH-treated patients with TS [132, 208, 215, 216] but data from GH registries do not suggest an increased risk of neoplasia in GH-treated subjects without underlying risk factors [152, 200, 203, 208, 217, 218]. There are no published data suggesting a direct cause and effect relationship between supranormal IGF-I concentrations during childhood and cancer in adulthood. Nevertheless, epidemiologic associations between high IGF-I and neoplasia have prompted guidance for IGF-I monitoring for patients receiving GH for all diagnoses [219]. Supranormal IGF-I concentrations (>+2 SD) during GH treatment in TS have been reported in some studies [126, 144], but not others [157, 220]. Therefore, as proposed by published guidelines [167], IGF-I should be measured at baseline and first follow-up (to assess initial response), then annually or following substantial GH dosage increases, with the general goal of maintaining IGF-I concentrations within the broad normal range [221]. GH dosage reduction is suggested if serum IGF-I is above +3 SD; for values in the +2 to +3 SD range, dosage adjustment should balance the need for growth stimulation against potential risks [167, 222, 223]. Continued surveillance of all GH-treated patients is needed, as neoplasia is rare in childhood and onset may be delayed for many years, so patient registries may not yet have accumulated adequate patient-years of follow-up in individuals with TS.

Glucose, Insulin, and Carbohydrate Metabolism

One issue requiring increased vigilance is glucose and insulin metabolism, as patients with TS are inherently at increased risk of insulin resistance, T2DM, dyslipidemia, and cardiovascular disease [224–227] and have a specific defect in glucose-stimulated insulin secretion [226]. Although most clinical trial data regarding effects of GH treatment in patients with TS have not raised concerns [191, 196, 228–231], one study reported persistently reduced insulin sensitivity 5 years after discontinuation of GH [194], underscoring the need for careful long-term follow-up. In contrast, another study found reduced abdominal adiposity and significantly better glucose tolerance in GH-treated vs. untreated girls with TS, suggesting that beneficial effects on body composition and regional fat deposition may outweigh GH-induced insulin antagonism [195]. Whereas results from clinical trials are hampered by limited patient numbers and varying analysis methods, the extended duration and statistical power of observational studies may provide more robust data. Analyses from two international observational studies reported clear increases in T2DM rates in TS vs. general population rates [203, 232]; diabetes data from a North American observational study are harder to interpret because standardized incidence ratios were not calculated for T2DM [200].

Overall, considering the increased risk of derangements of glucose and insulin metabolism in TS, as well as the often insidious onset of T2DM, and the fact that GH induces a physiologic state of (potentially reversible) insulin resistance, monitoring for changes in glucose/insulin metabolism is key. Therefore, current TS guidelines recommend obtaining blood glucose, preferably fasting, and HbA1c at least once per year [167]. An oral glucose tolerance test should be performed in patients whose results fulfill DM guidelines [233, 234]. The presence of other risk factors such as obesity, family history of T2DM or diabetes-prone ethnicity, concomitant treatment with oxandrolone, or other medication(s) potentially associated with insulin resistance [233, 235] should prompt closer scrutiny.

Contraindications to GH Treatment

According to the United States Food and Drug Administration prescribing information for somatropin (recombinant DNA-derived human GH), absolute contraindications to its use are acute critical illness, active malignancy, and active proliferative or severe nonproliferative diabetic retinopathy [236]. Similar guidance is provided by other pharmaceutical regulatory agencies. Conditions that may be considered relative contraindications, requiring increased vigilance during treatment, include: history of certain malignancies, particularly those treated with cranial irradiation, preexisting type 1 DM, severe scoliosis, and intracranial hypertension or papilledema.

Oxandrolone

Well-controlled studies have demonstrated modest synergistic increases in growth response with addition of the non-aromatizable anabolic steroid oxandrolone during GH treatment [133, 140–142, 237, 238]; a meta-analysis of four studies reported a mean incremental AH gain of 2 cm (95% CI, 0.1–4.1) when oxandrolone was added to GH [239]. However, the drug is not available in many countries and the potential for the unwanted effects of delayed breast development and dose-dependent virilization (e.g., clitoromegaly, voice deepening, hirsutism, acne) [240] prompts the need for caution. Furthermore, in one study six of seven girls with TS who developed DM had received oxandrolone, and in the study population as a whole oxandrolone (with or without GH) had significant effects on indices of carbohydrate metabolism, whereas GH alone did not [228]. However, oxandrolone may be considered if AH outcome is likely to be unsatisfactory, such as in situations of delayed diagnosis or delayed initiation of GH, or in girls with particularly short midparental height. In those for whom oxandrolone is felt necessary, this should be withheld until around 8–10 years of age and should be used at lowest effective dosages: initial dose 0.03 mg/kg/day, maintenance no greater than 0.05 mg/kg/day [167, 239].

Studies of oxandrolone effects on psychosocial and quality of life measures, although more recent and generally better designed than those of GH effects, provide little evidence of benefit or detriment for these nongrowth-related outcomes [241–243].

Low-Dose Estrogen During Childhood (Prepuberty)

As described in the section of this chapter detailing the etiology of the growth disturbance, girls with TS are estrogen-deficient from birth. Thus they lack not only the dramatic pubertal estradiol rise but also the more subtle increase in estradiol secretion of mid-childhood [40, 107, 244]. Building on this foundation, the dose-dependent effects of estrogen on the physiology of growth have been studied since the early 1980s, leading to a model of nonlinear response, in which estrogen stimulates growth at low dosages but not at high dosages [245]. These findings led to the hypothesis that ultra-low-dose estrogen might be useful as an adjunctive growth-promoting agent, quite distinct from the role of estrogen replacement in stimulating secondary sexual development and skeletal maturation at puberty. Following this concept, a unique double-blind clinical trial examined the effects of ultra-low dose estrogen from age 5, in addition to GH (Table 3.2, Ross 2011) [127]. During the "growth-promoting" phase from ages 5–12 years the estrogen regimen comprised slowly increasing dosages of oral ethinyl estradiol (EE2) starting at 25 ng/kg/day from age 5–8, then 50 ng/kg/day age 8–12. Pubertal induction began after age 12 with 100 ng/kg/day EE2 escalating to a mamimum of 800 ng/kg/day from age 16; progestin was added after onset of menses. An important aspect of the study was the individualization of the EE2 dosage by 50% reductions for any sign of early feminization, followed by slower age- and weight-based increments thereafter. This study demonstrated a modest synergistic increase in adult height with childhood EE2, thought to result from local estrogen action at the skeletal growth plate enhancing responsiveness to GH/IGF-I [127]. Additional outcomes of this specific childhood estrogen regimen included normalization of the timing of thelarche for about one quarter of the girls (Table 3.2, Quigley 2014) and improvements in cognition and memory [127, 147, 246, 247].

Other studies have explored the concept of childhood (relatively) low-dose estrogen replacement using different approaches. A UK study randomized 58 girls aged 5–15 years to 3 groups: EE2 at a starting dose of 50–75 ng/kg/day, GH alone, or the combination; after 1 year GH was added for girls initially receiving EE2 alone [146]. In the large multicenter US study previously described (Table 3.2, Quigley 2002), 232 girls aged 5 to ~14 years were randomized to 5 groups: GH at either 0.27 mg/kg/week. (39 ng/kg/day) or 0.36 mg/kg/week. (51 ng/kg/day) with or without EE2 (~25–50 ng/kg/day) from age 8; the fifth group received placebo injections with oral placebo (transitioned onto active therapy after 18 months) [124]. Unlike the NIH study (Table 3.2, Ross 2011), neither of these studies demonstrated a benefit of early EE2 in terms of height SDS gain from baseline to AH [124, 146]. The differences in height outcomes between these three studies highlight the fact that the addition of estrogen as a growth-promoting agent has not yet been optimized. The suggestive positive results from the NIH study using the lowest estrogen dosage at the youngest ages support the validity of the original hypothesis proposed in the 1980s that estrogen may contribute to the processes of normal childhood growth, but dosage and timing are critical and probably highly individual.

Overall, in addition to its obvious effects on secondary sexual development, estrogen deficiency appears to contribute to the growth (and possibly cognitive or behavioral) deficits of TS, but optimal physiological replacement strategies remain elusive, particularly for childhood (prepubertal) replacement. In view of the fact that oral estrogens decrease IGF-I serum concentrations, can have detrimental effects on the clotting profile, and suppress certain IGF-independent metabolic effects of GH, whereas transdermal estrogens do not, additional studies using lower estradiol dosages and transdermal or other parenteral form of administration are needed [248–252].

The more conventional use of estrogen as a feminizing agent rather than a growth-promoting agent has been studied extensively, as most girls with TS require estrogen replacement to either initiate or complete puberty (discussed in Chap. 5). The route, dosage, and escalation tempo of pubertal estrogen replacement influence the rate and duration of pubertal growth and, consequently, overall attained height.

Summary

Turner syndrome is characterized by a pattern of inexorable growth failure from intrauterine life to adulthood, culminating in adult heights of non-GH-treated women on average 20 cm below the mean heights of women in the general population (mean untreated TS adult height, 143–146 cm; range 132–155 cm). The etiology of the growth failure is complex and multifactorial: the primary deficiency appears to be a form of epiphyseal dysplasia, mainly as a result of haploinsufficiency of the X chromosomal *SHOX* gene. Estrogen deficiency and secondary disturbances of GH-IGF-I physiology likely interact to contribute to the growth disorder.

GH treatment (average dose approximately 50 μg/kg/day) stimulates catch-up growth, promptly and significantly increasing height velocity and height SDS in the first year of treatment. Early treatment initiation can preserve genetic growth potential, prevent ongoing growth failure, and maintain height within the normal range for age, reducing the potential for stature-related physical and social problems and allowing for physiologically timed puberty. Adult height following uninterrupted GH treatment is estimated from clinical trial data to be on average 5–8 cm greater than without treatment, allowing many women to attain heights within the lower part of the reference range for the population (above ~150 cm or −2.0 SD by North American standards; approximately 5 cm taller in Northern European cohorts). Younger age and taller height for age relative to population standards at the start of GH treatment are associated with taller AH.

Large observational studies have generally found no unexpected safety issues associated with GH treatment in children with TS. However, to reduce potential for excessive GH dosing serum IGF-I should be maintained, where possible, within the age-appropriate reference range. Women with TS have an increased risk of disturbances of carbohydrate metabolism and type 2 DM, which may be increased by GH treatment. Therefore, all girls and women with TS should be monitored according to published guidelines for development of insulin resistance and diabetes.

Dedicated to my father the wordsmith, my inspiration.

References

1. Turner HH. A syndrome of infantilism, congenital webbed neck, and cubitus valgus. Endocrinology. 1938;23(5):566–74.
2. Tesch LG, Rosenfeld RG. Morgagni, Ullrich and Turner: the discovery of gonadal dysgenesis. Endocrinology. 1995;5:327–8.
3. Ullrich O. Uber typische Kombinationsbilder multipler Abartung. Z Kinderheilkd. 1930;49:271–6.
4. Lyon AJ, Preece MA, Grant DB. Growth curve for girls with Turner syndrome. Arch Dis Child. 1985;60(10):932–5.
5. Ranke MB, Pfluger H, Rosendahl W, Stubbe P, Enders H, Bierich JR, et al. Turner syndrome: spontaneous growth in 150 cases and review of the literature. Eur J Pediatr. 1983;141(2):81–8.
6. Pelz L, Timm D, Eyermann E, Hinkel GK, Kirchner M, Verron G. Body height in Turner's syndrome. Clin Genet. 1982;22:62–6.
7. Lenko HL, Perheentupa J, Soderholm A. Growth in Turner's syndrome: spontaneous and fluoxymesterone stimulated. Acta Paediatr Scand Suppl. 1979;227:57–63.
8. Rosenberg D, Tell G. Syndrome de Turner. A propos d'une statistique de 60 observations. Pediatrie. 1972;27:831–50.
9. Garcia-Rudaz C, Martinez AS, Heinrich JJ, Lejarraga H, Keselman A, Laspiur M, et al. Growth of Argentinian girls with Turner syndrome. Ann Hum Biol. 1995;22(6):533–44.
10. Haeusler G, Schemper M, Frisch H, Blumel P, Schmitt K, Plochl E. Spontaneous growth in Turner syndrome: evidence for a minor pubertal growth spurt. Eur J Pediatr. 1992;151(4):283–7.
11. Massa G, Vanderschueren-Lodeweyckx M, Malvaux P. Linear growth in patients with Turner syndrome: influence of spontaneous puberty and parental height. Eur J Pediatr. 1990;149(4):246–50.
12. Park E, Bailey JD, Cowell CA. Growth and maturation of patients with Turner's syndrome. Pediatr Res. 1983;17:1–7.
13. Naeraa RW, Nielsen J. Standards for growth and final height in Turner's syndrome. Acta Paediatr Scand. 1990;79:182–90.

14. Rongen-Westerlaken C, Corel L, van den Broeck J, Massa G, Karlberg J, Albertsson-Wikland K, et al. Reference values for height, height velocity and weight in Turner's syndrome. Swedish Study Group for GH treatment. Acta Paediatr. 1997;86(9):937–42.

15. El-Bassyouni HT, Afifi HH, Aglan MS, Mahmoud WM, Zaki ME. Growth curves of Egyptian patients with Turner syndrome. Am J Med Genet Part A. 2012;158:2687–91.

16. Sempé M, Hansson Bondallaz C, Limoni C. Growth curves in untreated Ullrich-Turner syndrome: French reference standards 1–22 years. Eur J Pediatr. 1996;155:862–9.

17. Suwa S. Standards for growth and growth velocity in Turner's syndrome. Acta Paediatr Jpn. 1992;34(2):206–21.

18. Isojima T, Yokoya S, Ito J, Horikawa R, Tanaka T. New reference growth charts for Japanese girls with Turner syndrome. Pediatr Int. 2009;51(5):709–14.

19. Isojima T, Yokoya S, Ito J, Naiki Y, Horikawa R, Tanaka T. Proposal of new auxological standards for Japanese girls with Turner syndrome. Clin Pediatr Endocrinol. 2010;19(3):69–82.

20. Even L, Cohen A, Marbach N, Brand M, Kauli R, Sippell W, et al. Longitudinal analysis of growth over the first 3 years of life in Turner's syndrome. J Pediatr. 2000;137(4):460–4.

21. Bernasconi S, Larizza D, Benso L, Volta C, Vannelli S, Milani S, et al. Turner's syndrome in Italy: familial characteristics, neonatal data, standards for birth weight and for height and weight from infancy to adulthood. Acta Paediatr. 1994;83(3):292–8.

22. Davenport ML, Punyasavatsut N, Stewart PW, Gunther DF, Savendahl L, Sybert VP. Growth failure in early life: an important manifestation of Turner syndrome. Horm Res. 2002;57(5–6):157–64.

23. Woelfle J, Lindberg A, Aydin F, Ong KC, Camach-Hubner C, Gohlke B. Secular trends on birth parameters, growth, and pubertal timing in girls with Turner syndrome. Front Endocrinol. 2018;9:54.

24. Ranke MB, Stubbe P, Majewski F, Bierich JR. Spontaneous growth in Turner syndrome. Acta Paediatr Scand Suppl. 1988;343:22–30.

25. Brook CG, Murset G, Zachmann M, Prader A. Growth in children with 45, XO Turner's syndrome. Arch Dis Child. 1974;49(10):789–95.

26. Hausler G, Schemper M, Frisch H, Blümel P, Schmitt K, Plöchl E. Spontaneous growth in Turner syndrome: evidence for a minor pubertal growth spurt. In: Ranke MB, Rosenfeld RG, editors. Amsterdam: Elsevier Science BV; 1991. p. 67–73.

27. Rochiccioli P, David M, Malpuech G, Colle M, Limal JM, Battin J, et al. Study of final height in Turner's syndrome: ethnic and genetic influences. Acta Paediatr. 1994;83(3):305–8.

28. Tuschy U. Spontaneous growth in Turner's syndrome. Padiatr Grenzgeb. 1990;29(5):419–23.

29. Lenko HL, Perheentupa J, Soderholm A. Growth in Turner syndrome: spontaneous and fluoximesterone stimulated. Acta Paediatr Scand Suppl. 1979;277:57–63.

30. Ranke MG, Chavez-Meyer H, Blank B, Frisch H, Hausler G. Spontaneous growth and bone age development in Turner syndrome: results of a multicentric study 1990. In: Ranke MB, Rosenfeld RG, editors. Turner syndrome: growth promoting therapies. Amsterdam: Elsevier Science BV; 1991. p. 101–6.

31. Rochiccioli P, Pienkowsky C, Tauber MT. Spontaneous growth in Turner syndrome: a study of 61 cases. In: Ranke MB, Rosenfeld RG, editors. Turner syndrome: growth promoting therapies. Amsterdam: Elsevier Science BV; 1991. p. 107–12.

32. Lippe B, Frane J. Growth in Turner syndrome: the United States experience. In: Ranke MB, Rosenfeld RG, editors. Turner syndrome: growth promoting therapies. Amsterdam: Elsevier Science BV; 1991. p. 59–65.

33. FitzSimmons J, Fantel A, Shepard TH. Growth parameters in mid-trimester fetal Turner syndrome. Early Hum Dev. 1994;38(2):121–9.

34. Holl RW, Kunze D, Etzrodt H, Teller W, Heinze E. Turner syndrome: final height, glucose tolerance, bone density and psychosocial status in 25 adult patients. Eur J Pediatr. 1994;153(1):11–6.

35. Karlberg J, Albertsson-Wikland K, Nilsson KO, Ritzén EM, Westphal O. Growth in infancy and childhood in girls with Turner's syndrome. Acta Paediatr Scand. 1991;80(12):1158–65.

36. Karlberg J, Albertsson-Wikland K, Naeraa RW, on behalf of the Swedish Pediatric Study Group for GH Treatment. The infancy-childhood-puberty model of growth for Turner girls.

In: Ranke MB, Rosenfeld RG, editors. Turner syndrome: growth promoting therapies. Amsterdam: Elsevier Science; 1991. p. 89–94.

37. Bertapelli F, Barros-Filho A de A, Antonio MÂ, Barbeta CJ, de Lemos-Marini SH, Guerra-Junior G. Growth curves for girls with Turner syndrome. Biomed Res Int. 2014;2014:687978.

38. Gunther DF, Eugster E, Zagar AJ, Bryant CG, Davenport ML, Quigley CA. Ascertainment bias in Turner syndrome: fewer clinical manifestations in girls diagnosed incidentally in prenatal life. Pediatrics. 2004;114:640–4.

39. Karlberg J, Engstrom I, Karlberg P, Fryer JG. Analysis of linear growth using a mathematical model. I. From birth to three years. Acta Paediatr Scand. 1987;76:478–88.

40. Courant F, Aksglaede L, Antignac J-P, Monteau F, Sorensen K, Andersson A-M, et al. Assessment of circulating sex steroid levels in prepubertal and pubertal boys and girls by a novel ultrasensitive gas chromatography-tandem mass spectrometry method. J Clin Endocrinol Metab. 2010;95(82–92):2010.

41. Frane J, Sherman B, Genentech Collaborative Group. Predicted adult height in Turner syndrome. In: Rosenfeld RG, Grumbach MM, editors. Turner syndrome. New York: Marcel Dekker; 1990. p. 405–19.

42. Hamelin CE, Anglin DG, Quigley CA, Deal CL. Genomic imprinting in Turner syndrome: effects on response to growth hormone and on risk of sensorineural hearing loss. J Clin Endocrinol Metab. 2006;91(8):3002–10.

43. Ko JM, Kim JM, Kim GH, Lee BH, Yoo HW. Influence of parental origin of the X chromosome on physical phenotypes and GH responsiveness of patients with Turner syndrome. Clin Endocrinol. 2010;73(1):66–71.

44. Bondy CA, Hougen HY, Zhou J, Cheng CM. Genomic imprinting and Turner syndrome. Pediatr Endocrinol Rev. 2012;9(Suppl 2):728–32.

45. Naeraa RW, Eiken M, Legarth EG, Nielsen J. Prediction of final height in Turner's syndrome: a comparative study. Acta Paediatr Scand. 1990;79:776–83.

46. van Teunenbroek A, Stijnen T, Otten B, de Muinck Keizer-Schrama S, Naeraa RW, Rongen-Westerlaken C, et al. A regression method including chronological and bone age for predicting final height in Turner's syndrome, with a comparison of existing methods. Acta Paediatr. 1996;85(4):413–20.

47. Stephure DK. Impact of growth hormone supplementation on adult height in Turner syndrome: results of the Canadian randomized controlled trial. J Clin Endocrinol Metab. 2005;90(6):3360–6.

48. Rongen-Westerlaken C, Rikken B, Vastrick P, Jeuken AH, de Lange MY, Wit JM, et al. Body proportions in individuals with Turner syndrome. Eur J Pediatr. 1993;152(10):813–7.

49. Gravholt CH, Naeraa RW. Reference values for body proportions and body composition in adult women with Ullrich-Turner syndrome. Am J Med Genet. 1997;72(4):403–8.

50. Sas TC, Gerver WJ, de Bruin R, Stijnen T, de Muinck Keizer-Schrama SM, Cole TJ, et al. Body proportions during long-term growth hormone treatment in girls with Turner syndrome participating in a randomized dose-response trial. J Clin Endocrinol Metab. 1999;84(12):4622–8.

51. Uematsu A, Yorifuji T, Muroi J, Yamanaka C, Momoi T. Relatively longer hand in patients with Ullrich-Turner syndrome. Am J Med Genet. 1999;82(3):254–6.

52. Binder G, Fritsch H, Schweizer R, Ranke MB. Radiological signs of Leri-Weill dyschondrosteosis in Turner syndrome. Horm Res. 2001;55(2):71–6.

53. Saenger P, Wikland KA, Conway GS, Davenport M, Gravholt CH, Hintz R, et al. Recommendations for the diagnosis and management of Turner syndrome. J Clin Endocrinol Metab. 2001;86:3061–9.

54. Lubin MB, Gruber HE, Rimoin DL, Lachman RS. Skeletal abnormalities in the Turner syndrome. In: Rosenfeld RG, Grumbach MM, editors. Turner syndrome. New York: Marcel Dekker; 1990. p. 281–300.

55. Ricotti S, Petrucci L, Carenzio G, Klersy C, Calcaterra V, Larizza D, et al. Prevalence and incidence of scoliosis in Turner syndrome: a study in 49 girls followed-up for 4 years. Eur J Phys Rehabil Med. 2011;47:447–53.

56. Elder DA, Roper MG, Henderson RC, Davenport ML. Kyphosis in a Turner syndrome population. Pediatrics. 2002;109(6):e93.

57. Kim JY, Rosenfeld SR, Keyak JH. Increased prevalence of scoliosis in Turner syndrome. J Pediatr Orthop. 2001;21(6):765–6.
58. Hochberg Z. Endocrine control of skeletal maturation. Basel: Karger; 2002. p. 60–3.
59. Ross JL, Long LM, Loriaux DL, Cutler GB. Growth hormone secretory dynamics in Turner syndrome. J Pediatr. 1985;106:202–6.
60. Massarano AA, Brook CG, Hindmarsh PC, Pringle PJ, Teale JD, Stanhope R, et al. Growth hormone secretion in Turner's syndrome and influence of oxandrolone and ethinyl oestradiol. Arch Dis Child. 1989;64:587–92.
61. Massa G, Vanderschueren-Lodeweyckx M, Craen M, Vandeweghe M, Van VG. Growth hormone treatment of Turner syndrome patients with insufficient growth hormone response to pharmacological stimulation tests. Eur J Pediatr. 1991;150:460–3.
62. Reiter JC, Craen M, Van VG. Decreased growth hormone response to growth hormone-releasing hormone in Turner's syndrome: relation to body weight and adiposity. Acta Endocrinol. 1991;125:38–42.
63. Pirazzoli P, Mazzanti L, Bergamaschi R, Perri A, Scarano E, Nanni S, et al. Reduced spontaneous growth hormone secretion in patients with Turner's syndrome. Acta Paediatr. 1999;88:610–3.
64. Wit JM, Massarano AA, Kamp GA, Hindmarsh PC, van Es A, Brook CG, et al. Growth hormone secretion in patients with Turner's syndrome as determined by time series analysis. Acta Endocrinol. 1992;127:7–12.
65. Cianfarani S, Vaccaro F, Pasquino AM, Marchione SA, Passeri F, Spadoni GL, et al. Reduced growth hormone secretion in Turner syndrome: is body weight a key factor? Horm Res. 1994;41:27–32.
66. Ballabio A, Bardoni B, Carrozzo R, Andria G, Bick D, Campbell L, et al. Contiguous gene syndromes due to deletions in the distal short arm of the human X chromosome. Proc Natl Acad Sci U S A. 1989;86:10001–5.
67. Ogata T, Goodfellow P, Petit C, Aya M, Matsuo N. Short stature in a girl with a terminal Xp deletion distal to DXYS15: localisation of a growth gene(s) in the pseudoautosomal region. J Med Genet. 1992;29(7):455–9.
68. Ogata T, Petit C, Rappold G, Matsuo N, Matsumoto T, Goodfellow P. Chromosomal localisation of a pseudoautosomal growth gene(s). J Med Genet. 1992;29(9):624–8.
69. Ogata T, Matsuo N. Sex chromosome aberrations and stature: deduction of the principal factors involved in the determination of adult height. Hum Genet. 1993;91:551–62.
70. Ogata T, Matsuo N. Turner syndrome and female sex chromosome aberrations: deduction of the principal factors involved in the development of clinical features. Hum Genet. 1995;95:607–29.
71. Rao E, Weiss B, Fukami M, Mertz A, Meder J, Ogata T, et al. FISH-deletion mapping defines a 270-kb short stature critical interval in the pseudoautosomal region PAR1 on human sex chromosomes. Hum Genet. 1997;100:236–9.
72. Rao E, Weiss B, Fukami M, Rump A, Niesler B, Mertz A, et al. Pseudoautosomal deletions encompassing a novel homeobox gene cause growth failure in idiopathic short stature and Turner syndrome. Nat Genet. 1997;16(1):54–63.
73. Ellison JW, Wardak Z, Young MF, Robey PG, Webster M, Chiong W. PHOG, a candidate gene for involvement in the short stature of Turner syndrome. Hum Mol Genet. 1997;6:1341–7.
74. van der Eerden BC, Karperien M, Wit JM. Systemic and local regulation of the growth plate. Endocr Rev. 2003;24(6):782–801.
75. Manolagas SC, O'Brien CA, Almeida M. The role of estrogen and androgen receptors in bone health and disease. Nat Rev Endocrinol. 2013;9(12):699–712.
76. Kosho T, Muroya K, Nagai T, Fujimoto M, Yokoya S, Sakamoto H, et al. Skeletal features and growth patterns in 14 patients with haploinsufficiency of SHOX: implications for the development of Turner syndrome. J Clin Endocrinol Metab. 1999;84(12):4613–21.
77. Rappold G, Blum WF, Shavrikova EP, Crowe BJ, Roeth R, Quigley CA, et al. Genotypes and phenotypes in children with short stature: clinical indicators of SHOX haploinsufficiency. J Med Genet. 2007;44(5):306–13.
78. Ross JL, Kowal K, Quigley CA, Blum WF, Cutler GB, Crowe B, et al. The phenotype of short stature homeobox gene (SHOX) deficiency in childhood: contrasting children with Léri-Weill dyschondrosteosis and Turner syndrome. J Pediatr. 2005;147(4):499–507.

79. Andrade AC, Baron J, Manolagas SC, Shaw NJ, Rappold GA, Donaldson MD, et al. Hormones and genes of importance in bone physiology and their influence on bone mineralization and growth in Turner syndrome. Horm Res Paediatr. 2010;73(3):161–5.
80. Binder G. Short stature due to SHOX deficiency: genotype, phenotype, and therapy. Horm Res Paediatr. 2011;75(2):81–9.
81. Child CJ, Rappold GA, Blum WF. Short Stature Homeobox-containing (SHOX) gene deficiency: genetics and growth response to growth hormone treatment in comparison with Turner syndrome. In: Preedy VR, editor. The handbook of growth and growth monitoring in health and disease. New York: Springer Science+Business Media, LLC; 2012. p. 2299–318.
82. Blaschke RJ, Rappold G. The pseudoautosomal regions, *SHOX* and disease. Curr Opin Genet Dev. 2006;16:233–9.
83. Clement-Jones M, Schiller S, Rao E, Blaschke RJ, Zuniga A, Zeller R, et al. The short stature homeobox gene *SHOX* is involved in skeletal abnormalities in Turner syndrome. Hum Mol Genet. 2000;9:695–702.
84. Hristov G, Marttila T, Durand C, Niesler B, Rappold GA. SHOX triggers the lysosomal pathway of apoptosis via oxidative stress. Hum Mol Genet. 2014;23:1619–30.
85. Marchini A, Marttila T, Winter A, Caldeira S, Malanchi I, Blaschke RJ, et al. The short stature homeodomain protein SHOX induces cellular growth arrest and apoptosis and is expressed in human growth plate chondrocytes. J Biol Chem. 2004;279:37103–14.
86. Munns CJ, Haase HR, Crowther LM, Hayes MT, Blaschke R, Rappold G, et al. Expression of SHOX in human fetal and childhood growth plate. J Clin Endocrinol Metab. 2004;89:4130–5.
87. Marchini A, Hacker B, Marttila T, Hesse V, Emons J, Weiss B, et al. BNP is a transcriptional target of the short stature homeobox gene *SHOX*. Hum Mol Genet. 2007;16:3081–7.
88. Bondy CA. Care of girls and women with Turner syndrome: a guideline of the Turner Syndrome Study Group. J Clin Endocrinol Metab. 2007;92(1):10–25.
89. Haverkamp F, Wolfle J, Zerres K, Butenandt O, Amendt P, Hauffa BP, et al. Growth retardation in Turner syndrome: aneuploidy, rather than specific gene loss, may explain growth failure. J Clin Endocrinol Metab. 1999;84(12):4578–82.
90. Bakalov VK, Axelrod L, Baron J, Hanton L, Nelson LM, Reynolds JC, et al. Selective reduction in cortical bone mineral density in Turner syndrome independent of ovarian hormone deficiency. J Clin Endocrinol Metab. 2003;88:5717–22.
91. Brook CGD. Growth hormone deficiency in Turner's syndrome. N Engl J Med. 1978;298:1203–4.
92. Albertsson-Wikland K, Rosberg S. Growth hormone secretory dynamics in Turners. In: Rosenfeld R, Grumbach M, editors. Turner syndrome. New York: Marcel Dekker; 1990.
93. Ranke MB, Blum WF, Haug F, Rosendahl W, Attanasio A, Enders H, et al. Growth hormone, somatomedin levels and growth regulation in Turner's syndrome. Acta Endocrinol. 1987;116:305–13.
94. Hochberg Z, Aviram M, Rubin D, Pollack S. Decreased sensitivity to insulin-like growth factor I in Turner's syndrome: a study of monocytes and T lymphocytes. Eur J Clin Investig. 1997;27:543–7.
95. Foster CM, Borondy M, Markovs ME, Hopwood NJ, Kletter GB, Beitins IZ. Growth hormone bioactivity in girls with Turner's syndrome: correlation with insulin-like growth factor I. Pediatr Res. 1994;35:218–22.
96. Attie KM, Julius JR, Stoppani C, Rundle AC. National Cooperative Growth Study substudy VI: the clinical utility of growth-hormone binding protein, insulin-like growth factor I, and insulin-like growth factor-binding protein 3 measurements. J Pediatr. 1997;131:S56–60.
97. Leung K-C, Johannsson G, Leong GM, Ho KKY. Estrogen regulation of growth hormone action. Endocr Rev. 2004;25(5):693–721.
98. Bas F, Darendeliler F, Aycan Z, Çetinkaya E, Berberoğlu M, Sıklar Z, et al. The exon 3-deleted/full-length growth hormone receptor polymorphism and response to growth hormone therapy in growth hormone deficiency and Turner syndrome: a multicenter study. Horm Res Paediatr. 2012;77(2):85–93.
99. Ko JM, Kim JM, Cheon CK, Kim DH, Lee DY, Cheong WY, et al. The common exon 3 polymorphism of the growth hormone receptor gene and the effect of growth hormone therapy on growth in Korean patients with Turner syndrome. Clin Endocrinol. 2010;72(2):196–202.

100. Gravholt CH. Epidemiological, endocrine and metabolic features in Turner syndrome. Eur J Endocrinol. 2004;151:657–87.
101. Gravholt CH, Frystyk J, Flyvbjerg A, Orskov H, Christiansen JS. Reduced free IGF-I and increased IGFBP-3 proteolysis in Turner syndrome: modulation by female sex steroids. Am J Physiol Endocrinol Metab. 2001;280:E308–14.
102. Lebl J, Pruhova S, Zapletalova J, Pechova M. IGF-I resistance and Turner's syndrome. J Pediatr Endocrinol Metab. 2001;14:37–41.
103. Bannink EM, van Doorn J, Stijnen T, Drop SL, de Muinck Keizer-Schrama SM. Free dissociable insulin-like growth factor I (IGF-I), total IGF-I and their binding proteins in girls with Turner syndrome during long-term growth hormone treatment. Clin Endocrinol. 2006;65(3):310–9.
104. Weiss L. Additional evidence of gradual loss of germ cells in the pathogenesis of streak ovaries in Turner's syndrome. J Med Genet. 1971;8(4):540–4.
105. Couse JF, Korach KS. Estrogen receptor null mice: what have we learned and where will they lead us? Endocr Rev. 1999;20:358–417.
106. Nilsson O, Marino R, De Luca F, Phillip M, Baron J. Endocrine regulation of the growth plate. Horm Res. 2005;64(4):157–65.
107. Klein KO, Baron J, Colli MJ, McDonnell DP, Cutler GB Jr. Estrogen levels in childhood determined by an ultrasensitive recombinant cell bioassay. J Clin Invest. 1994;94:2475–80.
108. Weise M, De-Levi S, Barnes KM, Gafni RI, Abad V, Baron J. Effects of estrogen on growth plate senescence and epiphyseal fusion. Proc Natl Acad Sci U S A. 2001;98(12):6871–6.
109. Nilsson O, Weise M, Landman EB, Meyers IL, Barnes KM, Baron J. Evidence that estrogen hastens epiphyseal fusion and cessation of longitudinal bone growth by irreversibly depleting the number of resting zone progenitor cells in female rabbits. Endocrinology. 2014;155(8):2892–9.
110. Smith EP, Boyd J, Frank GR, Takahashi H, Cohen RM, Specker B, et al. Estrogen resistance caused by a mutation in the estrogen receptor gene in a man. N Engl J Med. 1994;331:1056–60.
111. Quaynor SD, Stradtman EW Jr, Kim H-G, Shen Y, Chorich LP, Schreihofer DA, Layman LC. Delayed puberty and estrogen resistance in a woman with estrogen receptor α variant. N Engl J Med. 2013;369(2):164–71.
112. Morishima A, Grumbach MM, Simpson ER, Fisher C, Qin K. Aromatase deficiency in male and female siblings caused by a novel mutation and the physiological role of estrogens. J Clin Endocrinol Metab. 1995;80(12):3689–98.
113. Grumbach MM, Auchus RJ. Estrogen: consequences and implications of human mutations in synthesis and action. J Clin Endocrinol Metab. 1999;84(12):4677–94.
114. Ross JL, Cassorla FG, Skerda MC, Valk IM, Loriaux DL, Cutler GB Jr. A preliminary study of the effect of estrogen dose on growth in Turner's syndrome. N Engl J Med. 1983;309(18):1104–6.
115. Ranke MB. Why treat girls with Turner syndrome with growth hormone: growth and beyond. Pediatr Endocrinol Rev. 2015;12(4):297–306.
116. Ranke MB, Lindberg A, Ferrández Longás A, Darendeliler F, Albertsson-Wikland K, Dunger D, et al. Major determinants of height development in Turner syndrome (TS) patients treated with GH: analysis of 987 patients from KIGS. Pediatr Res. 2007;61(1):105–10.
117. Baxter L, Bryant J, Cave CB, Milne R. Recombinant growth hormone for children and adolescents with Turner syndrome. Cochrane Database Syst Rev. 2007;1:CD003887.
118. Li P, Cheng F, Xiu L. Height outcome of the recombinant human growth hormone treatment in Turner syndrome: a meta-analysis. Endocr Connect. 2018;7(4):573–83.
119. Buchanan CR, Law CM, Milner RDG. Growth hormone in short, slowly growing children and those with Turner's syndrome. Arch Dis Child. 1987;62:912–6.
120. Underwood LE. Report of the conference on uses and possible abuses of biosynthetic human growth hormone. N Engl J Med. 1984;311(9):606–8.
121. Rosenfeld RG. Acceleration of growth in Turner syndrome patients treated with growth hormone: summary of three-year results. J Endocrinol Investig. 1989;12:49–51.

122. Vanderschueren-Lodeweyckx M, Massa G, Maes M, Craen M, van Vliet G, Heinrichs C, et al. Growth-promoting effect of growth hormone and low dose ethinyl estradiol in girls with Turner's syndrome. J Clin Endocrinol Metab. 1990;70:122–6.
123. Werther GA. A multi-centre double-blind study of growth hormone and low-dose estrogen in Turner syndrome: an interim analysis. In: Ranke MB, Rosenfeld RG, editors. Turner syndrome: growth promoting therapies. Philadelphia: Elsevier Science BV; 1991.
124. Quigley CA, Crowe BJ, Anglin DG, Chipman JJ, and the US Turner Syndrome Study Group. Growth hormone and low dose estrogen in Turner syndrome: results of a United States multi-center trial to near-final height. J Clin Endocrinol Metab. 2002;87(5):2033–41.
125. Kollmann F, Damm M, Reinhardt D, Stover B, Heinrich U, Brendel L, et al. Growth-promoting effects of human recombinant growth hormone in subjects with Ullrich-Turner syndrome (UTS). In: Ranke MB, Rosenfeld RG, editors. Turner syndrome: growth promoting therapies, vol. 924. Amsterdam: Elsevier Science BV; 1991. p. 201–7.
126. Davenport ML, Crowe BJ, Travers SH, Rubin K, Ross JL, Fechner PY, et al. Growth hormone treatment of early growth failure in toddlers with Turner syndrome: a randomized, controlled, multicenter trial. J Clin Endocrinol Metab. 2007;92(9):3406–16.
127. Ross JL, Quigley CA, Cao D, Feuillan P, Kowal K, Chipman JJ, et al. Growth hormone plus childhood low-dose estrogen in Turner's syndrome. N Engl J Med. 2011;364(13):1230–42.
128. Ranke MB, Lindberg A. Observed and predicted growth responses in prepubertal children with growth disorders: guidance of growth hormone treatment by empirical variables. J Clin Endocrinol Metab. 2010;95(3):1229–37.
129. Tanner JM, Davies PW. Clinical longitudinal standards for height and height velocity for North American children. J Pediatr. 1985;107(3):317–29.
130. Plotnick L, Attie KM, Blethen SL, Sy JP. Growth hormone treatment of girls with Turner syndrome: the National Cooperative Growth Study Experience. Pediatrics. 1998;102(2):479–81.
131. Wasniewska M, De Luca F, Bergamaschi R, Guarneri MP, Mazzanti L, Matarazzo P, et al. Early treatment with GH alone in Turner syndrome: prepubertal catchup growth and waning effect. Eur J Endocrinol. 2004;151(5):567–72.
132. Quigley CA, Fechner PY, Geffner ME, Eugster EA, Ross JL, Habiby RL, et al. Long-term results of early growth hormone treatment in the "Toddler Turner" cohort. J Clin Endocrinol Metab. 2020;
133. Rosenfeld RG, Attie KM, Frane J, Brasel JA, Burstein S, Cara JF, et al. Growth hormone therapy of Turner's syndrome: beneficial effect on adult height. J Pediatr. 1998;132(2):319–24.
134. Chernausek SD, Attie KM, Cara JF, Rosenfeld RG, Frane J. Growth hormone therapy of Turner syndrome; the impact of age of estrogen replacement on final height. Genentech Inc. Collaborative Study Group. J Clin Endocrinol Metab. 2000;85(7):2439–45.
135. Pasquino AM, Pucarelli I, Segni M, Tarani L, Calcaterra V, Larizza D. Adult height in sixty girls with Turner syndrome treated with growth hormone matched with an untreated group. J Endocrinol Investig. 2005;28:350–6.
136. Ranke MB, Partsch CJ, Lindberg A, Dorr HG, Bettendorf M, Hauffa BP, et al. Adult height after GH therapy in 188 Ullrich-Turner syndrome patients: results of the German IGLU Follow-up Study 2001. Eur J Endocrinol. 2002;147(5):625–33.
137. Carel JC, Mathivon L, Gendrel C, Ducret JP, Chaussain JL. Near normalization of final height with adapted doses of growth hormone in Turner's syndrome. J Clin Endocrinol Metab. 1998;83(5):1462–6.
138. Sas TC, de Muinck Keizer-Schrama SM, Stijnen T, Jansen M, Otten BJ, Hoorweg-Nijman JJ, et al. Normalization of height in girls with Turner syndrome after long-term growth hormone treatment: results of a randomized dose-response trial. J Clin Endocrinol Metab. 1999;84(12):4607–12.
139. van Pareren YK, de Muinck Keizer-Schrama SM, Stijnen T, Sas TC, Jansen M, Otten BJ, et al. Final height in girls with Turner syndrome after long-term growth hormone treatment in three dosages and low dose estrogens. J Clin Endocrinol Metab. 2003;88(3):1119–25.

140. Gault EJ, Perry RJ, Cole TJ, Casey SR, Paterson WF, Hindmarsh PC, et al. Effect of oxandrolone and timing of pubertal induction on final height in Turner's syndrome: randomised, double blind, placebo controlled trial. BMJ. 2011;342:d1980.

141. Menke LA, Sas TC, de Muinck Keizer-Schrama SM, Zandwijken GR, de Ridder MA, Odink RJ, et al. Efficacy and safety of oxandrolone in growth hormone-treated girls with Turner syndrome. J Clin Endocrinol Metab. 2010;95(3):1151–60.

142. Nilsson KO, Albertsson-Wikland K, Alm J, Aronson S, Gustafsson J, Hagenäs L, et al. Improved final height in girls with Turner's syndrome treated with growth hormone and oxandrolone. J Clin Endocrinol Metab. 1996;81(2):635–40.

143. Wasniewska M, Aversa T, Mazzanti L, Guarneri MP, Matarazzo P, De Luca F, et al. Adult height in girls with Turner syndrome treated from before 6 years of age with a fixed per kilogram GH dose. Eur J Endocrinol. 2013;169(4):439–43.

144. Linglart A, Cabrol S, Berlier P, Stuckens C, Wagner K, de Kerdanet M, et al. French Collaborative Young Turner Study Group. Growth hormone treatment before the age of 4 years prevents short stature in young girls with Turner syndrome. Eur J Endocrinol. 2011;164(6):891–7.

145. Vanderschueren-Lodeweyckx M, Massa G, Maes M, Craen M, van Vliet G, Heinrichs C, et al. Growth-promoting effect of growth hormone and low dose ethinyl estradiol in girls with Turner's syndrome. J Clin Endocrinol Metab. 1990;70(1):122–6.

146. Johnston DI, Betts P, Dunger D, Barnes N, Swift PGF, Buckler JMH, et al. A multicentre trial of recombinant growth hormone and low-dose oestrogen in Turner syndrome: near final height analysis. Arch Dis Child. 2001;84:76–81.

147. Quigley CA, Wan X, Garg S, Kowal K, Cutler GB Jr, Ross JL. Effects of low-dose estrogen replacement during childhood on pubertal development and gonadotropin concentrations in patients with Turner syndrome: results of a randomized, double-blind, placebo-controlled clinical trial. J Clin Endocrinol Metab. 2014;99(9):E1754–64.

148. Blum WF, Ross JL, Zimmermann AG, Quigley CA, Child CJ, Kalifa G, et al. GH treatment to final height produces similar height gains in patients with SHOX deficiency and Turner syndrome: results from a multicenter trial. J Clin Endocrinol Metab. 2013;98:E1383–92.

149. Pasquino AM, Pucarelli I, Segni M, Tarani L, Calcaterra V, Larizza D. Adult height in sixty girls with Turner syndrome treated with growth hormone matched with an untreated group. J Endocrinol Investig. 2005;28(4):350–6.

150. Reiter EO, Blethen SL, Baptista J, Price L. Early initiation of growth hormone treatment allows age-appropriate estrogen use in Turner's syndrome. J Clin Endocrinol Metab. 2001;86(5):1936–41.

151. Soriano-Guillen L, Coste J, Ecosse E, Léger J, Tauber M, Cabrol S, et al. Adult height and pubertal growth in Turner syndrome after treatment with recombinant growth hormone. J Clin Endocrinol Metab. 2005;90(9):5197–204.

152. Bolar K, Hoffman AR, Maneatis T, Lippe B. Long-term safety of recombinant human growth hormone in Turner syndrome. J Clin Endocrinol Metab. 2008;93:344.

153. Carel JC, Ecosse E, Bastie-Sigeac I, Cabrol S, Tauber M, Léger J, et al. Quality of life determinants in young women with Turner's syndrome after growth hormone treatment: results of the StaTur population-based cohort study. J Clin Endocrinol Metab. 2005;90(4):1992–7.

154. Concato J, Shah N, Horwitz RI. Randomized, controlled trials, observational studies and the hierarchy of research designs. NEJM. 2000;342(25):1887–92.

155. Ranke MB, Lindberg A, Chatelain P, Wilton P, Cutfield W, Albertsson-Wikland K, et al. Prediction of long-term response to recombinant human growth hormone in Turner syndrome: development and validation of mathematical models. KIGS International Board. Kabi International Growth Study. J Clin Endocrinol Metab. 2000;85(11):4212–8.

156. Ranke MB, Lindberg A, Brosz M, Kaspers S, Loftus J, Wollmann H, et al. Accurate long-term prediction of height during the first four years of growth hormone treatment in prepubertal children with growth hormone deficiency or Turner syndrome. Horm Res Paediatr. 2012;78(1):8–17.

157. Ranke MB, Schweizer R, Martin DD, Ehehalt S, Schwarze CP, Serra F, et al. Analyses from a centre of short- and long-term growth in Turner's syndrome on standard growth hormone doses confirm growth prediction algorithms and show normal IGF-I levels. Horm Res Paediatr. 2012;77(4):214–21.
158. Ross JL, Lee PA, Gut R, Germak J. Impact of age and duration of growth hormone therapy in children with Turner syndrome. Horm Res Pediatr. 2011;76:392–9.
159. Prader A, Largo RH, Molinari L, Issler C. Physical growth of Swiss children from birth to 20 years of age First Zurich longitudinal study of growth and development. Helv Paediatr Acta. 1989;52(suppl S2):1–25.
160. Stevens A, Murray P, Wojcik J, Raelson J, Koledova E, Chatelain P, et al. Validating genetic markers of response to recombinant growth hormone in children with growth hormone deficiency and Turner syndrome: the PREDICT validation study. Eur J Endocrinol. 2016;175:633–43.
161. Braz AF, Costalonga EF, Trarbach EB, Scalco RC, Malaquias AC, Guerra-Junior G, et al. Genetic predictors of long-term response to growth hormone (GH) therapy in children with GH deficiency and Turner syndrome: the influence of a SOCS2 polymorphism. J Clin Endocrinol Metab. 2014 Sep;99(9):E1808–13.
162. Wit JM, Ranke MB, Albertsson-Wikland K, Carrascosa A, Rosenfeld RG, Van Buuren S, et al. Personalized approach to growth hormone treatment: clinical use of growth prediction models. Horm Res Paediatr. 2013;79(5):257–70.
163. Ranke MB, Lindberg A, KIGS International Board. Observed and predicted growth responses in prepubertal children with growth disorders: guidance of growth hormone treatment by empirical variables J Clin Endocrinol Metab 2010;95:1229–1237.
164. Ranke MB, Lindberg A. Observed and predicted total pubertal growth during treatment with growth hormone in adolescents with idiopathic growth hormone deficiency, Turner syndrome, short stature, born small for gestational age and idiopathic short stature: KIGS analysis and review. Horm Res Paediatr. 2011;75:423–32.
165. Carel JC, Mathivon L, Gendrel C, Chaussain JL. Growth hormone therapy for Turner syndrome: evidence for benefit. Horm Res. 1997;48(Suppl 5):31–4.
166. Hofman P, Cutfield WS, Robinson EM, Clavano A, Ambler GR, Cowell C. Factors predictive of response to growth hormone therapy in Turner's syndrome. J Pediatr Endocrinol Metab. 1997;10(1):27–33.
167. Gravholt CH, Andersen NH, Conway GS, Dekkers OM, Geffner ME, Klein KO, et al. Clinical practice guidelines for the care of girls and women with Turner syndrome: proceedings from the 2016 Cincinnati International Turner syndrome meeting. Eur J Endocrinol. 2017;177:G1–G70.
168. Hughes IP, Choong CS, Harris M, Ambler GR, Cutfield WS, Hofman PL, et al. Growth hormone treatment for Turner syndrome in Australia reveals that younger age and increased dose interact to improve response. Clin Endocrinol. 2011;74(4):473–80.
169. Bettendorf M, Inta IM, Doerr HG, Hauffa BP, Mehls O, Ranke MB. Height gain in Ullrich-Turner syndrome after early and late growth hormone treatment start: results from a large retrospective German study and potential basis for an individualized treatment approach. Horm Res Paediatr. 2013;80(5):356–62.
170. van Teunenbroek A, de Muinck Keizer-Schrama SM, Stijnen T, Jansen M, Otten BJ, Delemarre-van de Waal HA, et al. Yearly stepwise increments of the growth hormone dose results in a better growth response after 4 years in girls with Turner syndrome. J Clin Endocrinol Metab. 1996;81(11):4013–21.
171. Coelho R, Brook CGD, Preece MA, Stanhope RG, Dattani MT, Hindmarsh PC. A randomised study of two doses of biosynthetic human growth hormone on final height of pubertal children with growth hormone deficiency. Horm Res. 2008;70:85–8.
172. Schrier L, de Kam ML, McKinnon R, Che Bakri A, Oostdijk W, Sas TC, et al. Comparison of body surface area versus weight-based growth hormone dosing for girls with Turner syndrome. Horm Res Paediatr. 2014;81(5):319–30.

173. Cohen P, Weng W, Rogol AD, Rosenfeld RG, Kappelgaard AM, Germak J. Dose-sparing and safety-enhancing effects of an IGF-I-based dosing regimen in short children treated with growth hormone in a 2-year randomized controlled trial: therapeutic and pharmacoeconomic considerations. Clin Endocrinol. 2014;81(1):71–6.
174. Cohen P, Germak J, Rogol AD, Weng W, Kappelgaard A-M, Rosenfeld RG. Variable degree of growth hormone (GH) and insulin-like growth factor (IGF) sensitivity in children with idiopathic short stature compared with GH-deficient patients: evidence from an IGF-based dosing study of short children. J Clin Endocrinol Metab. 2010;95:2089–98.
175. Albertsson-Wikland K. The effect of human growth hormone injection frequency on linear growth rate. Acta Paediatr Scand Suppl. 1987;337:110–6.
176. Kastrup KW, Christiansen JS, Andersen JK, Orskov H. Increased growth rate following transfer to daily sc administration from three weekly im injections of hGH in growth hormone deficient children. Acta Endocrinol. 1983;104(2):148–52.
177. Hopwood NJ, Hintz RL, Gertner JM, Attie KM, Johanson AJ, Baptista J, et al. Growth response of children with non-growth-hormone deficiency and marked short stature during three years of growth hormone therapy. J Pediatr. 1993;123(2):215–22.
178. Sas TC, de Muinck Keizer-Schrama SM, Stijnen T, van Teunenbroek A, Hokken-Koelega AC, Waelkens JJ, et al. Final height in girls with Turner's syndrome treated with once or twice daily growth hormone injections. Dutch Advisory Group on Growth Hormone. Arch Dis Child. 1999;80(1):36–41.
179. Otero SC, Eiser C, Wright NP, Butler G. Implications of parent and child quality of life assessments for decisions about growth hormone treatment in eligible children. Child Care Health Dev. 2013;39(6):782–8.
180. Bannink EM, Raat H, Mulder PG, de Muinck Keizer-Schrama SM. Quality of life after growth hormone therapy and induced puberty in women with Turner syndrome. J Pediatr. 2006;148(1):95–101.
181. van Pareren YK, Duivenvoorden HJ, Slijper FM, Koot HM, Drop SL, de Muinck Keizer-Schrama SM. Psychosocial functioning after discontinuation of long-term growth hormone treatment in girls with Turner syndrome. Horm Res. 2005;63(5):238–44.
182. Lagrou K, Xhrouet-Heinrichs D, Heinrichs C, Craen M, Chanoine JP, Malvaux P, et al. Age-related perception of stature, acceptance of therapy, and psychosocial functioning in human growth hormone-treated girls with Turner's syndrome. J Clin Endocrinol Metab. 1998;83(5):1494–501.
183. Rovet JF, Ireland L. Behavioral phenotype in children with Turner syndrome. J Pediatr Psychol. 1994;19(6):779–90.
184. Rovet JF, Holland J. Psychological aspects of the Canadian randomised controlled trial of human growth hormone and low-dose ethinyl oestradiol in children with Turner syndrome. Horm Res. 1993;39(Suppl 2):60–4.
185. Rovet JF, Van Vliet G. Growth hormone supplementation and psychosocial functioning to adult height in Turner syndrome: a questionnaire study of participants in the Canadian Randomized Trial. Front Endocrinol. 2019;10:125.
186. Krantz E, Landin-Wilhelmsen K, Trimpou P, Bryman I, Wide U. Health-related quality of life in Turner syndrome and the influence of growth hormone therapy: a 20-year follow-up. J Clin Endocrinol Metab. 2019;104(11):5073–83.
187. Ross JL, Feuillan P, Kushner H, Roeltgen D, Cutler GB Jr. Absence of growth hormone effects on cognitive function in girls with Turner syndrome. J Clin Endocrinol Metab. 1997;82(6):1814–7.
188. Reis CT, de Assumpção MS, Guerra-Junior G, de Lemos-Marini SHV. Systematic review of quality of life in Turner syndrome. Qual Life Res. 2018;27(8):1985–2006.
189. Bakker B, Frane J, Anhalt H, Lippe B, Rosenfeld RG. Height velocity targets from the National Cooperative Growth Study for first-year growth hormone responses in short children. J Clin Endocrinol Metab. 2008;93(2):352–7.
190. Bannink EM, van der Palen RL, Mulder PG, de Muinck Keizer-Schrama SM. Long-term follow-up of GH-treated girls with Turner syndrome: BMI, blood pressure, body proportions. Horm Res. 2009;71(6):336–42.

191. Van Pareren YK, De Muinck Keizer-Schrama SM, Stijnen T, Sas TC, Drop SL. Effect of discontinuation of long-term growth hormone treatment on carbohydrate metabolism and risk factors for cardiovascular disease in girls with Turner syndrome. J Clin Endocrinol Metab. 2002;87(12):5442–8.
192. Radetti G, Crepaz R, Milanesi O, Paganini C, Cesaro A, Rigon F, et al. Cardiac performance in Turner's syndrome patients on growth hormone therapy. Horm Res. 2001;55(5):240–4.
193. Sas TC, Cromme-Dijkhuis AH, de Muinck Keizer-Schrama SM, Stijnen T, van Teunenbroek A, Drop SL. The effects of long-term growth hormone treatment on cardiac left ventricular dimensions and blood pressure in girls with Turner's syndrome. Dutch Working Group on Growth Hormone. J Pediatr. 1999;135(4):470–6.
194. Bannink EM, van der Palen RL, Mulder PG, de Muinck Keizer-Schrama SM. Long-term follow-up of GH-treated girls with Turner syndrome: metabolic consequences. Horm Res. 2009;71(6):343–9.
195. Wooten N, Bakalov VK, Hill S, Bondy CA. Reduced abdominal adiposity and improved glucose tolerance in growth hormone-treated girls with Turner syndrome. J Clin Endocrinol Metab. 2008;93(6):2109–14.
196. Mazzanti L, Bergamaschi R, Castiglioni L, Zappulla F, Pirazzoli P, Cicognani A. Turner syndrome, insulin sensitivity and growth hormone treatment. Horm Res. 2005;64(Suppl 3):51–7.
197. Ari M, Bakalov VK, Hill S, Bondy CA. The effects of growth hormone treatment on bone mineral density and body composition in girls with Turner syndrome. J Clin Endocrinol Metab. 2006;91(11):4302–5.
198. Davenport ML, Roush J, Lui C, Zagar AJ, Eugster E, Travers SH, et al. Growth hormone treatment does not affect incidences of middle ear disease or hearing loss in infants and toddlers with Turner syndrome. Horm Res Paediatr. 2010;74(1):23–32.
199. Quigley CA, Gill AM, Crowe BJ, Robling K, Chipman JJ, Rose SR, et al. Safety of growth hormone treatment in pediatric patients with idiopathic short stature. J Clin Endocrinol Metab. 2005;90:5188–96.
200. Bell J, Parker KL, Swinford RD, Hoffman AR, Maneatis T, Lippe B. Long-term safety of recombinant human growth hormone in children. J Clin Endocrinol Metab. 2010;95(1):167–77.
201. Darendeliler F, Karagiannis G, Wilton P. Headache, idiopathic intracranial hypertension and slipped capital femoral epiphysis during growth hormone treatment: a safety update from the KIGS database. Horm Res. 2007;68(Suppl 5):41–7.
202. Child CJ, Zimmermann AG, Scott RS, Cutler GB Jr, Battelino T, Blum WF, et al. Prevalence and incidence of diabetes mellitus in GH-treated children and adolescents: analysis from the GeNeSIS observational research program. J Clin Endocrinol Metab. 2011;96(6):E1025–34.
203. Child CJ, Zimmermann AG, Chrousos GP, Cummings E, Deal CL, Hasegawa T, et al. Safety outcomes during pediatric GH therapy: final results from the prospective GeNeSIS observational program. J Clin Endocrinol Metab. 2019;104(2):379–89.
204. Allen DB. Safety of human growth hormone therapy: current topics. J Pediatr. 1996;128(5 Pt 2):S8–13.
205. Blethen SL, Rundle AC. Slipped capital femoral epiphysis in children treated with growth hormone. A summary of the National Cooperative Growth Study experience. Horm Res. 1996;46(3):113–6.
206. Lowenstein EJ, Kim KH, Glick SA. Turner's syndrome in dermatology. J Am Acad Dermatol. 2004;50(5):767–76.
207. Wyatt D. Melanocytic nevi in children treated with growth hormone. Pediatrics. 1999;104(4Pt 2):1045–50.
208. Gravholt CH, Jund S, Naeraa RW, Hansen J. Morbidity in Turner syndrome. J Clin Epidemiol. 1998;51(2):147–58.
209. Shoemaker MJ, Swerdlow AJ, Higgins CD, Wright AF, Jacobs PA, United Kingdom Clinical Cytogenetics Group. Mortality in women with Turner syndrome in Great Britain: a national cohort study. J Clin Endocrinol Metab. 2008;93:4735–42.
210. Quigley CA, Child CJ, Zimmermann AG, Rosenfeld RG, Blum WF, Robison L. Mortality in children receiving growth hormone treatment for growth disorders: data from the GeNeSIS observational program. J Clin Endocrinol Metab. 2017;102(9):3195–205.

211. Bondy CA, Van PL, Bakalov VK, Ho VB. Growth hormone treatment and aortic dimensions in Turner syndrome. J Clin Endocrinol Metab. 2006;91(5):1785–8.
212. Lin AE, Silberbach M. Focus on the heart and aorta in Turner syndrome. J Pediatr. 2007;150(6):572–4.
213. Lopez L, Arheart KL, Colan SD, Stein NS, Lopez-Mitnik G, Lin AE, et al. Turner syndrome is an independent risk factor for aortic dilation in the young. Pediatrics. 2008;121(6):e1622–7.
214. van den Berg J, Bannink EM, Wielopolski PA, Pattynama PM, de Muinck Keizer-Schrama SM, Helbing WA. Aortic distensibility and dimensions and the effects of growth hormone treatment in the Turner syndrome. Am J Cardiol. 2006;97(11):1644–9.
215. Cabanas P, García-Caballero T, Barreiro J, Castro-Feijóo L, Gallego R, Arévalo T, et al. Papillary thyroid carcinoma after recombinant GH therapy for Turner syndrome. Eur J Endocrinol. 2005;153(4):499–502.
216. Morotti RA, Killackey M, Shneider BL, Repucci A, Emre S, Thung SN. Hepatocellular carcinoma and congenital absence of the portal vein in a child receiving growth hormone therapy for Turner syndrome. Semin Liver Dis. 2007;27(4):427–31.
217. Tuffli GA, Johanson A, Rundle AC, Allen DB. Lack of increased risk for extracranial, nonleukemic neoplasms in recipients of recombinant deoxyribonucleic acid growth hormone. J Clin Endocrinol Metab. 1995;80(4):1416–22.
218. Raman S, Grimberg A, Waguespack SG, Miller BS, Sklar CA, Meacham LR, et al. Risk of neoplasia in pediatric patients receiving growth hormone therapy—a report from the Pediatric Endocrine Society Drug and Therapeutics Committee. J Clin Endocrinol Metab. 2015;100:2192–203.
219. Park P, Cohen P. The role of insulin-like growth factor I monitoring in growth hormone-treated children. Horm Res. 2004;62(Suppl 1):59–65.
220. Blum WF, Crowe BJ, Quigley CA, Jung H, Cao D, Ross JL, et al. Growth hormone is effective in treatment of short stature associated with short stature homeobox-containing gene deficiency: two-year results of a randomized, controlled, multicenter trial. J Clin Endocrinol Metab. 2007;92(1):219–28.
221. Clayton PE, Banerjee I, Murray PG, Renehan AG. Growth hormone, the insulin-like growth factor axis, insulin and cancer risk. Nat Rev Endocrinol. 2011;7(1):11–24.
222. Albertsson-Wikland K, Mårtensson A, Sävendahl L, Niklasson A, Bang P, Dahlgren J, et al. Mortality is not increased in recombinant human growth hormone-treated patients when adjusting for birth characteristics. J Clin Endocrinol Metab. 2016;101(5):2149–59.
223. Cutfield WS, Lundgren F. Insulin-like growth factor I and growth responses during the first year of growth hormone treatment in KIGS patients with idiopathic growth hormone deficiency, acquired growth hormone deficiency, Turner syndrome and born small for gestational age. Horm Res. 2009;71(Suppl 1):39–45.
224. Nielsen J, Johansen K, Yde H. The frequency of diabetes mellitus in patients with Turner's syndrome and pure gonadal dysgenesis. Blood glucose, plasma insulin and growth hormone level during an oral glucose tolerance test. Acta Endocrinol. 1969;62(2):251–69.
225. Caprio S, Boulware D, Tamborlane V. Growth hormone and insulin interactions. Horm Res. 1992;38(Suppl 2):47–9.
226. Bakalov VK, Cooley MM, Quon MJ, Luo ML, Yanovski JA, Nelson LM, et al. Impaired insulin secretion in the Turner metabolic syndrome. J Clin Endocrinol Metab. 2004;89(7):3516–20.
227. Radetti G, Pasquino B, Gottardi E, Boscolo Contadin I, Aimaretti G, Rigon F. Insulin sensitivity in Turner's syndrome: influence of GH treatment. Eur J Endocrinol. 2004;151(3):351–4.
228. Wilson DM, Frane JW, Sherman B, Johanson AJ, Hintz RL, Rosenfeld RG. Carbohydrate and lipid metabolism in Turner syndrome: effect of therapy with growth hormone, oxandrolone, and a combination of both. J Pediatr. 1988;112:210–7.
229. Weise M, James D, Leitner CH, Hartmann KK, Bohles HJ, Attanasio A. Glucose metabolism in Ullrich Turner syndrome: long-term effects of therapy with human growth hormone. German Lilly UTS Study Group. Horm Res. 1993;39(1–2):36–41.
230. Saenger P, Attie KM, Martino-Nardi J, Fine RN. Carbohydrate metabolism in children receiving growth hormone for 5 years. Chronic renal insufficiency compared with growth hormone

deficiency, Turner syndrome, and idiopathic short stature. Genentech Collaborative Group. Pediatr Nephrol. 1996;10(3):261–3.

231. Sas TC, de Muinck Keizer-Schrama SM, Stijnen T, Aanstoot HJ, Drop SL. Carbohydrate metabolism during long-term growth hormone (GH) treatment and after discontinuation of GH treatment in girls with Turner syndrome participating in a randomized dose-response study. Dutch Advisory Group on Growth Hormone. J Clin Endocrinol Metab. 2000;85(2): 769–75.

232. Cutfield WS, Wilton P, Bennmarker H, Albertsson-Wikland K, Chatelain P, Ranke MB, et al. Incidence of diabetes mellitus and impaired glucose tolerance in children and adolescents receiving growth-hormone treatment. Lancet. 2000;355(9204):610–3.

233. American Diabetes Association. 2. Classification and diagnosis of diabetes. Diabetes Care. 2016;39(Suppl 1):S13–22.

234. Zeitler P, Fu J, Tandon N, Nadeau K, Urakami T, Barrett T, et al. ISPAD Clinical Practice Consensus Guidelines 2014. Type 2 diabetes in the child and adolescent. Pediatr Diabetes. 2014;15(Suppl 20):26–46.

235. Growth Hormone Research Society. Critical evaluation of the safety of recombinant human growth hormone administration: statement from the Growth Hormone Research Society. J Clin Endocrinol Metab. 2001;86(5):1868–70.

236. https://www.accessdata.fda.gov/drugsatfda_docs/label/2008/021426s004lbl.pdf.

237. Zeger MP, Shah K, Kowal K, Cutler GB Jr, Kushner H, Ross JL. Prospective study confirms oxandrolone-associated improvement in height in growth hormone-treated adolescent girls with Turner syndrome. Horm Res Paediatr. 2011;75(1):38–46.

238. Sas TC, Gault EJ, Bardsley MZ, Menke LA, Freriks K, Perry RJ, et al. Safety and efficacy of oxandrolone in growth hormone-treated girls with Turner syndrome: evidence from recent studies and recommendations for use. Horm Res Paediatr. 2014;81(5):289–97.

239. Sheanon NM, Backeljauw PF. Effect of oxandrolone therapy on adult height in Turner syndrome patients treated with growth hormone: a meta-analysis. Int J Pediatr Endocrinol. 2015;2015:18.

240. Freriks K, Sas TC, Traas MA, Netea-Maier RT, den Heijer M, Hermus AR, et al. Long-term effects of previous oxandrolone treatment in adult women with Turner syndrome. Eur J Endocrinol. 2012;168(1):91–9.

241. Ross JL, Mazzocco MM, Kushner H, Kowal K, Cutler GB Jr, Roeltgen D. Effects of treatment with oxandrolone for 4 years on the frequency of severe arithmetic learning disability in girls with Turner syndrome. J Pediatr. 2009;155(5):714–20.

242. Menke LA, Sas TC, Visser M, Kreukels BP, Stijnen T, Zandwijken GR, et al. The effect of the weak androgen oxandrolone on psychological and behavioural characteristics in growth hormone-treated girls with Turner syndrome. Horm Behav. 2010;57(3):297–305.

243. Freriks K, Verhaak CM, Sas TC, Menke LA, Wit JM, Otten BJ, et al. Long-term effects of oxandrolone treatment in childhood on neurocognition, quality of life and social-emotional functioning in young adults with Turner syndrome. Horm Behav. 2015;69(5):59–67.

244. Cutler GB Jr. The role of estrogen in bone growth and maturation during childhood and adolescence. J Steroid Biochem Mol Biol. 1997;61(3–6):141–4.

245. Ross JL, Cassorla FG, Skerda MC, Valk IM, Loriaux DL, Cutler GB Jr. A preliminary study of the effect of estrogen dose on growth in Turner's syndrome. N Engl J Med. 1983;309:1104–6.

246. Ross JL, Roeltgen D, Feuillan P, Kushner H, Cutler GB Jr. Effects of estrogen on nonverbal processing speed and motor function in girls with Turner's syndrome. J Clin Endocrinol Metab. 1998;83(9):3198–204.

247. Ross JL, Roeltgen D, Feuillan P, Kushner H, Cutler GB. Use of estrogen in young girls with Turner syndrome: effects on memory. Neurology. 2000;54(1):164–70.

248. Davenport ML. Approach to the patient with Turner syndrome. J Clin Endocrinol Metab. 2010;95:1487–95.

249. Rosenfield RL, Devine N, Hunold JJ, Mauras N, Moshang T Jr, Root AW. Salutary effects of combining early very low-dose systemic estradiol with growth hormone therapy in girls with Turner syndrome. J Clin Endocrinol Metab. 2005;90:6424–30.

250. Torres-Santiago L, Mericq V, Taboada M, Unanue N, Klein KO, Singh R, et al. Metabolic effects of oral versus transdermal 17β-estradiol (E2): a randomized clinical trial in girls with Turner syndrome. J Clin Endocrinol Metab. 2013;98:2716–24.
251. Nabhan ZM, DiMeglio LA, Qi R, Perkins SM, Eugster EA. Conjugated oral *versus* transdermal estrogen replacement in girls with Turner syndrome: a pilot comparative study. J Clin Endocrinol Metab. 2009;94:2009–14.
252. Davenport ML. Evidence for early initiation of growth hormone and transdermal estradiol therapies in girls with Turner syndrome. Growth Hormon IGF Res. 2006;16(Suppl):91–7.

Chapter 4
Fertility Preservation for Turner Syndrome

Courtney Finlayson, Lia Bernardi, and Reema Habiby

Premature ovarian insufficiency leading to ovarian failure is a major concern for women with Turner syndrome (TS) as well as for parents of girls with TS. While spontaneous pubertal development can occur in up to 38% of girls with TS and up to 16% may have spontaneous menarche [1, 2], most will go on to have premature ovarian failure [3]. Spontaneous pregnancy occurs in only 2–5% of women with TS and generally occurs in those with a mosaic karyotype [4].

Under normal circumstances, women are born with a fixed supply of germ cells. The maximum number of germ cells is present in a fetus at mid-gestation, with a total of 6–7 million germ cells [5]. After this time, the number of germ cells declines, and no further gametogenesis occurs. At birth, the number of germ cells is estimated to be 1–2 million, and by the onset of puberty, the germ cell number has declined to ~ 300,000–400,000 [6, 7]. The premature ovarian insufficiency (POI) that occurs in TS is due to accelerated follicular apoptosis. Girls with TS have normal ovarian follicular counts early in gestation, but undergo rapid follicular loss, as early as 18 weeks gestation, resulting in POI and reduced fertility potential [8, 9]. While there is a subset of girls with TS who may have a reduced but present ovarian follicle reserve, further loss of ovarian follicles is expected later in childhood and early puberty, eventually leading to POI [10]. The challenge is to identify these girls as early as possible so they may benefit from existing fertility preservation options. Though the physiologic role of anti-Müllerian hormone (AMH) has not been fully elucidated, it appears to be the best hormonal marker of the size of the follicular

C. Finlayson (✉) · R. Habiby
Division of Endocrinology, Department of Pediatrics, Ann & Robert H. Lurie Children's Hospital of Chicago, Northwestern University Feinberg School of Medicine, Chicago, IL, USA
e-mail: cfinlayson@luriechildrens.org; rhabiby@luriechildrens.org

L. Bernardi
Division of Reproductive Endocrinology, Department of Obstetrics and Gynecology, Northwestern University Feinberg School of Medicine, Chicago, IL, USA
e-mail: Lia.bernardi@northwestern.edu

© Springer Nature Switzerland AG 2020
P. Y. Fechner (ed.), *Turner Syndrome*,
https://doi.org/10.1007/978-3-030-34150-3_4

ovarian reserve [11, 12]. AMH is a member of the TGF-β family and is secreted by granulosa cells of the primary and small antral follicles [13] and may reflect ovarian follicular reserve. In adult women of reproductive age, serum AMH levels correlate strongly with antral follicle counts. Over time, AMH levels decline, and by menopause, AMH levels are undetectable. The decline in serum AMH levels precedes more traditional markers of ovarian reserve, such as follicle stimulation hormone (FSH), estradiol, and inhibin B [14]. In children, AMH levels increase from birth and plateau at adolescence. It is not until after the age of 25 years that there is a correlation between increasing age and declining AMH levels. Visser et al. studied 270 girls and adolescents with Turner syndrome. AMH was measurable in only 21.9% of patients. When compared with healthy controls, AMH levels in TS were generally lower, though there was some overlap. Serum levels of AMH were strongly correlated with karyotype. Measurable levels of AMH were only found in 10% of TS patients with a 45, X karyotype. In contrast, 77% of TS patients with 45, X/46, XX and 25% with other TS karyotypes had measurable AMH levels. There was a strong negative correlation between FSH and AMH levels. A similar negative correlation between luteinizing hormone (LH) and AMH levels was seen. There was no significant relationship between serum estradiol or inhibin B levels and AMH. Hagen et al. studied AMH levels in 926 healthy women and 172 subjects with TS longitudinally and found that AMH may be a promising marker of ovarian function in TS patients. Lunding et al. [15] studied 120 Turner syndrome patients longitudinally and found that AMH levels < −2 SD predicted failure to enter puberty in young girls and imminent POI in adolescent girls and adult women with TS. Additionally, karyotype, low FSH, high AMH, spontaneous menarche, and spontaneous onset of puberty have been identified as discriminating factors for finding remaining follicles in girls with TS [16]. Because the timing of POI is variable in TS, the optimal timing and methods of fertility preservation remain unknown.

Nonexperimental Fertility Options

Adoption

Adoption has been pursued by many women with TS. Domestic adoptions in the United States can occur through state-licensed public agencies, private adoption agencies, or by independent adoptions that directly place a child through an attorney or mediating agency [10, 17]. Agencies typically assess the capabilities of the prospective parents, including conducting interviews, home studies, and background checks, though the processes, policies, and requirements can vary between agencies. There are no documented cases of adoption being denied to a woman due to her diagnosis of Turner syndrome.

International adoption is another option available to women with TS. The intercountry adoption process varies significantly between countries. Intercountry adoptions have declined since 2004 [18] likely attributable to economic, social, and political factors within each country as well as changing policies toward adoption and social change.

Spontaneous Pregnancy

Spontaneous pregnancy occurs in only 2–5% of women with TS, most often in those with a mosaic karyotype [4]. Women with TS become pregnant as easily as women with other causes of infertility, with varying reports of miscarriage rate [10, 19]; however, they have a higher rate of maternal complications as discussed later in this chapter. Women with TS are often small in size, and thus many need to deliver by cesarean section. TS women have increased rates of maternal hypertension and diabetes and, most critically, are at increased risk of aortic dilation and dissection during pregnancy (see risks). Offspring of women with TS also have a greater risk of chromosomal aberrations [19–22]. It is recommended that any woman with TS considering pregnancy be referred to a reproductive endocrinologist and in vitro fertilization with autologous oocytes should be considered.

Oocyte Donation

Historically, the only option for women with TS who had POI and wanted to carry a pregnancy was to use donated oocytes or embryos [5, 11, 23], an option which has been available to women since the first delivery in 1984 [24]. Although clinical pregnancy rates after oocyte donation are fairly high, with a general range of 17–40% [25], data suggest that patients with TS do have lower pregnancy rates and increased rates of implantation failure after oocyte donation compared to other recipients of donor oocytes. This may be due to issues with endometrial receptivity in the TS population [26]. Due to increased risks of first trimester bleeding, hypertension, and preeclampsia, when women with TS conceive, they should be followed in a high-risk obstetrical setting [11], and only single embryo transfer is recommended.

Gestational Surrogacy

Given the medical and cardiac comorbidities that may be associated with pregnancy in women with TS, gestational surrogacy is an option that should be considered in those who desire children. Gestational surrogacy occurs when a woman carries a pregnancy for another woman who has a medical condition where pregnancy is contraindicated. The gestational surrogate undergoes transfer of an embryo that has been created from another individual's oocyte. In the setting of TS, the embryo could be created from an oocyte from the woman with TS or from an oocyte donor. The American Society for Reproductive Medicine recommends that all women with TS should be counseled on the option of using a gestational surrogate [5].

Oocyte Cryopreservation Following Ovarian Stimulation

The process of oocyte cryopreservation requires 10–15 days of hormonal stimulation followed by transvaginal oocyte retrieval under anesthesia [5, 10]. This procedure is performed for females who are facing medical diagnoses or treatment that will likely result in gonadal toxicity and failure (e.g., cancer). The American Society for Reproductive Medicine no longer considers this procedure experimental [27]. Ovarian stimulation followed by oocyte retrieval and cryopreservation has been reported in adults with TS. There are few reported cases of successful harvesting of oocytes following hormonal stimulation in post-menarchal girls (ages 13–16 years) with mosaic TS [10, 28–30]. In most reported cases, the ovaries were stimulated using recombinant or highly purified FSH, as well as recombinant LH or human menopausal gonadotropins to provide supplementation of LH and achieve adequate steroidogenesis [10]. Serial abdominal ultrasound examinations and measurement of serum estradiol levels were obtained to monitor ovarian response to stimulation. Oocyte maturation was triggered using recombinant human chorionic gonadotropin, highly purified human chorionic gonadotropin, or leuprolide acetate. The oocyte retrieval was performed transvaginally using ultrasound guidance, under general anesthesia. In Oktay et al. [29], an average of 13.3 oocytes was retrieved (range 7–19), of which an average of 8.5 was mature (range 4–10) and cryopreserved [10]. One 14-year-old girl underwent two cycles of oocyte cryopreservation, 1 year apart. It is notable that the mature oocyte yield decreased from eight to four in the second cycles, perhaps due to a rapidly declining ovarian reserve. It is unknown whether these harvested and cryopreserved oocytes will lead to successful embryos or pregnancies. This procedure is limited to post-menarchal females as prepubertal girls have an immature hypothalamic-pituitary-gonadal axis and therefore cannot produce mature oocytes. In addition, it is unclear if exposure to high levels of estrogen which result from ovarian stimulation, albeit briefly, has an impact on final adult height in these girls, where short stature is already a major issue. The challenge remains in identifying those girls who would be the best candidates for this procedure and the proper timing of intervention. Oktay et al. has proposed an algorithm for identification and timing using serial anti-Müllerian hormone, FSH, LH, estradiol and inhibin B levels, and antral follicle counts obtained by abdominal ultrasonography (Fig. 4.1). Questions remain regarding the psychosocial impact of this procedure on prepubertal girls.

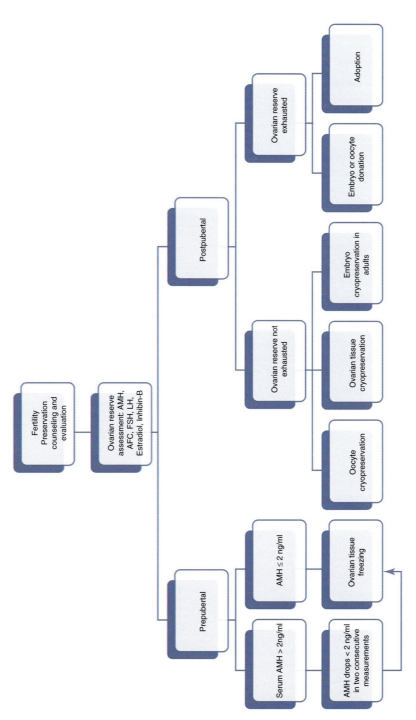

Fig. 4.1 A proposed algorhythmic approach to decision-making for fertility preservation in females diagnosed with Turner syndrome. For prepubertal girls with sufficient ovarian reserve, expert experience dictates utility of serial serum anti-Müllerian hormone (AMH) assessments to delay intervention to a postpubertal age so that oocyte cryopreservation can be considered. Serum AMH level of less than 2 ng/mL corresponds to levels in the lower quartile for girls aged 5–13 years of age [23]. In postpubertal girls, because the risk of follicle loss is extremely high and can proceed at a fast pace, we recommend fertility preservation regardless of the initial AMH. (Oktay et al. [10]. Copyright © 2016 North American Society for Pediatric and Adolescent Gynecology)

Experimental Fertility Options

Ovarian Tissue Cryopreservation

Ovarian tissue cryopreservation (OTC) was first described by Hovatta et al. in 1996 and involves laparoscopically removing ovarian cortical tissue that is cryopreserved for potential future fertility. No hormonal stimulation is required prior to this procedure, and it is typically performed as an outpatient procedure. Pieces of the outer layer of the ovary, where the primordial follicles are present, are then cryopreserved. Because ovarian reserve is already reduced in girls with TS, it is recommended to remove as much ovarian tissue as possible, typically the entire ovary [5, 10] as well. The cryopreserved ovarian tissue is available for transplantation to restore ovarian endocrine function and fertility at the time it is desired. The cryopreserved tissue is then thawed, followed by autotransplantation back into the patient. Autotransplantation sites include the ovarian fossae in the pelvis or under the skin in the forearm [10]. While OTC remains an experimental procedure, it is currently the only option available for prepubertal girls. This procedure has been offered on an experimental basis to patients with a variety of cancer, genetic, endocrine, and rheumatologic conditions in which patients may be exposed to gonadotoxic therapies that result in a high likelihood of ovarian failure. There are now over 60 reported cases of successful pregnancies resulting in live births following ovarian tissue transplant after OTC in adult patients [31], 1 live birth following transplant of tissue preserved from a peri-pubertal patient [32] and a recent news report of 1 live birth from OTC that was performed in a prepubertal patient [33]. Primordial follicles have been identified in ovarian tissue harvested for cryopreservation in girls with both mosaic and non-mosaic TS up to 17 years of age [34], and there are larger ongoing trials of ovarian tissue cryopreservation in girls with TS 1–25 years of age [35]. It is important to note that there are currently no reports of successful pregnancies following OTC in patients with Turner syndrome. Therefore, the safety and promise of success for this technology remain uncertain. It should therefore be performed under an institutional review board-approved experimental protocol.

Risks of Ovarian Tissue Cryopreservation Procedures

As with any surgical procedure, ovarian tissue cryopreservation is associated with risks of both surgery and anesthesia. Although general surgical risks, including blood loss, infection, and injury to surrounding organs, are low in procedures relevant to FP, additional procedure-specific risks exist. Ovarian tissue may be damaged during the removal process as a result of coagulation for hemostasis. Due to the high risk of POI and low density of follicles in TS, it is therefore recommended that the entire ovary be removed [5, 10]. Anesthesia risks are also important to consider, particularly given that those with TS who are undergoing FP are generally young. The US Food and Drug Administration (FDA) recently issued a warning that "repeated or lengthy use of general anesthetic and sedation drugs during surgeries or procedures in children younger than 3 years … may affect the development of children's brains" [36] and experts have recommended avoiding nonurgent procedures requiring general anesthesia in this age group. As fertility preservation in this population is considered, the fact that success with oocyte cryopreservation may be highest in the youngest aged individuals must be weighed against these potential surgical and anesthesia risks.

Risks to Offspring

Offspring of women with TS are reported to have higher rates of chromosomal aberrations. The four large pregnancy studies in TS were reviewed [19–22], but conclusions are limited because preimplantation genetic testing was not pursued in all pregnancies nor was karyotyping completed in all offspring. The Bernard et al. study of 52 spontaneous pregnancies reported (1) 2 pregnancies were terminated due to Trisomy 21 and Trisomy 13 and (2) 11/17 female infant offspring underwent karyotyping in which 2 were found to have Turner syndrome (from mothers with X chromosome structural abnormalities). Hadnott et al. reported that of 13 pregnancies to 10 women (5 spontaneous, 5 with ART), none of the offspring had chromosomal aberrations. Birkebaek et al. reported outcomes of 64 offspring in which 25 were tested and 6 were found to have chromosomal aberrations. Bryman et al. did not report on karyotype. In addition to chromosomal aberrations, concerns have been raised by these studies about additional abnormalities in the infants, including prematurity, low birth weight, cardiac abnormalities, brain abnormalities, and genital ambiguity.

There are methods of determining whether chromosomal abnormalities are present in offspring, as both pre- and postimplantation evaluations are available to screen for chromosomal aberrations like aneuploidy. Preimplantation genetic testing can be performed to ensure that only chromosomally normal embryos are transferred following in vitro fertilization (IVF). Onalan et al. described a case in which a 29-year-old woman with 45,X/46,XX TS underwent preimplantation genetic diagnosis in which 2/4 blastomeres were found to be normal and pregnancy was achieved [37]. Postimplantation techniques include evaluation by newer methods like cell-free DNA as well as traditional chorionic villous sampling and amniocentesis.

Obstetrical and Maternal Complications of Pregnancy in Turner Syndrome

Miscarriage rates are significantly higher in this population, reported at up to 50% [10]. While the reasons for this are not elucidated, a likely etiology is an increased rate of fetal aneuploidy. Uterine factors such as small uterine size and altered development and receptivity of the endometrium may also contribute to the increased rate of miscarriage. Rates of cesarean section are also approximately double the rate for women without TS [20].

Maternal mortality has been reported as high as 2%, which is 100–200 times greater than in the general population [10]. This is attributed to increased cardiac load during pregnancy and cardiovascular and connective tissue disorders with subsequent aortic dissection. At highest risk are those with baseline progressive aortic root dilation, coarctation of the aorta, and hypertension [38]. This has led the Practice Committee of the American Society for Reproductive Medicine to conclude that TS is a relative contraindication to pregnancy, that appropriate screening must be conducted, and that an aortic size index greater than 2 cm/m^2 is an absolute contraindication to pregnancy in TS. The French College of Obstetrics and Gynecology has issued similar guidelines [39]. Dissections may also occur after pregnancy; thus, ongoing surveillance is recommended.

Rates of pregnancy-induced hypertensive disorders, including hypertension, preeclampsia, and eclampsia, are also higher in TS. They are reported in 13–63% of TS pregnancies [11, 20, 40, 41]. While the rates reported in all of these studies are greater than the rate of pregnancy-induced hypertension in non-TS pregnancies, the discrepancy from 13% to 63% may be related to spontaneous pregnancies (13% [20]) versus those achieved with oocyte donation (38% [40], 63% [41]). Bernard et al. noted that their cohort with spontaneous pregnancy was younger than the oocyte donation cohorts and may have had a less severe phenotype, allowing spontaneous pregnancy.

Women with TS also have higher rates of other conditions complicating pregnancy, including thyroid dysfunction, diabetes and other autoimmune disease, obesity, and renal anomalies.

Ethical Considerations

Pregnancy in TS, whether spontaneous, through use of FP, or by ART using donor oocytes, raises many ethical questions. As described above, there are significant risks of maternal morbidity and mortality. These must be balanced against the desire for a biological child [42], and women with TS considering pregnancy must be evaluated and counseled appropriately. Further discussion in this chapter focuses on ethical issues of fertility preservation procedures in the pediatric population.

Timing

Optimal timing of FP is a complicated issue as we lack reliable data to accurately predict ovarian reserve in an individual in infancy. While we know that in the TS population as a whole, factors including karyotype and AMH levels are predictive of ovarian status [15], it remains challenging to extrapolate this data for an individual. An individual with a mosaic karyotype has a higher likelihood of ovarian reserve and may have greater fertility potential through proven postpubertal techniques for oocyte cryopreservation, but POI prior to that time remains likely. Oktay et al. employ serial AMH measurements, but we await long-term studies on the efficacy and ideal protocol for such a strategy. Ovarian reserve is likely greatest at the youngest ages, but should we remove ovarian tissue in infancy or early childhood? This subjects a child to a surgical procedure at a young age, and the choice to cryopreserve immature ovarian tissue results in removal of an entire ovary. Removal of this tissue may have the unwanted effect of decreasing the likelihood of spontaneous pubertal development, menarche, and fertility. Thus, for any provider weighing options for FP with an individual family, many questions remain.

Consent and Assent

An ethical issue in all pediatric practice is a child's ability to provide assent and consent for medical treatment. While parents are generally trusted as proxy decision-makers, with their children's best interests and values in mind, reproductive decisions are seen as more personal than other healthcare decisions [43]. It may be difficult for parents to distinguish their own best interests from those of their children [44]; thus, ideally choices about reproduction would be delayed until the child reached the age of majority. In some pediatric conditions including TS, however, the child's greatest likelihood of successful FP may be as a minor, thus compelling transgenerational reproductive decision-making. If the child is mature enough, she should be included in the decision-making process and give assent if possible [45, 46]. However, even with assent, decisional regret may occur because young patients cannot always predict their future wishes [47].

Experimental Treatment and False Hope

Decisions regarding FP in TS are complicated by the experimental nature of some techniques. While postpubertal girls with TS may benefit from established FP methods, prepubertal patients only have the option for experimental ovarian tissue cryopreservation [48]. Technologies and research are rapidly advancing so that experimental treatments on cryopreserved tissue may be successful in the future [49], but it is unknown whether any patients who choose to undergo this procedure will directly benefit. This also raises concern about the concept of "false hope," a type of psychological risk that occurs when patients are misled about the possibility of success for a particular treatment [50, 51]. The risks involved with FP, including surgical, psychological, and lack of autonomy, must be weighed against the potential benefits of future fertility potential.

Cost and Insurance Coverage

FP is expensive (ranging from thousands to tens of thousands of dollars) and requires storage of frozen gametes [52]. Insurance coverage for FP in many conditions is variable [52], but often these procedures are considered elective and thus not covered, and storage is always the financial responsibility of the individual. In addition to ethical arguments about whether these types of procedures should be considered elective, we must also consider that the distributive justice concerns that only children from families who can afford these procedures will have access to FP.

Transmitting Genetic Condition to Offspring

There is also concern about transmission of aneuploidy to offspring, raising ethical arguments about whether there is an obligation to produce the "best" children versus the assertion that this is a eugenic viewpoint [53–55]. As discussed above, for women concerned about having children with aneuploidy, preimplantation genetic testing or postimplantation techniques can screen embryos for chromosomal aberrations.

Additional Considerations in Turner Syndrome with Y Chromosome

Additional ethical questions arise for girls with Turner syndrome with Y chromosome because they face an increased risk of gonadal germ cell cancer (GCC). The risk of gonadoblastoma, estimated from many studies, is 12–35% [56, 57], and gonadectomy is recommended as prophylaxis [2]. The clinical perception has long been that such gonads, without usual hormone function and fertility potential, lack purpose and that, given GCC risk, should be removed. However, there is increasing evidence that a small percentage of these individuals have ovarian reserve, and spontaneous pregnancy is reported [20], calling into question the assumption that these gonads lack purpose. Controversy surrounding prophylactic gonadectomy is increasing for those with disorders (differences) in sex development. While gonadoblastoma may be present at young ages, it may take years to progress to invasive malignancy, which is generally localized, and highly curable; thus, some argue observation protocols may be reasonable for select individuals [58]. On the other hand, gonadectomy with concurrent efforts for fertility preservation may also be a reasonable approach [55]. The role of fertility potential and preservation is important to consider in the management of these patients.

Conclusion

Women with TS cite infertility as their major concern in qualitative analysis of challenges they face in their condition [59]. To serve the needs and concerns of girls and women with TS, counseling about fertility options including fertility preservation is important. Ideally this discussion should begin at the time of diagnosis, to afford patients and parents the most opportunity and time to consider options for fertility preservation. Choices about whether and when to pursue fertility preservation are complicated by the gaps in knowledge, experimental nature of some of the procedures, and ethical considerations. Some of this uncertainty will improve if we can establish better predictors of fertility potential and with the establishment of proven techniques for the prepubertal population. This necessitates adherence to proper experimental protocols, collaboration among centers and through international groups like the Oncofertility Consortium, and continuing ethical interrogation.

References

1. Pasquino AM, et al. Spontaneous pubertal development in Turner's syndrome. Italian Study Group for Turner's syndrome. J Clin Endocrinol Metab. 1997;82(6):1810–3.
2. Negreiros LP, Bolina ER, Guimaraes MM. Pubertal development profile in patients with Turner syndrome. J Pediatr Endocrinol Metab. 2014;27(9–10):845–9.
3. Abir R, et al. Turner's syndrome and fertility: current status and possible putative prospects. Hum Reprod Update. 2001;7(6):603–10.
4. Hovatta O. Pregnancies in women with Turner's syndrome. Ann Med. 1999;31(2):106–10.
5. Grynberg M, et al. Fertility preservation in Turner syndrome. Fertil Steril. 2016;105(1):13–9.
6. Mamsen LS, et al. Germ cell numbers in human embryonic and fetal gonads during the first two trimesters of pregnancy: analysis of six published studies. Hum Reprod. 2011;26(8):2140–5.
7. Modi DN, Sane S, Bhartiya D. Accelerated germ cell apoptosis in sex chromosome aneuploid fetal human gonads. Mol Hum Reprod. 2003;9(4):219–25.
8. Weiss L. Additional evidence of gradual loss of germ cells in the pathogenesis of streak ovaries in Turner's syndrome. J Med Genet. 1971;8(4):540–4.
9. Singh RP, Carr DH. The anatomy and histology of XO human embryos and fetuses. Anat Rec. 1966;155(3):369–83.
10. Oktay K, et al. Fertility preservation in women with turner syndrome: a comprehensive review and practical guidelines. J Pediatr Adolesc Gynecol. 2016;29(5):409–16.
11. Hagman A, et al. Obstetric and neonatal outcome after oocyte donation in 106 women with Turner syndrome: a Nordic cohort study. Hum Reprod. 2013;28(6):1598–609.
12. Broer SL, et al. Anti-Mullerian hormone: ovarian reserve testing and its potential clinical implications. Hum Reprod Update. 2014;20(5):688–701.
13. Weenen C, et al. Anti-Mullerian hormone expression pattern in the human ovary: potential implications for initial and cyclic follicle recruitment. Mol Hum Reprod. 2004;10(2):77–83.
14. Visser JA, et al. Anti-Mullerian hormone levels in girls and adolescents with Turner syndrome are related to karyotype, pubertal development and growth hormone treatment. Hum Reprod. 2013;28(7):1899–907.
15. Lunding SA, et al. AMH as predictor of premature ovarian insufficiency: a longitudinal study of 120 turner syndrome patients. J Clin Endocrinol Metab. 2015;100(7):E1030–8.

16. Borgstrom B, et al. Fertility preservation in girls with turner syndrome: prognostic signs of the presence of ovarian follicles. J Clin Endocrinol Metab. 2009;94(1):74–80.
17. Kleinman E. Caring for our own: why American adoption law and policy must change. Columbia J Law Soc Probl. 1997;30:327.
18. State, U.S.D.o., Annual report on intercountry adoption, U.S.D.o. State, Editor. 2015.
19. Hadnott TN, et al. Outcomes of spontaneous and assisted pregnancies in turner syndrome: the U.S. National Institutes of Health experience. Fertil Steril. 2011;95(7):2251–6.
20. Bernard V, et al. Spontaneous fertility and pregnancy outcomes amongst 480 women with Turner syndrome. Hum Reprod. 2016;31(4):782–8.
21. Birkebaek NH, et al. Fertility and pregnancy outcome in Danish women with Turner syndrome. Clin Genet. 2002;61(1):35–9.
22. Bryman I, et al. Pregnancy rate and outcome in Swedish women with Turner syndrome. Fertil Steril. 2011;95(8):2507–10.
23. Foudila T, Soderstrom-Anttila V, Hovatta O. Turner's syndrome and pregnancies after oocyte donation. Hum Reprod. 1999;14(2):532–5.
24. Lutjen P, et al. The establishment and maintenance of pregnancy using in vitro fertilization and embryo donation in a patient with primary ovarian failure. Nature. 1984;307(5947):174–5.
25. Alvaro Mercadal B, et al. Pregnancy outcome after oocyte donation in patients with Turner's syndrome and partial X monosomy. Hum Reprod. 2011;26(8):2061–8.
26. Yaron Y, et al. Patients with Turner's syndrome may have an inherent endometrial abnormality affecting receptivity in oocyte donation. Fertil Steril. 1996;65(6):1249–52.
27. Practice Committees of American Society for Reproductive, M. and T. Society for Assisted Reproductive. Mature oocyte cryopreservation: a guideline. Fertil Steril. 2013;99(1):37–43.
28. Oktay K, Rodriguez-Wallberg KA, Sahin G. Fertility preservation by ovarian stimulation and oocyte cryopreservation in a 14-year-old adolescent with Turner syndrome mosaicism and impending premature ovarian failure. Fertil Steril. 2010;94(2):753 e15–9.
29. Oktay K, Bedoschi G. Oocyte cryopreservation for fertility preservation in postpubertal female children at risk for premature ovarian failure due to accelerated follicle loss in Turner syndrome or cancer treatments. J Pediatr Adolesc Gynecol. 2014;27(6):342–6.
30. Huang JY, et al. Cryopreservation of ovarian tissue and in vitro matured oocytes in a female with mosaic Turner syndrome: case report. Hum Reprod. 2008;23(2):336–9.
31. Donnez J, Dolmans MM. Ovarian cortex transplantation: 60 reported live births brings the success and worldwide expansion of the technique towards routine clinical practice. J Assist Reprod Genet. 2015;32(8):1167–70.
32. Demeestere I, et al. Live birth after autograft of ovarian tissue cryopreserved during childhood. Hum Reprod. 2015;30(9):2107–9.
33. Donnelly L. Woman gives birth to baby using ovary frozen in her childhood in 'world first', in The Telegraph. 2016.
34. Hreinsson JG, et al. Follicles are found in the ovaries of adolescent girls with Turner's syndrome. J Clin Endocrinol Metab. 2002;87(8):3618–23.
35. Schleedoorn MJ, et al. To freeze or not to freeze? An update on fertility preservation in females with Turner syndrome. Pediatr Endocrinol Rev. 2019;16(3):369–82.
36. Rappaport BA, et al. Anesthetic neurotoxicity–clinical implications of animal models. N Engl J Med. 2015;372(9):796–7.
37. Onalan G, et al. Successful pregnancy with preimplantation genetic diagnosis in a woman with mosaic Turner syndrome. Fertil Steril. 2011;95(5):1788 e1–3.
38. Practice Committee of American Society For Reproductive, M. Increased maternal cardio-vascular mortality associated with pregnancy in women with Turner syndrome. Fertil Steril. 2012;97(2):282–4.
39. Cabanes L, et al. Turner syndrome and pregnancy: clinical practice. Recommendations for the management of patients with Turner syndrome before and during pregnancy. Eur J Obstet Gynecol Reprod Biol. 2010;152(1):18–24.

40. Bodri D, et al. Poor outcome in oocyte donation after elective transfer of a single cleavage-stage embryo in Turner syndrome patients. Fertil Steril. 2009;91(4 Suppl):1489–92.
41. Chevalier N, et al. Materno-fetal cardiovascular complications in Turner syndrome after oocyte donation: insufficient prepregnancy screening and pregnancy follow-up are associated with poor outcome. J Clin Endocrinol Metab. 2011;96(2):E260–7.
42. Wasserman D, Asch A. Reproductive medicine and Turner syndrome: ethical issues. Fertil Steril. 2012;98(4):792–6.
43. Rodriguez SB, Campo-Engelstein L. Conceiving wholeness: women, motherhood, and ovarian transplantation, 1902 and 2004. Perspect Biol Med. 2011;54(3):409–16.
44. Johnson EK, Finlayson C. Preservation of fertility potential for sex diverse individuals. Transgend Health. 2016;1(1):41–4.
45. Gracia CR, et al. Ovarian tissue cryopreservation for fertility preservation in cancer patients: successful establishment and feasibility of a multidisciplinary collaboration. J Assist Reprod Genet. 2012;29(6):495–502.
46. Ginsberg JP, et al. An experimental protocol for fertility preservation in prepubertal boys recently diagnosed with cancer: a report of acceptability and safety. Hum Reprod. 2010;25(1):37–41.
47. Campo-Engelstein L. Gametes or organs? How should we legally classify ovaries used for transplantation in the USA? J Med Ethics. 2011;37(3):166–70.
48. Johnson EK, Finlayson C. Preservation of fertility potential for gender and sex diverse individuals. Transgend Health. 2016;1(1):41–4.
49. Informed consent, parental permission, and assent in pediatric practice. Committee on Bioethics, American Academy of Pediatrics. Pediatrics. 1995;95(2):314–7.
50. Loren AW, et al. Fertility preservation for patients with cancer: American Society of Clinical Oncology clinical practice guideline update. J Clin Oncol. 2013;31(19):2500–10.
51. Luyckx V, et al. Evaluation of cryopreserved ovarian tissue from prepubertal patients after long-term xenografting and exogenous stimulation. Fertil Steril. 2013;100(5):1350–7.
52. McDougall R. The ethics of fertility preservation for paediatric cancer patients: from offer to rebuttable presumption. Bioethics. 2015;29(9):639–45.
53. Quinn GP, et al. Frozen hope: fertility preservation for women with cancer. J Midwifery Womens Health. 2010;55(2):175–80.
54. Basco D, Campo-Engelstein L, Rodriguez S. Insuring against infertility: expanding state infertility mandates to include fertility preservation technology for cancer patients. J Law Med Ethics. 2010;38(4):832–9.
55. Campo-Engelstein L, et al. The ethics of fertility preservation for pediatric patients with differences (disorders) of sex development. J Endocr Soc. 2017;1(6):638–45.
56. Abaci A, Catli G, Berberoglu M. Gonadal malignancy risk and prophylactic gonadectomy in disorders of sexual development. J Pediatr Endocrinol Metab. 2015;28(9–10):1019–27.
57. Zelaya G, et al. Gonadoblastoma in patients with Ullrich-Turner syndrome. Pediatr Dev Pathol. 2015;18(2):117–21.
58. Albers P, et al. Guidelines on testicular cancer: 2015 update. Eur Urol. 2015;68(6):1054–68.
59. Sutton EJ, et al. Turner syndrome: four challenges across the lifespan. Am J Med Genet A. 2005;139A(2):57–66.

Chapter 5
Estrogen Replacement in Turner Syndrome

Karen O. Klein, Robert L. Rosenfield, Richard J. Santen, Aneta M. Gawlik, Philippe Backeljauw, Claus H. Gravholt, Theo C. J. Sas, and Nelly Mauras

K. O. Klein (✉)
University of California, San Diego & Rady Children's Hospital, San Diego, CA, USA

R. L. Rosenfield
The University of Chicago Pritzker School of Medicine, Chicago, IL, USA
e-mail: rrosenfi@peds.bsd.uchicago.edu

R. J. Santen
University of Virginia, Charlottesville, VA, USA
e-mail: rjs5y@hscmail.mcc.virginia.edu

A. M. Gawlik
Department of Pediatrics and Pediatric Endocrinology, School of Medicine in Katowice, Medical University of Silesia, Katowice, Poland
e-mail: agawlik@mp.pl

P. Backeljauw
The Cincinnati Center for Pediatric and Adult Turner Syndrome Care, Cincinnati Children's Hospital Medical Center, University of Cincinnati College of Medicine, Cincinnati, OH, USA
e-mail: philippe.backeljauw@cchmc.org

C. H. Gravholt
Department of Endocrinology and Internal Medicine, Aarhus University Hospital, Aarhus, Denmark

Department of Molecular Medicine, Aarhus University Hospital, Aarhus, Denmark

Department of Endocrinology and Internal Medicine and Medical Research Laboratories, Aarhus University Hospital, Aarhus, Denmark
e-mail: ch.gravholt@dadlnet.dk

T. C. J. Sas
Albert Schweitzer Hospital Dordrecht and Sophia Children's Hospital Rotterdam, Rotterdam, The Netherlands
e-mail: t.c.j.sas@asz.nl

N. Mauras
Nemours Children's Health System, Jacksonville, FL, USA
e-mail: nelly.mauras@nemours.org

© Springer Nature Switzerland AG 2020   93
P. Y. Fechner (ed.), *Turner Syndrome*,
https://doi.org/10.1007/978-3-030-34150-3_5

Background

The most recent guidelines from the International Turner Syndrome Consensus Group were published in 2017 in the European Journal of Endocrinology [1]. This chapter updates the detailed review of hormone replacement therapy undertaken by the estrogen subcommittee of the international consensus group [2].

Turner syndrome (TS) defines phenotypic females who have one X chromosome and complete or partial absence of the second X chromosome. TS is characterized by physical features including a classic facial appearance, neck webbing, short stature, and lymphedema, as well as ovarian insufficiency, sensorineural hearing loss, congenital cardiovascular disease, renal anomalies, some neurodevelopmental disorders, and increased risk of thyroid and celiac disease. TS affects 25–50 per 100,000 females, and there is a very broad clinical spectrum of presentation. Some individuals have all the features mentioned above, and others have minimal features, with or without short stature and ovarian insufficiency. The karyotype in TS ranges from complete 45,X to forms of mosaicism in which there is a normal (46,XX or 46,XY) cell line and an abnormal second (or third) cell line [3].

Turner syndrome is usually accompanied by hypergonadotropic hypogonadism due to gonadal dysgenesis and ensuing primary or secondary amenorrhea. Most TS patients will therefore need hormonal replacement therapy – first for induction of puberty and then for maintaining secondary sex characteristics, attaining peak bone mass, and normalizing uterine growth for possible pregnancy later.

Spontaneous Puberty in Girls with Turner Syndrome

Approximately one-third of girls with Turner syndrome have spontaneous breast development that may progress to menarche, occurring most often in girls with mosaicism [4, 5]. Regular menstrual cycles occur in ~6% [6] of these young women.

Laboratory Markers of Ovarian Function

Elevated gonadotropins, luteinizing hormone (LH), and particularly follicle-stimulating hormone (FSH) indicate ovarian failure [7, 8]. FSH concentrations are higher in girls with 45,X karyotype compared to those with mosaic karyotype from the neonatal period [7, 9] (Fig. 5.1). FSH and LH in girls with TS then decline to levels marginally greater than those of girls with normal ovarian function during mid-childhood, and rise again in the peripubertal years (Fig. 5.2) [7, 9] or at the time of loss of previous ovarian function. Low anti-Müllerian hormone levels and undetectable inhibin B levels have been reported to predict ovarian failure in TS [7, 10]. Seventy girls with TS and 2406 girls without TS had LH, FSH, and inhibin B

Fig. 5.1 Differences in FSH between 45,X, mosaic 45X/46XX, and other karyotypes. Dotted line shows upper limit of normal range for age. (*Reproduced with permission from Fechner 2006 JCEM* [8])

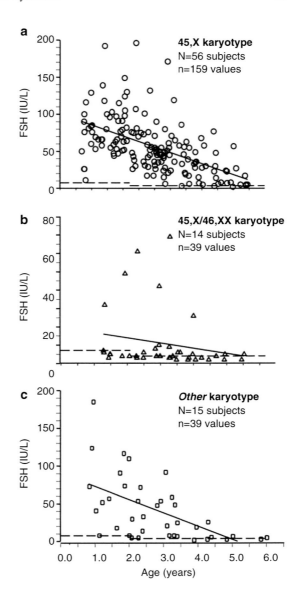

measured prior to estrogen treatment [7]. Ovarian function was related to whether girls had 45X or a mosaic karyotype. According to these data, undetectable inhibin B may predict the absence of spontaneous puberty, but the specificity was low. Anti-Müllerian hormone in 120 girls with TS predicted no ovarian function when <4 pmol/L and predicted ovarian function when >19 pmol/L [10].

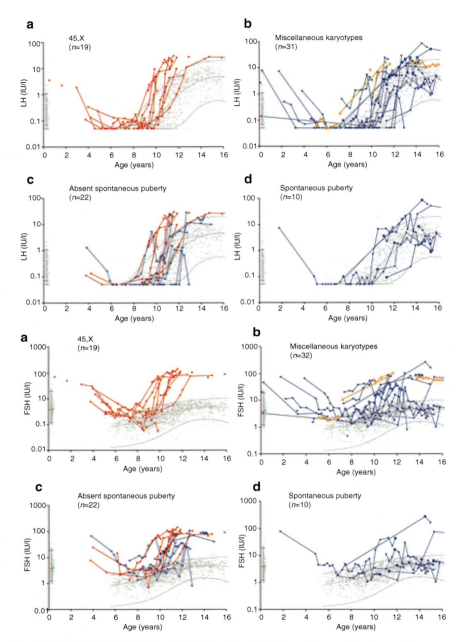

Fig. 5.2 Serum FSH and LH levels (IU/l) in girls with TS (*n* = 51) according to age, karyotype, and spontaneous puberty onset compared with a reference range based on 2406 healthy Danish girls (gray dots). Lines represent geometric means and 95% prediction interval (±2 SD). Girls with 45,X monosomy (red, **a**), miscellaneous TS karyotypes before (blue) and after gonadectomy (orange) (**b**), TS patients with absent spontaneous puberty (**c**), and spontaneous puberty (**d**) are shown according to karyotype. Age at spontaneous pubertal onset is illustrated by filled circles. (*Reproduced with permission from Hagen 2010 JCEM* [7])

Treatment Options for Induction of Puberty and Maintenance of Feminization

Estrogen Forms Available for Replacement

Estradiol (E_2) is the natural form of estrogen that is secreted and binds to the estrogen receptor in humans [11]. Ethinyl estradiol (EE) is a very potent synthetic E_2 analogue that is not metabolized to E_2. It binds to both estrogen receptors α and β. EE has an ethinyl group covalently attached at the 17α-position. EE is taken up in unmodified form and retained by estrogen target tissues for a longer time than is E_2. The E_2 precursor estrone acts after being metabolized to E_2. Equine estrogens, the major components of the widely used conjugated equine estrogens (CEE), consist of over 100 forms of estrogens of different receptor affinity and potency. Estrogens are metabolized in the liver by microsomal cytochrome P-450 with aromatic hydroxylation at either C2 or C4 position as the major route. Other pathways include formation of glucuronide conjugates and sulfation [12–14].

Table 5.1 lists commonly available, lower-dose estrogen treatments for pubertal induction, and considerations for their use. Table 5.2 lists some common progestin and estrogen/progestin combination replacement options after pubertal induction is complete. The reader should be aware that availability and trade names differ among countries. The list is not all-inclusive. We present data from various routes and preparations, but list other preparations for reference, with the caution that studies have not been done in TS with each preparation listed. Table 5.3 summarizes published low-dose estrogen treatments for puberty induction in TS.

Timing and Dose of Estrogen Replacement for the Induction of Pubertal Feminization

The optimal estrogen replacement therapy regimen to induce pubertal development and maintain beneficial effects in adults is still being evaluated. A substantial body of literature to date supports the effectiveness and theoretical benefits of starting pubertal estrogen replacement with low-dose transdermal estrogen (E_2) although, to our knowledge, there is no study to date of transdermal use from initiation of puberty until adulthood. Theoretical benefits of transdermal use include the more physiologic route of delivery, avoiding first-pass effects in the liver that include the accumulation of unphysiologic estrogens observed after the oral route [15] and avoiding effects associated with a pro-coagulation state [16] and increased risk of stroke [17].

The goals of replacement are to mimic the normal progression of puberty in girls while maximizing growth potential and minimizing risks. Delaying estrogen replacement may be deleterious to bone, uterine, and psychosocial health parameters [18]. To mimic normal physical and social development, initiation of treatment should begin at 11–12 years of age if gonadotropins are elevated, or AMH is low. LH and FSH may be measured yearly starting at age 11, based on average age of

Table 5.1 Some common low-dose estrogen treatment options for pubertal induction in TS and considerations for use

Preparation[a]	Doses available, frequency, route	Starting dose at puberty	Dose increase approximately every 6 m to adult dosing	Considerations for use
Transdermal options (some brands)		3–7 µg/day	25–100 µg/day	See text on applying patches
Menostar (Bayer) (matrix)	14 µg weekly TD	½ patch weekly	Only used for low dosing, not full replacement	Easiest way to give low dose; once a week dosing
Vivelle Dot (Novartis) (matrix)	25, 37.5, 50, 75, 100 µg twice weekly	¼ patch weekly, or 1 patch per month (no patch other 3 weeks)	25–100 µg twice weekly	Designed for twice weekly, but can give once per week to increase dose slower
Vivelle Mini (matrix)	25, 37.5, 50, 75, 100 µg twice weekly	Too small to consistently cut	25–100 µg twice weekly	Smaller size patch, but not smaller dosing
Generic (different brands in different countries)	25, 37.5, 50, 75, 100 µg twice weekly	¼ patch weekly, or 1 patch per month (no patch other 3 weeks)	25–100 µg twice weekly	Once a week dosing can be used
Estraderm (matrix)	50, 100 µg twice weekly	Not small enough to initiate puberty	50–100 µg twice weekly	Can't use to initiate puberty
E_2 gel Estrogel (Ascend) 0.06% Divigel (Vertical) (0.1%)	0.75 mg E_2/pump 0.25, 0.5, 0.1 mg E_2/pump	0.25 mg/pump	1 pump daily	Only available in some countries at the low dose
Oral options				
17β-estradiol (E_2) (ex: Estrace (Allergen), Cetura (ACE))	0.5, 1, 2, 4 mg daily	½ pill daily	1–4 mg/day	Cheapest option, brands vary by country
Ethinyl Estradiol (EE)		2 µg/day	10–20 µg/day	Not available in many countries
Premarin (CEE)	0.3, 0.625, 0.9, 1.25 mg daily	½ pill daily	0.625–1.25 mg/day	Not available in many countries, not recommended based on safety
Depot options				
Depot E_2 (cypionate)	5 mg/ml	0.2 mg/m	2 mg/m	Not available in Europe
Adding Gestagen options		Not needed to initiate puberty		Add once bleeding occurs or after 2 years

Medroxyprogesterone acetate	10 mg daily for 10 days		Give with TD E_2, or alone for 10 days	
Micronized progesterone (Prometrium)	100 mg daily		Give continuously with TD E_2	Less breast cancer risk long term
Combined E_2/Gestagen sequential patch		Do not use to initiate puberty		
Climara Pro	E_2 0.045 mg/levonorgestrel 0.015 mg/24 h		1 patch weekly	
Combipatch	E_2 0.045 mg/norethidrone 0.14 or 0.25 mg/24 h		1 patch weekly	
Evo-Sequi	E_2 50 µg /norethisterone acetate 170 µg/24 h		2 patches weekly	
Femoston	1–2 mg E_2/10 mg dydrogesterone		E_2 patch for 2 weeks; then combined patch for 2 weeks	
Combined E_2/Gestagen sequential pills		Do not use to initiate puberty		
Trisequens	E_2 2 mg/norethisterone acetate 1 mg		1 pill/day	
Divina plus	Estradiolvalerate 2 mg/ Medroxyprogesterone acetate 10 mg		1 pill/day	
Oral contraceptive pills	Ethinyl estradiol and progestins		Do not use to initiate puberty	
Loestrin (norethindrone)				Less progestational, less androgenic, low estrogenic
Lo-ovral (norgestrel)				More progestational, intermediate androgenic, low estrogenic
Orthotricylcen (norgestimate)				Less androgenic but progestational and more estrogenic

Reprinted from: Klein et al. [2]

[a]The reader should be aware that availability and trade names differ among countries. The list is not all-inclusive

Table 5.2 Some common progestin and estrogen/progestin combination replacement options after pubertal induction is complete

Adding progestin options	Doses available, frequency and route	Not needed to initiate puberty	Add once bleeding occurs or after 2 years	Notes
Medroxyprogesterone acetate	10 mg daily for 10 days		Give with TD E_2, or alone for 10 days	
Micronized progesterone (Prometrium)(AbbVie)	100 mg daily		Give continuously with TD E_2	Less breast cancer risk long term
Combined E_2/Progestin sequential patch – some brand options		Do not use to initiate puberty		
Climara Pro (Bayer)	E_2 0.045 mg/ levonorgestrel 0.015 mg/24 h		1 patch weekly	
Combipatch (Noven)	E_2 0.045 mg/norethidrone 0.14 or 0.25 mg/24 h		1 patch weekly	
Evo-Sequi (Janssen)	E_2 50 µg /norethisterone acetate 170 µg/24 h		2 patches weekly	
Combined E_2/Progestin sequential pills		Do not use to initiate puberty		
Trisequens (NovoNordisk)	E_2 2 mg /norethisterone acetate 1 mg		1 pill/day	
Divina plus	Estradiol valerate 2 mg/ Medroxyprogesterone acetate 10 mg		1 pill/day	
Femoston (Mylan)	E_2 and dydrogesterone 1/10 or 2/10 mg		1 pill/day	
Oral contraceptive pills[a]		Do not use to initiate puberty		

Reprinted from: Klein et al. [2]

[a]There are multiple types of oral contraceptive pills, which differ in estrogen dose, sequential vs continuous, and type and dose of progestin. The reader is referred to the text to outline general principles

Table 5.3 Summary of published low-dose estrogen treatment for puberty induction in TS

Author, Journal, Year	Subjects	Estrogen treatment, route and dose	Outcomes	Height
Ankarberg-Lindgren, JCEM, 2001 [24]	8 girls with TS (12–16 years) and 7 with other hypogonadism	TD E$_2$ 6 µg – 18 µg given just 12 h overnight	B2 in 3–6 m in 75% of girls on low dose, and B3 in 2 years on higher dose; TD dose correlated with serum E$_2$ ($p < 0.001$)	No height data
Van Pareren, JCEM, 2003 [22]	60 girls with TS, ± spontaneous puberty	Oral E$_2$ 5 µg/kg X 2 year → 7.5 µg/kg X 1 year → 10 µg/kg after 4 years GH	B2 onset in 0.2 year avg	No neg effect on height or growth velocity vs spontaneous puberty
Piippo, JCEM 2004 [39]	23 girls with TS	E$_2$ gel 0.1 mg X1 year → 0.2 mg X1 year → 0.5 mg X1 year → 1 mg X1 year → 1.5 mg X1 year	Pubertal advance about 1 stage per year treatment with 50% ≥B2 at 6 m	Adult height 153.1 ± 4.8 cm
Soriano-Guillen, JCEM 2005 [26]	704 girls with TS ± spontaneous puberty	Oral EE 1–5 µg/day; oral E$_2$ 0.5 mg/day; TD ¼ of a 25 µg/day patch	No data on rate of pubertal progression	TD E$_2$ taller than oral by 2.1 cm avg.; but shorter than spontaneous
Rosenfield, JCEM, 2005 [19]	14 girls with TS, compared with NCGS registry, 12–15 years	Depot E$_2$ 0.2 mg/mo with increase of 0.2 mg every 0.5 years; GH also given 0.05 mg/kg/day	Half of girls B1 – >B2 in 0.5 years; and increased one stage per 0.5 years with each 0.2 mg increase in dose; On 1 mg – 100% B3–B5 by 2 years and menarche in 62.5% by 2.5 years	Lowest dose had greatest GV; FH > PAH at start of Rx; FH > GH alone, growth not as good as in TS with spontaneous puberty
Nabhan, JCEM, 2009 [21]	12 girls with TS, 11.3–17 years	Oral CEE (0.3–0.45 mg/day) vs. TD (25 µg/day for 6 m – >37.5 µg/day for 6 m)	B3–4 by 1 years in 83%; no change in 17%; TD group had greatest increase in spine density, BMD, uterine length and volume	No height data

(continued)

Table 5.3 (continued)

Author, Journal, Year	Subjects	Estrogen treatment, route and dose	Outcomes	Height
Bannink, Clin Endocrinol, 2009 [23]	56 girls with TS, 11–18 yo	Oral E_2 (5 μg/kg/day) × 2 years; with progression to 7.5 and 10 μg/kg/day	Breast stage progressed in same timing as average Dutch population: B1 – >B2 in 0.2 years; B1 – >B4 in 2.1 years	No height data
Torres-Santiago, JCEM, 2013 [16]	40 girls with TS, 13–20 years	Oral E_2 (avg 2 mg) vs. TD E_2 (avg 0.1 mg) – dose titrated to plasma E_2	No difference in body composition, BMD, or lipids between groups	No height data
Ross, NEJM, 2011 [29]; and Quigley, JCEM, 2014 [50]	144 girls with TS analyzed for growth; 123 girls with TS analyzed for puberty, 5–12.5 years	Oral EE: 25 ng/kg/day, 5–8 years; 50 ng/kg/day, >8–12 years; >12 years, escalating from 100 ng/kg/day; ± GH	EE dose decreased for breast before 12 years or vaginal bleeding before 14 years; Age of menarche similar to general population; Earlier breasts for girls who received the early low dose	GH + EE group height SDS increase of 0.58 compared to increase of 0.26 in GH alone
Perry, Hormone Res in Pediatr, 2014 [49]	92 girls with TS, 7–13 years	Oral EE: 2 μg/day Y 1; 4 μg/day Y 2; 6/8/10 μg/day increases every 4 m in Y 3	B1->B2 in 0.65 years and to B4 in 2.25 years	Growth not as good as with depot E_2 reported
Cakir, J Pediatr Endocrinol Metab, 2015 [20]	13 girls with TS, 11–17 years	Oral E_2 (0.5 mg/day) vs. TD (4.5 μg/day)	B1->B3–4 in 1 year	BA advance less with TD (ΔCA/ΔBA 2.2 vs. 0.58, $p = 0.005$); GV greater on TD at 1 year (4.35 vs. 3.8, $p = 0.022$)

Reprinted from: Klein et al. [2]
Legend: *B2 (3, 4)* breast stage 2 (3, 4), *BA* bone age, *CA* chronologic age, *GV* growth velocity, *FH* final height, *PAH* predicted adult height, *GH* growth hormone

pubertal onset. If gonadotropins are normal for age, observation for spontaneous puberty is appropriate, with future replacement therapy if gonadal failure occurs.

Some parents raise the question of whether a girl's readiness socially and psychologically can be considered an indication for delaying the initiation of pubertal feminization. We do not recommend this, as it may lead to the deleterious effects of prolonged hypoestrogenism. The optimal estrogen dose to initiate pubertal feminization approximates 10% of the adult replacement dose [19].

Incremental dose increases at approximately 6-month intervals can mimic the normal pubertal tempo until adult dosing is reached over a 2–3 year period. This theoretically translates into 25–100% increase in dose every 6 months for 4–6 dose changes between the initiation and adult doses portrayed in the Table 5.1. However, no studies to date have rigorously studied outcomes in relation to the rate of dose increase for the different preparations.

In general, the studies summarized in Table 5.3 report onset of breast buds within 6 months in most girls [20–24]. Each of these regimens results in pubertal stage 4 breasts in an average of 2.25 years, which is similar to that in TS girls with spontaneous puberty (1.9 years), as well as in the general population [23].

Girls with TS are very short and have a very short adult height potential, typically 20 cm less than the average female population in all countries studied. Growth hormone (GH) treatment is an FDA-approved therapy to promote growth in these girls, and the earlier it is started, the better the growth promotion. However, the expectations of intervention are modest; in general GH therapy results in a net gain of 1 cm/year of treatment [25, 26]. In girls in whom GH treatment has been delayed, consideration of initiation of GH prior to low-dose estrogen is particularly important to optimize growth. There are no data to support the specifics of timing in such cases, but rather an individualized judgment, balancing the desire for taller height versus the desire for more rapid feminization. When height is a greater concern, often GH treatment can be initiated prior to low-dose E_2; however, we recommend that E_2 not be delayed past 14 years of age. When feminization is a greater concern, GH and E_2 can be started simultaneously.

Initiation with low doses of E_2 is crucial to preserve growth potential even if growth hormone treatment has already been initiated. Very low-dose EE and E_2 do not interfere with growth response to growth hormone therapy when started ≤ 12 years of age [19, 27].

Progestin Replacement

TS patients have a normal uterus anatomy, so progestin must be added once breakthrough bleeding occurs, or after 2 years of E_2 treatment, to minimize the risks of endometrial hyperplasia, namely, irregular bleeding and endometrial cancer associated with prolonged unopposed estrogen [28, 29].

Progestins are divided into several classes (Table 5.4), and individual agents can bind to the progesterone receptor as well as the androgen, glucocorticoid, and

Table 5.4 Classification of progestins

Classification	Progestin
Natural	Progesterone
Synthetic	
Pregnane derivatives	
Acetylated	Medroxyprogesterone acetate
	Megestrol acetate
	Cyproterone acetate
Nonacetylated	Chlormadinone acetate
	Dydrogesterone
	Medrogestone
19-Norpregnane derivatives	
Acetylated	Nomegestrol acetate
	Nesterone
Nonacetylated	Demegestone
	Promegestone
	Trimegestone
Nor-testosterone	
Ethinylated estranes	Norethindrone (norethisterone)
	Norethindrone acetate
	Ethynodiol diacetate
	Norethynodrel
	Lynestrenol
	Tibolone
13-Ethylgonanes	Levonorgestrel
	Desogestrel
	Norgestimate
	Gestodene
Nonethinylated	Dienogest
	Drospirenone

Reprinted from: Klein et al. [2]

mineralocorticoid receptors [30]. Each progestin exerts differential effects on these various receptors and accordingly, unique, nonclass action effects. In addition to the progestational effects, the 19-nor-derivatives are associated with androgenic, medroxyprogesterone acetate with glucocorticoid agonistic, and drospirenone with anti-androgenic and anti-mineralocorticoid actions, whereas progesterone is more specific to progestational effects. The combined oral contraceptives (OCs) containing progestins are divided into first-, second-, third-, and fourth-generation OCs. First-generation OCs contain 50 mcg of the estrogen mestranol and the progestogen norethynodrel (e.g., Enovid[R]). Most later generation pills utilize 20–35 mcg of EE as the estrogen. Second-generation progestogens include norethindrone, and its acetate, ethynodiol diacetate, and levonorgestrel. Third-generation progestogens include desogestrel, norgestimate, and gestodene. Fourth-generation pills include drospirenone. All OCs increase the risk of venothrombotic episodes (VTEs). A recent guideline [31] concludes that combinations of EE with the third-generation (desogestrel, norgestimate, gestodene) or fourth-generation (drospirenone) progestogens have a slightly higher risk of VTE than those containing first and second generation. Micronized progesterone is associated with a lesser risk [32].

Regimens of estrogen plus a progestin can be either combined sequential with an estrogen for 21–25 days and the progestin for only 10–14 days or combined continuous with both sex steroids continuously. The estrogen is given for up to 21–25 days to cause the endometrium to become proliferative, and the progestin in combination with the estrogen induces the luteal phase of the endometrium. Ten days of a progestin each month protects against estrogen-induced endometrial hyperplasia, and 3 months of combined continuous estrogen plus a progestin is also protective [33]. The combined sequential regimens are associated with menstruation and are preferred in younger women, whereas the combined continuous prevent uterine bleeding, an attractive factor in older women. Intrauterine devices containing a progestin block endometrial hyperplasia and unwanted bleeding, can be used along with an estrogen, and can be especially attractive for women with bleeding problems on either transdermal or oral combined formulations. Availability of products varies by country (see Table 5.2).

Route of Estradiol Administration: Oral vs. Transdermal (TD) Comparisons

E_2 is normally secreted into the systemic circulation, the liver receives the same dose as other somatic tissues, and a systemic route of estrogen delivery is physiologic [11]. In contrast, estrogen given orally reaches the systemic circulation only after absorption into the portal venous system and metabolism by the liver, thus exposing the liver to a greater dose of estrogen than the rest of the body.

Transdermal E_2 is the most widely used of these physiologic E_2 options, but the commercially available forms (patches and gels) are designed for the adult female market, and thus the lowest dose forms are four–tenfold greater than are appropriate to deliver early pubertal E_2 blood levels. The main strategies that have been advocated to fractionate transdermal E_2 in a manner that is appropriate for early puberty are based on different perspectives on normal pubertal E_2 physiology.

Currently, the lowest dose patch commercially available delivers 14 µg/day of E_2, and the most widely used low-dose patches deliver 25 µg/day. One method to deliver lower doses is to cut the patch in smaller pieces. Patches with a matrix design can be easily cut, while patches with a reservoir technology should not be cut. The disadvantages of cutting patches are that handling the smaller pieces may be difficult and that this is not recommended by the products' labels. However, there is clinical experience with this, especially in Scandinavia. There a group showed that a fractionated patch dose (one-quarter patch of 25 µg dose = approximately 6.2 µg or even less) applied overnight mimicked the normal early morning serum E_2 peak and fell back to baseline within a few hours of patch removal [22]. If one does not want to cut the patches, it has also been proposed that cyclic administration of patches, commencing with the application of a 14–25 µg patch for 1 week monthly, may achieve similar results, although we have no data at this time with this method [19, 34]. This proposal comes from an expert committee of the Pediatric Endocrine Society, which recommended initiating cyclic therapy with 25 µg/day of transdermal E_2 for 1 week and then gradually increasing the duration of patch application to 3 weeks per month before increasing the patch size. Support for this recommendation includes not only considerations of convenience and manufacturer recommendations against patch fractionation, but evidence of efficacy of cyclic administration of depot systemically delivered E_2 [19]. Evidence also exists that estrogenization of the vaginal mucosa lags behind changes in serum E_2 by about 1 week [16, 35] suggesting that the pituitary-ovarian axis activity normally commences with attenuated cyclicity [36]. Expert discussion of this method, however, suggests that 1 week with and 3 weeks without E_2 would cause such variable changes in plasma E_2 concentrations during these 4 weeks that may not mimic physiology. Further data are needed before conclusions can be made regarding the optimum mode of patch application recommendation.

Two studies in the Mauras' group have directly compared the transdermal and oral routes of E_2 administration in teenagers [16, 37]. The pharmacokinetics and pharmacodynamics of different doses of E_2 given orally vs. transdermally were examined in a group of girls with TS. Transdermal E_2 results in E_2, E_1, and bio-estrogen concentrations closer to normal and achieves greater suppression of LH/FSH in lower doses compared with normally menstruating girls without TS (Fig. 5.3) [38]. The metabolic effects of oral vs. transdermal E_2 were further compared in 40 late-teen girls with TS followed for 1 year [16]. The study found no differences in body composition, bone mineralization, or plasma lipids when the plasma E_2 levels were titrated to those of normally menstruating adolescents. Although no metabolic differences were observed, oral estrogen was associated with a marked increase in conjugated estrogen precursors such as estrone sulfate and increased serum estrogenic bioactivity. This is concerning in the context of the increased thromboembolic risk observed with oral estrogen in epidemiological studies, although there are no data to suggest that such problems are present in TS (see section "Estrogens/Progestin Therapy and Cardiovascular Risk"). Some European countries use an E_2 gel (Table 5.1), but it is very difficult to give a small enough dose for pubertal induction, and there is only one study with data from girls with TS [39].

Depot Route of Estradiol Administration

A randomized controlled trial showed that early, very low-dose, depot E_2 monthly injections stimulated normal pubertal growth and development in conjunction with growth hormone treatment [19]. This remains a viable alternative in the USA, although less attractive due to the pain of injection.

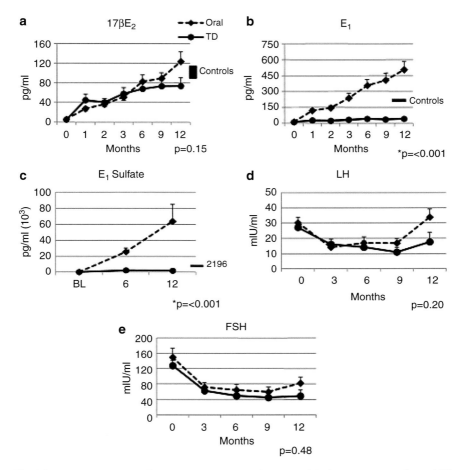

Fig. 5.3 Hormone concentrations: oral vs. transdermal. Mean ± SE plasma concentrations of E2 (**a**), E1 (**b**), E1S (**c**), LH (**d**), FSH (**e**) after oral or transdermal (TD) estradiol treatment (Rx) over 12 months. E2 levels achieved were comparable between the groups ($p = 0.15$) and similar to healthy age-matched controls averaged from follicular and luteal phase values (bar on the right). E1 and E1S concentrations were much higher after oral E2 than TD ($p < 0.001$). Gonadotropins decreased comparably over 12 months between groups ($p > 0.20$ for both), although there was an increase in both oral and TD LH at 12 mo. Black bars represent controls. Analysis done by mixed model repeated measures ANOVA. To convert to SI units, multiply by E2, 3.67; E1, 3.699; E1S, 2.73. (*Reproduced with permission from Torres-Santiago 2013 JCEM* [16])

Practical Considerations

Estrogen treatment is crucial for girls with TS, first to induce puberty and then to maintain healthy levels for all the reasons described here. Individualizing treatment to optimize compliance is important, and helping girls understand how easy it is to help them have breast development consistent with their peers should be encouraged. Based on literature and theoretical principles presented here, we suggest the following practical approach to feminize girls with TS: initiate puberty with low dose TD E_2, when available, starting with half of a 14 µg patch applied weekly or a whole 14 or 25 µg patch for 1 week per month at 11–12 years of age (Table 5.1) and increase every 6–12 months based on response and growth potential. Add a progestin when bleeding begins or after 2–3 years of estrogen treatment if no bleeding occurs. See Fig. 5.4 for flow diagram. When TD E_2 is not available, or for physician or patient alternative preference, consider approaches discussed above as well as in Tables 5.1 and 5.2.

For the adult patient with TS, no long-term studies have assessed the optimal dose, route, or duration of E_2 treatment. Our recommendations are based on available data in both women with TS as well as other hypogonadal patients. The effects of hormone treatment in TS may be different from what is observed in other patient populations, and caution is needed when extrapolating data from postmenopausal studies [38]. With those cautions, the type and route must be negotiated with the patient taking into account the preference of the patient, the size of the uterus (for possible oocyte donation), bone and body composition assessed by DEXA, blood pressure and quality of life, as well as other considerations (see sections below "Outcomes and Risks of Sex Hormone Therapy: Growth, Lipids, Liver, Bone Health, Uterine Health, and Thrombosis Risk"). Adult transdermal replacement doses of 50–150 µg/day or oral replacement doses of 2–4 mg of E_2 will often be sufficient. Oral progestin for 10 days per month (combined sequential approach) or continuous progestin regimens are suggested (analogous to the combined/continu-

Fig. 5.4 Flow diagram for initiating estrogens and progestins

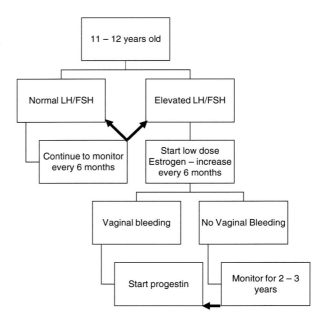

ous methodology commonly used for menopausal hormone therapy [40]). If bleeding irregularities occur or if the patient prefers, an intrauterine progestin-coated device can be used together with either continuous oral or transdermal E_2. This will reduce bleeding irregularities and often abolish bleedings and the need for systemic progestin use. Close collaboration with a gynecologist with knowledge of TS is very useful.

Duration of Sex Hormone Replacement Therapy

Once adult replacement doses are reached, treatment should continue until the time of usual menopause around age 51–53 years, when the risks versus benefits of continuing should be assessed, individualized, and reassessed annually [33, 40]. Combined estrogen and progestin treatment duration is limited by increased risk of breast cancer [41]; however, there are no clinical or epidemiological data among TS to suggest that breast cancer is a problem. Actually, breast cancer seems to occur less frequently among women with TS [1], although diminished overall estrogen exposure may be a factor. Estrogen therapy alone after menopausal age has a more favorable risk/benefit ratio allowing more flexibility in duration but is only indicated in women having undergone hysterectomy [42]. There will often be a continued need for education of the TS patient in order to explain the beneficial effects of hormonal replacement therapy on multiple organ systems, in order to maintain adherence to therapy.

Monitoring Sex Hormone Replacement Treatment

Routine monitoring of serum LH or FSH is not recommended during estrogen treatment as levels remain elevated in agonadal women until higher levels of estrogen are given [43]. The suppression of gonadotropins was comparable after oral and TD E_2 when doses were titrated to similar serum E_2 levels [16]. Estradiol measurement using a sensitive assay (e.g., liquid or gas chromatography with tandem mass spectrometry) allows titrating dosage if desired, though E_2 levels for optimal linear growth remain to be determined. Clinical assessment, patient satisfaction, patient age, and, often, residual growth potential are the primary determinants for dose increase. If potential for taller stature is still possible, girls may remain on lower estrogen doses longer. If girls are already older at initiation, the duration of time until adult dosing may be shortened.

Adult replacement transdermal doses of 50–200 µg/day typically allow women to reach normal adult plasma E_2 concentrations. The normal range of estradiol in cycling women is very wide with early follicular phase levels as low as 20–40 pg/mL (75–150 pmol/L) and midcycle peak of 200–600 pg/mL (730–2200 pmol/L), and some experts replace to these levels [16]. When oral estrogen is used, adult replacement doses of 2–4 mg of E_2 will result in normal circulating E_2 levels (i.e., approximately 100–155 pg/mL (367–568 pmol/L)) [43] and may lead to normal levels of FSH and LH in some women [43, 44]. However, women with TS lack inhibin [45], so normalizing LH and FSH is not the goal per se [46, 47]. Optimizing all the health benefits and minimizing the risks is the goal, and it is important to remember that this must be individualized.

Outcomes and Risks of Sex Hormone Therapy: Growth, Lipids, Liver, Bone Health, Uterine Health, and Thrombosis Risk

Estrogens and Linear Growth

Low-dose estrogen regimens do not appear to interfere with growth response to growth hormone therapy when begun at 11–12 years of age at low doses [19, 27, 48, 49]. Ultralow-dose oral EE (starting at 25 ng/kg/day, ages 5–12 years) in childhood TS has been reported but is not currently recommended based on an increased risk of earlier thelarche and no proven benefit to growth or pubertal outcome [50].

A consistent effect of physiologic E_2 replacement on IGF-1 concentration has not been established [3]. IGF-1 concentrations tended to be lower on oral than TD E_2 (-16 ± 12 vs. 28 ± 12 ng/mL at 12 months ($p = 0.059$), while an earlier study from the same group showed no change in IGF1 concentration after oral or TD therapy [51]. TD application caused a decrease in IGF binding protein-3 and GH binding protein compared with an increase of IGFBP3 and unchanged level of GHBP after oral administration [52]. In contrast, contraceptive doses of oral EE are known to suppress IGF-1 [53, 54]. In a small study (13 girls), bone age advanced less on TD E_2 than oral E_2 (Δchronological age/Δbone age 2.2 vs. 0.58, $p = 0.005$). At the same time, growth velocity was greater on TD E_2 than oral E_2 at 1 year (4.35 vs. 3.8 cm/year, $p = 0.022$), suggesting overall better growth [24].

Estrogens and Metabolism

Lipids

Although there are theoretical reasons to be concerned about the relative systemic and hepatic hyperestrogenism of low-dose oral estrogens vs low-dose transdermal E_2, evidence thus far does not indicate that the hepatic effects on lipids or binding proteins causes an appreciable clinical difference between the two forms of treatment (Table 5.5) [16, 37, 55]. With the exception of one study reporting significantly higher

Table 5.5 Estrogen treatment and metabolic outcome data

Author, journal, year	(n)	Treatment	Main metabolic measure outcome
Jospe, J Pediatr Endocrinol Metab, 1995 [56]	8	Oral E_2: 100 ng/kg/day vs. TD E_2: 0.0125 mg/kg/day	Oral, but not TD, increased serum HDL
Gravholt, Diabetes Care, 1998 [81], J Clin Endocrinol Metab, 1997 [52]	15 (oral) 8 (TD)	Oral: 2 mg/day E_2 days 1–22, + 1 mg/day norethisterone acetate days 13–22, and 1 mg/d E_2 days 23–28 vs. TD E_2 50 mg/day for 28 days + oral 1 mg norethisterone days 13–22	No difference between oral and TD in insulin sensitivity, body composition changes, 24 h ambulatory blood pressure, IGF-I, liver function tests and lipids
Gussinyé, Horm Res, 2000 [69]	12	TD E_2: 100 μg/day	BMD and BMD z-score values significantly increased; no significant differences in BMI, calcium intake and physical activity habits
Guttmann, Clin Endocrinol (Oxf) 2001 [64]	17	CEE: 0.625 mg/day vs. EE: 30 μg/day	Hyperinsulinemia was suppressed to normal by both EE and CEE Lipid profiles were normal on both regimens. PTH and 1,25-dihydroxyvitamin D levels increased on HRT (EE > CEE), and phosphorus decreased Alkaline phosphatase, osteocalcin and urinary deoxypyridinoline cross-links (DPD) were high off therapy; the former two suppressed to high-normal levels on the EE regimen, but not on CEE.
Naeraa, Acta Paediatr, 2001 [67]	9	Morning Oral E_2 6–11 μg/kg/day vs. Evening Oral E_2 6–11 μg/kg/day	During OGTT in the morning, glucagon and insulin were lower following evening E_2 administration as well as insulin resistance tended to be lower
Alves, Gyncecol Endocrinol, 2006 [65]	9	CEE: 0.625 mg/day vs. TD E_2 (gel): 1.5 mg/day	No difference in BMI, WHR, or insuline tolerance between CEE and TD E_2 During TD: Tendency to increased total lean mass

(continued)

Table 5.5 (continued)

Author, journal, year	(n)	Treatment	Main metabolic measure outcome
Mauras, JCEM, 2007 [51] Taboada, JCEM, 2011 [37]	11 10	Low dose Oral E_2: 0.5 mg/day Low dose TD E_2: 0.0375 mg/day High dose Oral E_2: 2.0 mg/day High dose TD E_2: 0.075 mg Oral E_2 0.5, 1, 2 mg/day for 2 weeks each vs. TD E_2 0.025, 0.0375, 0.05 mg/day for 2 weeks each	LDL/HDL cholesterol responses were variable among groups Neither Oral nor TD E_2 adversely affected rates of protein turnover, lipolysis, and lipid oxidation rates or plasma lipids, fibrinogen, or fasting insulin concentrations
Torres-Santiago, JCEM, 2013 [16]	40	Oral E_2: 2 mg vs. TD E_2: 0.1 mg	Similar fat-free mass, %fat mass, bone mineral density accrual, lipid oxidation, resting energy expenditure rates No significant changes in lipids, glucose, osteocalcin, hs-CRP
Reinehr, Clin Endocrinol (Oxf), 2016 [66]	490	Oral vs. TD (no details availabe)	The duration and dose of estrogens, its route of administration did not correlate significantly to changes of BMI-SDS

Reprinted from: Klein et al. [2]
Legend: E_2 estradiol, *TD* transdermal, *CE* conjugated estrogen, *EE* ethinyl estradiol, *OGTT* oral glucose tolerance test, *BMI* body mass index, *WHR* waist to hip ratio, *BMD* bone mineral density, *SDS* standard deviation score

HDL-cholesterol after oral estradiol [56], there were no significant differences in lipids between groups with different routes of estrogen administration [16, 37].

Estrogen deficiency in TS is associated with elevated intrahepatocellular lipids [57]. Notably, while liver enzymes are elevated in untreated TS [44, 52, 58, 59], exogenous estrogen-progestin administered orally or transdermally reduces these levels [44, 53, 60]. However, withdrawal of estrogen substitution did not influence liver enzymes [61, 62]. There was no evidence of liver toxicity from estrogen replacement therapy [55].

Glucose and Insulin

The risk of both type 1 and type 2 diabetes mellitus is increased in patients with TS across all ages [63]. However, there were no significant differences in glucose [16], insulin tolerance [64, 65] fasting insulin concentration, protein turnover and lipolysis [51], osteocalcin or highly sensitive C-reactive protein [16], BMI, or waist to hip ratio [65, 66] between groups with transdermal versus oral estrogen treatment (Table 5.5). Glucagon and insulin (during oral glucose tolerance testing) as well as insulin resistance tended to be lower following evening oral E_2 administration (0.3–0.5 mg/day) [67]. Hyperinsulinemia was suppressed to normal by both EE and CEE. A recent study in 104 girls with TS followed up to 7 years after GH therapy showed no negative influence of GH treatment on β cell function, which is also reassuring as most of these girls continued on estrogen therapy [68].

Estrogens and Bone Density

Maintenance of bone health is crucial for women with TS. Delaying estrogen replacement is deleterious to bone health. Initiating and maintaining estrogen therapy as outlined above during puberty and adulthood is important for bone density accrual and prevention of fractures. In girls with TS, transdermal E_2 administration (25–37.5 μg/day) has been reported as better than CEE (0.3–0.45 mg/day) for spine bone mineral density in one study (0.12 ±0.01 vs. 0.06 ± 0.01 g/cm^2, $p = 0.004$) [21, 69]. A recent study suggests that a higher than usual oral dose (4 vs 2 mg) during early adulthood improves body composition (increased muscle mass) and increases bone formation markers, which, although bone mineral density (BMD) was not increased during the study period, in the long run could improve overall bone health [70].

Some adult women with Turner syndrome prefer combined estrogen and progestin pill options for convenience sake [71]. Few studies have directly compared transdermal estrogen regimens with oral regimens in women with premature ovarian insufficiency including patients with Turner syndrome. The better powered studies indicated improved lumbar spine density on a physiologic sex steroid replacement regimen (100–150 μg E_2 daily + 400 mg vaginal progesterone 2 week/mo) [47].

On the basis of these studies, the guidelines written by the European Society of Human Reproduction and Embryology favored transdermal estradiol in women with premature ovarian failure and commented that oral contraceptive pills may be appropriate for some women but effects on BMD are less favorable [72–74]. More comprehensive long-term studies will be necessary to confirm these results and to examine fracture rates.

Estrogens and Uterine Growth

Data concerning the influence of different routes of estrogen therapy on uterine volume is still inconclusive because route, dose, age at onset of treatment, and duration of treatment all influence uterine growth [21, 23, 75–79]. However, it is clear that the longer the duration of treatment and the higher the dose of estrogen, the better the chances of normalizing uterine size, which is important only if pregnancy options are pursued. One study in 12 girls with TS reported uterine length significantly greater with TD E_2 (25–37.5 µg/day) compared to CEE (0.3–0.45 mg/day) (4.13 ±0.39 vs. 1.98 ± 0.39 cm, $p = 0.003$) and uterine volume greater (22.2 ± 4.4 vs. 4.0 ± 4.4 mL, $p = 0.02$) [78]. Higher than usual doses are often necessary before oocyte donation, where oral doses up to 8 mg have been used for up to 2 years in order to achieve satisfactory uterine growth [80].

Estrogens/Progestin Therapy and Cardiovascular Risk

Although there have been no studies in children, or women with TS, we recommend against CEE use in view of thromboembolic and cardiovascular disease risks reported in postmenopausal women, especially in the first year of treatment using oral estrogen, and in women with existing risk factors like obesity [16, 17, 81–83].

E_2 replacement therapy, oral or transdermal, lowers blood pressure [81–83], although E_2 causes salt and water retention [84]. This contrasts with EE-containing contraceptives, which raise blood pressure significantly unless containing an anti-mineralocorticoid progestin [85].

Recent publications showed no increased risk of stroke with progesterone, pregnane derivatives, or nortestosterone derivatives [17, 86]. However, norpregnane derivatives were found to increase risk [17]. Studies have not been done in TS comparing various progestin options.

Several studies examining both oral E_2 and oral conjugated estrogens vs. transdermal E_2 replacement in the postmenopausal setting have shown increased thromboembolic risk, especially in the first year of treatment in the oral group, more pronounced in women with existing risk factors such as obesity [17, 43, 87]. Studies directly comparing thromboembolic risk in women with Turner syndrome have not been done.

Screening for thromboembolic risk, through measurement of Factor V Leiden and prothrombinase levels, should be done in girls with a personal or family history of VTE; however, routine screening is not recommended, and screening is done only to educate the family on risks, not to postpone estrogen therapy [88]. Transdermal estrogen is the preferred treatment in these girls.

Socialization and Neurocognitive Benefits

Estrogen replacement in TS girls may improve motor speed and verbal and nonverbal processing time compared to placebo-treated TS patients [89, 90]. In TS adolescents, oral estrogen therapy improved self-reported self-esteem and psychological well-being over time. At the same time, their parents reported improvement in problem behaviors [91]. Data concerning adults with TS have not been so optimistic. TS adults had relative difficulty with measures of spatial/perceptual skills, visual-motor integration, affect recognition, visual memory, attention, and executive function. These deficits were apparent in TS women despite evidently adequate estrogen treatment [92, 93]. Age of onset of puberty influenced sexual experience in one study [94] but not in another [95]. A more recent follow-up report suggests that women with TS face more challenges in areas of sexual confidence and self-esteem [96].

The young women with TS who reached normal height and had age-appropriate pubertal development reported normal health-related quality of life (HRQoL); satisfaction with breast development (and height) had a positive influence on several HRQoL scales [97]. Puberty should be induced at a physiologically appropriate age in patients with Turner syndrome to optimize self-esteem, social adjustment, and timing of initiation of the patient's sex life. However, one study showed that neither estrogen use nor age of puberty influenced sexual function in TS patients [95].

Oxandrolone Effect on Puberty

Oxandrolone is a non-aromatizable weak androgen with direct growth-promoting effects. Low-dose oxandrolone has been shown to act synergistically with GH to increase linear growth in several well-controlled studies [47, 98–100]. However, oxandrolone may also increase hirsutism and clitoral size slightly and modestly slow pubertal progression (by 1.3 years) and delay menarche in response to estrogen replacement [101]. These effects are usually minor and/or transient. One study indicates that normal adult breast size is subsequently attained as oxandrolone is discontinued and adult estrogen replacement is instituted [102]. Pubic hair stage was not affected. Therefore, a reasonable suggestion is that treatment with oxandrolone 0.03–0.05 mg/kg/day (maximum 2.5 mg/day) starting from the age of 10 years onward be considered as adjunctive therapy only in very short TS girls [101, 103].

Summary and Conclusion

In summary, we suggest that estrogen replacement should mimic normal physical and social development for timing and progression of puberty, starting between 11 and 12 years of age and increasing over 2–3 years. This regimen improves socialization and growth and optimizes uterine and bone health. Neurocognitive benefits are inconclusive.

When available, low-dose E_2 administered by a systemic route is preferred, and evidence supports its effectiveness and theoretical benefits. When transdermal E_2 is not available, or compliance is an issue, evidence supports use of oral micronized E_2 or depot E_2 preparations. Only when these forms of E_2 are unavailable should other forms of estrogen be prescribed. Progestin should be added once vaginal bleeding occurs or after 2 years of estrogen treatment. At that time, some women prefer the ease of use of an oral combination of estrogen and progestin. Some preparations are safer than others, and availability varies by country, but ordinarily the benefit of good compliance to a chosen regimen outweighs the risks. Treatment is monitored by patient satisfaction and growth and development measures.

References

1. Gravholt CH, Andersen NH, Conway GS, Dekkers OM, Geffner ME, Klein KO, Lin AE, Mauras N, Quigley CA, Rubin K, Sandberg DE, Sas TCJ, Silberbach M, Söderström-Anttila V, Stochholm K, van Alfen-van derVelden JA, Woelfle J, Backeljauw PF, International Turner Syndrome ConsensusGroup. Clinical practice guidelines for the care of girls and women with Turner syndrome: proceedings from the 2016 Cincinnati International Turner Syndrome Meeting. Eur J Endocrinol. 2017;177(3):G1–G70.
2. Klein KO, Rosenfield RL, Santen RJ, Gawlik AM, Backeljauw PF, Gravholt CH, Sas TCJ, Mauras N. Estrogen replacement in Turner syndrome: literature review and practical considerations. J Clin Endocrinol Metab. 2018;103:1–14.
3. Canonico M, Carcaillon L, Plu-Bureau G, Oger E, Singh-Manoux A, Tubert-Bitter P, Elbaz A, Scarabin P-Y. Postmenopausal hormone therapy and risk of stroke impact of the route of estrogen administration and type of progestogen. Stroke. 2016;47:1734–41.
4. Tanaka T, Igarashi Y, Ozono K, Ohyama K, Ogawa M, Osada H, Onigata K, Kanzaki S, Kohno H, Seino Y, Takahashi H, Tajima T, Tachibana K, Tanaka H, Nishi Y, Hasegawa T, Fujita K, Yorifuji T, Horikawa R, Yokoya S. Frequencies of spontaneous breast development and spontaneous menarche in Turner syndrome in Japan. Clin Pediatr Endocrinol. 2015;24(4):167–73.
5. Negreiros LP, Bolina ER, Guimarães MM. Pubertal development profile in patients with Turner syndrome. J Pediatr Endocrinol Metab. 2014;27(9–10):845–9.
6. Pasquino AM, Passeri F, Pucarelli I, et al. Spontaneous pubertal development in Turner's syndrome. Italian Study Group for Turner's Syndrome. J Clin Endocrinol Metab. 1997;82:1810–3.
7. Hagen CP, Main KM, Kjaergaard S, Juul A. FSH, LH, inhibin B and estradiol levels in Turner syndrome depend on age and karyotype: longitudinal study of 70 Turner girls with or without spontaneous puberty. Hum Reprod. 2010;25(12):3134–41.
8. Fechner PY, Davenport ML, Qualy RL, Ross JL, Gunther DF, Eugster EA, Huseman C, Zagar AJ, Quigley CA, Toddler Turner Study Group. Differences in follicle-stimulating hormone secretion between 45,X monosomy Turner syndrome and 45,X/46,XX mosaicism are evident at an early age. J Clin Endocrinol Metab. 2008;91(12):4896–902.

9. Conte FA, Grumbach MM, Kaplan SL. A diphasic pattern of gonadotropin secretion in patients with the syndrome of gonadal dysgenesis. J Clin Endocrinol Metab. 1975;40(4):670–4.
10. Lunding SA, Aksglaede L, Anderson RA, Main KM, Juul A, Hagen CP, Pedersen AT. AMH as predictor of premature ovarian insufficiency: a longitudinal study of 120 Turner syndrome patients. J Clin Endocrinol Metab. 2015;100(7):E1030–8.
11. Rosenfield RL, Perovic N, Devine N, Mauras N, Moshang T, Root AW, Sy JP. Optimizing estrogen replacement treatment in Turner syndrome. Pediatr. 1998;102:486–8.
12. Lee AJ, Cai MX, Thomas PE, Conney AH, Zhu BT. Characterization of the oxidative metabolites of 17beta-estradiol and estrone formed by 15 selectively expressed human cytochrome p450 isoforms. Endocrinology. 2003;144(8):3382–98.
13. Lepine J, Bernard O, Plante M, Tetu B, Pelletier G, Labrie F, Belanger A, Guillemette C. Specificity and regioselectivity of the conjugation of estradiol, estrone, and their catecholestrogen and methoxyestrogen metabolites by human uridine diphospho-glucuronosyltransferases expressed in endometrium. J Clin Endocrinol Metabol. 2004;89(10):5222–32.
14. Levesque E, Turgeon D, Carrier JS, Montminy V, Beaulieu M, Belanger A. Isolation and characterization of the UGT2B28 cDNA encoding a novel human steroid conjugating UDP glucuronosyltransferase. Biochemistry. 2001;40(13):3869–81.
15. Cameron-Pimblett A, La Rosa C, King TFJ, Davies MC, Conway GS. The Turner syndrome life course project: karyotype-phenotype analyses across the lifespan. Clin Endocrinol. 2017;87:532–8.
16. Torres-Santiago L, Mericq V, Taboada M, Unanue N, Klein K, Singh R, Hossain J, Santen R, Ross J, Mauras N. Metabolic effects of oral vs. transdermal 17 beta estradiol (E_2): a randomized clinical trial in girls with Turner syndrome. J Clin Endocrinol Metab. 2013;98:2716–24.
17. Mohammed K, Dabrh AMA, Benkhadra K, Al Nofal A, Carranza Leon BG, Prokop LJ, Montori VM, Faubion SS, Murad MH. Oral vs transdermal estrogen therapy and vascular events: a systematic review and meta-analysis. J Clin Endocrinol Metab. 2015;100(11):4012–20.
18. Misra M, Katzman D, Miller KK, Mendes N, Snelgrove D, Russell M, Goldstein MA, Ebrahimi S, Clauss L, Weigel T, Mickley D, Schoenfeld DA, Herzog DB, Klibanski A. Physiologic estrogen replacement increases bone density in adolescent girls with anorexia nervosa. J Bone Miner Res. 2011;26:2430–8.
19. Rosenfield RL, Devine N, Hunold JJ, Mauras N, Moshang T Jr, Root AW. Salutary effects of combining early very low-dose systemic estradiol with growth hormone therapy in girls with Turner syndrome. J Clin Endocrinol Metab. 2005;90:6424–30.
20. Cakir ED, Saglam H, Eren E, Ozgur T, Tarim OF. Retrospective evaluation of pubertal development and linear growth of girls with Turner syndrome treated with oral and transdermal estrogen. J Pediatr Endocrinol Metab. 2015;28:1219–26.
21. Nabhan ZM, Dimeglio LA, Qi R, Perkins SM, Eugster EA. Conjugated oral versus transdermal estrogen replacement in girls with Turner syndrome: a pilot comparative study. J Clin Endocrinol Metab. 2009;94:2009–14.
22. van Pareren YK, de Muinck Keizer-Schrama SM, Stijnen T, Sas TC, Jansen M, Otten BJ, Hoorweg-Nijman JJ, Vulsma T, Stokvis-Brantsma WH, Rouwe CW, Reeser HM, Gerver WJ, Gosen JJ, Rongen-Westerlaken C, Drop SL. Final height in girls with Turner syndrome after long-term growth hormone treatment in three dosages and low dose estrogens. J Clin Endocrinol Metab. 2003;88:1119–25.
23. Bannink EM, van Sassen C, van Buuren S, de Jong FH, Lequin M, Mulder PG, de Muinck Keizer-Schrama SM. Puberty induction in Turner syndrome: results of oestrogen treatment on development of secondary sexual characteristics, uterine dimensions and serum hormone levels. Clin Endocrinol. 2009;70:265–73.
24. Ankarberg-Lindgren C, Elfving M, Wikland KA, Norjavaara E. Nocturnal application of transdermal estradiol patches produces levels of estradiol that mimic those seen at the onset of spontaneous puberty in girls. J Clin Endocrinol Metab. 2001;86:3039–44.
25. Bondy CA. Care of girls and women with Turner syndrome: a guideline of the Turner syndrome study group. J Clin Endocrinol Metab. 2007;92:10–25.

26. Soriano-Guillen L, Coste J, Ecosse E, Leger J, Tauber M, Cabrol S, Nicolino M, Brauner R, Chaussain JL, Carel JC. Adult height and pubertal growth in Turner syndrome after treatment with recombinant growth hormone. J Clin Endocrinol Metab. 2005;90:5197–204.

27. Ross JL, Quigley CA, Cao D, Feuillan P, Kowal K, Chipman JJ, Cutler GB Jr. Growth hormone plus childhood low-dose estrogen in Turner's syndrome. N Engl J Med. 2011;364:1230–42.

28. Shifren JL. Gass MLS the North American Menopause Society recommendations for clinical care of midlife women. Menopause. 2014;21(10):1–25.

29. Fournie A, Berrino F, Clavel-Chapelon. Unequal risks for breast cancer associated with different hormone replacement therapies: results from the E3N cohort study. [Erratum Appears in Breast Cancer Res Treat. 2008; Jan;107(2):307–8]. Breast Cancer Res Treat. 2008;107(1):103–11.

30. Stanczyk FZ, Hapgood JP, Winder S, Mishell DR Jr. Progestogens used in postmenopausal hormone therapy: differences in their pharmacological properties, intracellular actions, and clinical effects. Endocr Rev. 2013;34(2):171–208.

31. Practice Committee of the American Society for Reproductive Medicine. Combined hormonal contraception and the risk of venous thromboembolism: a guideline. Fertil Steril. 2017;107(1):43–51.

32. Devineni D, Skee D, Vaccaro N, Massarella J, Janssens L, LaGuardia KD, Leung AT. Pharmacokinetics and pharmacodynamics of a transdermal contraceptive patch and an oral contraceptive. J Clin Pharmacol. 2007;47(4):497.

33. Santen RJ, Allred DC, Ardoin SP, Archer DF, Boyd N, Braunstein GD, Burger HG, Colditz GA, Davis SR, Gambacciani M, Gower BA, Henderson VW, Jarjour WN, Karas RH, Kleerekoper M, Lobo RA, Manson JE, Marsden J, Martin KA, Martin L, Pinkerton JV, Rubinow DR, Teede H, Thiboutot DM, Utian WH. Executive summary: postmenopausal hormone therapy: an endocrine society scientific statement. J Clin Endocrinol Metab. 2010;95(Suppl 1):S1–S66.

34. Rosenfield RL, DiMeglio LA, Mauras N, Ross J, Shaw ND, Greeley SA, Haymond M, Rubin K, Rhodes ET. Commentary: launch of a quality improvement network for evidence-based management of uncommon pediatric endocrine disorders: Turner syndrome as a prototype. J Clin Endocrinol Metab. 2015;100:1234–6.

35. Rosenfield RL, Fang VS, Dupon C, Kim MH, Refetoff S. The effects of low doses of depot estradiol and testosterone in teenagers with ovarian failure and Turner's syndrome. J Clin Endocrinol Metab. 1973;37:574–80.

36. Rosenfield RL, Bordini B, Yu C. Comparison of detection of normal puberty in girls by a hormonal sleep test and a gonadotropin-releasing hormone agonist test. J Clin Endocrinol Metab. 2013;98(4):1591–601.

37. Taboada M, Santen R, Lima J, Hossain J, Singh R, Klein KO, Mauras N. Pharmacokinetics and pharmacodynamics of oral and transdermal 17β estradiol in girls with Turner syndrome. J Clin Endocrinol Metab. 2011;96(11):3502–10.

38. Trolle C, Hjerrild B, Cleemann L, Mortensen KH, Gravholt CH. Sex hormone replacement in Turner syndrome. Endocrine. 2012;41(2):200–19.

39. Piippo S, Lenko H, Kainulainen P, Sipilä I. Use of percutaneous estrogen gel for induction of puberty in girls with Turner syndrome. J Clin Endocrinol Metab. 2004;89:3241–7.

40. Stuenkel CA, Davis SR, Gompel A, Lumsden MA, Murad MH, Pinkerton JV, Santen RJ. Treatment of symptoms of the menopause: an endocrine society clinical practice guideline. J Clin Endocrinol Metab. 2015;100(11):3975–4011.

41. Morch LS, Skovlund CW, Hannaford PC, Iversen L, Fielding S, Lidegaard O. Contemporary hormonal contraception and the risk of breast cancer. N Engl J Med. 2017;377:2228–39.

42. The NAMS 2017 Hormone Therapy Position Statement Advisory Panel. The 2012 hormone therapy position statement of the North American Menopause Society. Menopause. 2012;19(3):257–71.

43. Ostberg JE, Storry C, Donald AE, Attar MJN, Halcox JPJ, Conway GS. A dose response study of hormone replacement in young hypogonadal women: effect on intima media thickness and metabolism. Clin Endocrinol. 2007;66:557–64.

44. Koulouri O, Ostberg J, Conway GS. Liver dysfunction in Turner's syndrome: prevalence, natural history and effect of exogenous oestrogen. Clin Endocrinol (Oxf). 2008;69(2):306–10.
45. Gravholt CH, Naeraa RW, Andersson AM, Christiansen JS, Skakkebaek NE. Inhibin A and B in adolescents and young adults with Turner's syndrome and no sign of spontaneous puberty. Hum Reprod. 2002;17(8):2049–53.
46. Taylor AE, Adams JM, Mulder JE, Martin KA, Sluss PM, Crowley WF Jr. A randomized, controlled trial of estradiol replacement therapy in women with hypergonadotropic amenorrhea. J Clin Endocrinol Metab. 1996;81(10):3615–21.
47. Crofton PM, Evans N, Bath LE, Warner P, Whitehead TJ, Critchley HO, et al. Physiological versus standard sex steroid replacement in young women with premature ovarian failure: effects on bone mass acquisition and turnover. Clin Endocrinol. 2010;73(6):707–14.
48. Gault EJ, Perry RJ, Cole TJ, Casey S, Paterson WF, Hindmarsh PC, Betts P, Dunger DB, Donaldson MD. Effect of oxandrolone and timing of pubertal induction on final height in Turner's syndrome: randomised, double blind, placebo controlled trial. BMJ. 2011;342:d1980.
49. Perry RJ, Gault EJ, Paterson WF, Dunger DB, Donaldson MD. Effect of oxandrolone and timing of oral ethinylestradiol initiation on pubertal progression, height velocity and bone maturation in the UK Turner study. Horm Res Paediatr. 2014;81:298–308.
50. Quigley CA, Wan X, Garg S, Kowal K, Cutler GB Jr, Ross JL. Effects of low-dose estrogen replacement during childhood on pubertal development and gonadotropin concentrations in patients with Turner syndrome: results of a randomized, double-blind, placebo-controlled clinical trial. J Clin Endocrinol Metab. 2014;99:E1754–64.
51. Mauras N, Shulman D, Hsiang HY, et al. Metabolic effects of oral versus transdermal estrogen in growth hormone-treated girls with Turner syndrome. J Clin Endocrinol Metab. 2007;92:4154–60.
52. Gravholt CH, Naeraa RW, Fisker S, Christiansen JS. Body composition and physical fitness are major determinants of the growth hormone-insulin-like growth factor axis aberrations in adult Turner's syndrome, with important modulations by treatment with 17 beta-estradiol. J Clin Endocrinol Metab. 1997;82(8):2570–7.
53. Kam GY, Leung KC, Baxter RC. Ho KK Estrogens exert route- and dose-dependent effects on insulin-like growth factor (IGF)-binding protein-3 and the acid-labile subunit of the IGF ternary complex. J Clin Endocrinol Metab. 2000;85:1918–22.
54. Weissberger AJ, Ho KK, Lazarus L. Contrasting effects of oral and transdermal routes of estrogen replacement therapy on 24-hour growth hormone (GH) secretion, insulin-like growth factor I, and GH-binding protein in postmenopausal women. JCEM. 1991;72:374–81.
55. Roulot D, Degott C, Chazouillères O, Oberti F, Calès P, Carbonell N, Benferhat S, Bresson-Hadni S, Valla D. Vascular involvement of the liver in Turner's syndrome. Hepatology. 2004;39(1):239–47.
56. Jospe N, Orlowski CC, Furlanetto RW. Comparison of transdermal and oral estrogen therapy in girls with Turner's syndrome. J Pediatr Endocrinol Metab. 1995;8(2):111–6.
57. Ostberg JE, Thomas EL, Hamilton G, Attar MJ, Bell JD, Conway GS. Excess visceral and hepatic adipose tissue in Turner syndrome determined by magnetic resonance imaging: estrogen deficiency associated with hepatic adipose content. J Clin Endocrinol Metab. 2005;90(5):2631–5.
58. Gravholt CH, Poulsen HE, Ott P, Christiansen JS, Vilstrup H. Quantitative liver functions in Turner syndrome with and without hormone replacement therapy. Eur J Endocrinol. 2007;156(6):679–86.
59. Larizza D, Locatelli M, Vitali L, Viganò C, Calcaterra V, Tinelli C, Sommaruga MG, Bozzini A, Campani R, Severi F. Serum liver enzymes in Turner syndrome. Eur J Pediatr. 2000;159(3):143–8.
60. Elsheikh M, Hodgson HJ, Wass JA, Conway GS. Hormone replacement therapy may improve hepatic function in women with Turner's syndrome. Clin Endocrinol (Oxf). 2001;55(2):227–31.
61. El-Mansoury M, Berntorp K, Bryman I, Hanson C, Innala E, Karlsson A, Landin-Wilhelmsen K. Elevated liver enzymes in Turner syndrome during a 5-year follow-up study. Clin Endocrinol (Oxf). 2008;68(3):485–90.

62. Albareda MM, Gallego A, Enríquez J, Rodríguez JL, Webb SM. Biochemical liver abnormalities in Turner's syndrome. Eur J Gastroenterol Hepatol. 1999;11(9):1037–9.
63. Gravholt CH, Juul S, Naeraa RW, Hansen J. Morbidity in Turner syndrome. J Clin Epidemiol. 1998;51:147–58.
64. Guttmann H, Weiner Z, Nikolski E, Ish-Shalom S, Itskovitz-Eldor J, Aviram M, Reisner S, Hochberg Z. Choosing an oestrogen replacement therapy in young adult women with Turner syndrome. Clin Endocrinol (Oxf). 2001;54(2):159–64.
65. Alves ST, Gallichio CT, Guimarães MM. Insulin resistance and body composition in Turner syndrome: effect of sequential change in the route of estrogen administration. Gynecol Endocrinol. 2006;22:590–4.
66. Reinehr T, Lindberg A, Toschke C, Cara J, Chrysis D, Camacho-Hübner C. Weight gain in Turner syndrome: association to puberty induction? – Longitudinal analysis of KIGS data. Clin Endocrinol. 2016;85(1):85–91.
67. Naeraa RW, Gravholt CH, Kastrup KW, Svenstrup B, Christiansen JS. Morning versus evening administration of estradiol to girls with Turner syndrome receiving growth hormone: impact on growth hormone and metabolism. A randomized placebo-controlled crossover study. Acta Paediatr. 2001;90(5):526–31.
68. Baronio F, Mazzanti L, Girtler Y, Tamburrino F, Lupi F, Longhi S, Fanolla A, Radetti G. The influence of GH treatment on glucose homeostasis in girls with Turner syndrome: a 7-year study. J Clin Endocrinol Metab. 2017;102(3):878–83. 3179.
69. Gussinyé M, Terrades P, Yeste D, Vicens-Calvet E, Carrascosa A. Low areal bone mineral density values in adolescents and young adult Turner syndrome patients increase after long-term transdermal estradiol therapy. Horm Res. 2000;54(3):131–55.
70. Cleemann L, Holm K, Kobbernagel H, Kristensen B, Skouby SO, Jensen AK, Gravholt CH. Dosage of estradiol, bone and body composition in Turner syndrome: a 5-year randomized controlled clinical trial. Eur J Endocrinol. 2017;176(2):233–42.
71. Cartwright B, Robinson J, Seed PT, Fogelman I, Rymer J. Hormone replacement therapy versus the combined oral contraceptive pill in premature ovarian failure: a randomized controlled trial of the effects on bone mineral density. J Clin Endocrinol Metab. 2016;101(9):3497–505.
72. European Society for Human Reproduction and Embryology (ESHRE) Guideline Group on POI, Webber L, Davies M, Anderson R, Bartlett J, Braat D, et al. ESHRE guideline: management of women with premature ovarian insufficiency. Hum Reprod. 2016;31(5):926–37.
73. Herrmann M, Seibel MJ. The effects of hormonal contraceptives on bone turnover markers and bone health. Clin Endocrinol. 2010;72(5):571–83.
74. Lopez LM, Grimes DA, Schulz KF, Curtis KM, Chen M. Steroidal contraceptives: effect on bone fractures in women. Cochrane Database of Syst Rev. 2014;2014(6):CD006033.
75. Paterson WF, Hollman AS, Donaldson MD. Poor uterine development in Turner syndrome with oral oestrogen therapy. Clin Endocrinol (Oxf). 2002;56(3):359–65.
76. Bakalov VK, Shawker T, Ceniceros I, Bondy CA. Uterine development in Turner syndrome. J Pediatr. 2007;151(5):528–31, 531.e1.
77. Rodrigues EB, Braga J, Gama M, Guimarães MM. Turner syndrome patients' ultrasound profile. Gynecol Endocrinol. 2013;29(7):704–6.
78. Elsedfy HH, Hamza RT, Farghaly MH, Ghazy MS. Uterine development in patients with Turner syndrome: relation to hormone replacement therapy and karyotype. J Pediatr Endocrinol Metab. 2012;25(5–6):441–5.
79. Cleemann L, Holm K, Fallentin E, Skouby SO, Smedegaard H, Møller N, Borch-Christensen H, Jeppesen EM, Wieslander SB, Andersson AM, Cohen A, Højbjerg Gravholt C. Uterus and ovaries in girls and young women with Turner syndrome evaluated by ultrasound and magnetic resonance imaging. Clin Endocrinol (Oxf). 2011;74(6):756–61.
80. Foudila T, Söderström-Anttila V, Hovatta O. Turner's syndrome and pregnancies after oocyte donation. Hum Reprod. 1999;14(2):532–5.
81. Gravholt CH, Naeraa RW, Nyholm B, Gerdes LU, Christiansen E, Schmitz O, Christiansen JS. Glucose metabolism, lipid metabolism, and cardiovascular risk factors in adult Turner's syndrome: the impact of sex hormone replacement. Diabetes Care. 1998;21:1062–70.

82. Langrish JP, Mills NL, Bath LE, Warner P, Webb DJ, Kelnar CJ, Critchley HOD, Newby DE, Wallace WHB. Cardiovascular effects of physiological and standard sex steroid replacement regimens in premature ovarian failure. Hypertension. 2009;53:805–11.
83. Mortensen KH, Anderson AH, Gravholt CH. Cardiovascular phenotype in Turner syndrome—integrating cardiology, genetics, and endocrinology. Endocr Rev. 2012;33:677–714.
84. Stachenfeld NS, DiPietro L, Palter SF, Nadel ER. Estrogen influences osmotic secretion of AVP and body water balance in postmenopausal women. Am J Phys. 1998;274:R187–95.
85. Oelkers W, Foidart JM, Dombrovicz N, Welter A, Heithecker R. Effects of a new oral contraceptive containing an antimineralocorticoid progestogen, drospirenone, on the renin-aldosterone system, body weight, blood pressure, glucose tolerance, and lipid metabolism. J Clin Endocrinol Metab. 1995;80:1816–21.
86. Renoux C, Dell'aniello S, Garbe E, Suissa S. Transdermal and oral hormone replacement therapy and the risk of stroke: a nested case-control study. BMJ. 2010;340:c2519.
87. Sweetland S, Beral V, Balkwill A, Liu B, Benson VS, Canonico M, Green J, Reeves GK, Million Women Study Collaborators. Venous thromboembolism risk in relation to use of different types of postmenopausal hormone therapy in a large prospective study. J Thromb Haemost. 2012;10(11):2277–86.
88. Baber RJ, Panay N, Fenton A, The IMS Writing Group. 2016 IMS recommendations on women's midlife health and menopause hormone therapy. Climacteric. 2016;19(2):109–50.
89. Ross JL, Roeltgen D, Feuillan P, Kushner H, Cutler GB Jr. Effects of estrogen on nonverbal processing speed and motor function in girls with Turner's syndrome. J Clin Endocrinol Metab. 1998;83(9):3198–204.
90. Ross JL, Roeltgen D, Feuillan P, Kushner H, Cutler GB Jr. Use of estrogen in young girls with Turner syndrome: effects on memory. Neurology. 2000;54(1):164–70.
91. Ross JL, McCauley E, Roeltgen D, Long L, Kushner H, Feuillan P, Cutler GB Jr. Self-concept and behavior in adolescent girls with Turner syndrome: potential estrogen effects. J Clin Endocrinol Metab. 1996;81(3):926–31.
92. Ross JL, Stefanatos GA, Kushner H, Zinn A, Bondy C, Roeltgen D. Persistent cognitive deficits in adult women with Turner syndrome. Neurology. 2002;58(2):218–25.
93. Ross JL, Stefanatos GA, Kushner H, Bondy C, Nelson L, Zinn A, Roeltgen D. The effect of genetic differences and ovarian failure: intact cognitive function in adult women with premature ovarian failure versus Turner syndrome. J Clin Endocrinol Metab. 2004;89(4):1817–22.
94. Carel JC, Elie C, Ecosse E, Tauber M, Léger J, Cabrol S, Nicolino M, Brauner R, Chaussain JL, Coste J. Self-esteem and social adjustment in young women with Turner syndrome–influence of pubertal management and sexuality: population-based cohort study. J Clin Endocrinol Metab. 2006;91(8):2972–9.
95. Sheaffer AT, Lange E, Bondy CA. Sexual function in women with Turner syndrome. J Womens Health. 2008;17(1):27–33.
96. Fjermestad KW, Naess EE, Bahr D, Gravholt CH. A 6-year follow-up survey of health status in middle-aged women with Turner syndrome. Clin Endocrinol. 2016;85:423–9.
97. Bannink EM, Raat H, Mulder PG, de Muinck Keizer-Schrama SM. Quality of life after growth hormone therapy and induced puberty in women with Turner syndrome. J Pediatr. 2006;148(1):95–101.
98. Nilsson KO, Albertsson Wikland K, Alm J, Aronson S, Gustafsson J, Hagenas L, Hager A, Ivarsson SA, Karlberg J, Kristrom B, Marcus C, Moell C, Ritzen M, Tuvemo T, Wattsgard C, Westgren U, Westphal O, Aman J. Improved final height in girls with Turner's syndrome treated with growth hormone and oxandrolone. J Clin Endocrinol Metab. 1996;81:635–40.
99. Menke LA, Sas TC, de Muinck Keizer-Schrama SM, Zandwijken GR, de Ridder MA, Odink RJ, Jansen M, Delemarre-van de Waal HA, Stokvis-Brantsma WH, Waelkens JJ, Westerlaken C, Reeser HM, van Trotsenburg AS, Gevers EF, van Buuren S, Dejonckere PH, Hokken-Koelega AC, Otten BJ, Wit JM. Efficacy and safety of oxandrolone in growth hormone-treated girls with Turner syndrome. J Clin Endocrinol Metab. 2010;95:1151–60.
100. Zeger MP, Shah K, Kowal K, Cutler GB Jr, Kushner H, Ross JL. Prospective study confirms oxandrolone-associated improvement in height in growth hormone-treated adolescent girls with Turner syndrome. Horm Res Paediatr. 2011;75:38–46.

101. Sas TC, Gault EJ, Bardsley MZ, Menke LA, Freriks K, Perry RJ, Otten BJ, de Muinck Keizer-Schrama SM, Timmers H, Wit JM, Ross JL, Donaldson MD. Safety and efficacy of oxandrolone in growth hormone-treated girls with Turner syndrome: evidence from recent studies and recommendations for use. Horm Res Paediatr. 2014;81:289–97.
102. Freriks K, Sas TC, Traas MA, Netea-Maier RT, den Heijer M, Hermus AR, Wit JM, van Alfen-van der Velden JA, Otten BJ, de Muinck Keizer-Schrama SM, Gotthardt M, Dejonckere PH, Zandwijken GR, Menke LA, Timmers HJ. Long-term effects of previous oxandrolone treatment in adult women with Turner syndrome. Europ J Endocrinol. 2013;168:91–9.
103. Sheanon NM, Backeljauw PF. Effect of oxandrolone therapy on adult height in Turner syndrome patients treated with growth hormone: a meta-analysis. Int J Pediatr Endocrinol. 2015;2015:18.

Chapter 6
The Heart and Vasculature in Turner Syndrome: Development, Surveillance, and Management

Luciana T. Young and Michael Silberbach

Introduction

Cardiovascular disease is the leading cause of early morbidity and mortality in girls and women with Turner syndrome (TS), accounting for a threefold higher mortality compared to the general population [1–3]. Congenital heart abnormalities occur in up to 50% of individuals and frequently include left-sided obstructive lesions of varying severity, such as bicuspid aortic valve, coarctation of the aorta, and hypoplastic left heart syndrome [4]. Progressive aortic enlargement may lead to aneurysm formation, dissection, and rupture, a potentially fatal complication [5, 6]. The risk for aortic dissection may be further aggravated by an increased incidence of hypertension. Acquired cardiovascular complications include coronary artery disease, myocardial infarction, and stroke [7]. These factors may be further aggravated by additional comorbidities, such as dyslipidemia, diabetes, and obesity [8].

Given the broad spectrum of cardiovascular concerns affecting individuals with Turner syndrome, these patients require a continuum of care, counseling, and preventive management into their adult years. It is therefore particularly relevant that the primary care provider has a good understanding of potential risks involved and how to manage them in order to deliver the best care for these patients and assure their best long-term outcomes.

This chapter is intended to provide an overview of the important cardiovascular issues facing girls and women who live with TS and to highlight important aspects of TS heart disease management, particularly where it diverges from the standards

L. T. Young (✉)
Seattle Children's Hospital/University of Washington, Division of Cardiology, Seattle, WA, USA
e-mail: Luciana.young@seattlechildrens.org

M. Silberbach
Doernbecher Children's Hospital, Oregon Health & Sciences University, Portland, OR, USA

© Springer Nature Switzerland AG 2020
P. Y. Fechner (ed.), *Turner Syndrome*,
https://doi.org/10.1007/978-3-030-34150-3_6

123

recommended for the general population. For those interested in a more depth and detailed review, the American Heart Association has recently published a review that includes comprehensive suggestions for TS surveillance and medical and operative management [9].

Origin of Heart Disease

Genetic Factors

A deficiency of the sex chromosome(s) in TS is necessary by definition to cause the predominance of left heart obstructive disease in TS. However, a deficiency of the second sex chromosome alone is not enough to cause the cardiac phenotype since up to 50% of individuals with TS have no heart disease [10]. In addition, the wide spectrum of cardiac malformations precludes the possibility that only sex chromosomal factors cause heart disease in TS. Taken together, this suggests that both sensitized autosomal genes and additional environmental factors (discussed below) are required to breach the heart disease threshold in TS [11]. Still, the origins of heart disease in TS remain poorly understood. While it is established that the frequency of affected males with left ventricular outflow and aortic arch obstruction is three times that of 46,XX females [12], it is unlikely that parental origin of the active X chromosome can explain the relatively huge effect size in the TS setting [13]. Several genotype-phenotype correlation studies have narrowed the search for gene candidates by comparing cohorts with pure X monosomy to individuals with deleted segments of the second X chromosome and then performing DNA sequencing or microarray studies to identify X-chromosome deletion breakpoints, the idea being that heart disease is more likely to occur in those with critical deletions that lack a cardiac-specific segment of the second sex chromosome. In such cases, cardioprotective "escape" genes from the entirely absent or deleted portion are predicted to have causal significance. Such studies have shown that TS individuals with short arm deletions (Xp-) are more likely to have heart disease [14, 15]. Corbitt et al. [16] performed such a study using molecular karyotyping in participants with or without bicuspid aortic valve (BAV) and found that hemizygosity of the X-linked gene *TIMP*1 (tissue inhibitor of matrix metalloproteinase, Xp11.3), in combination with a *TIMP*3 variant on chromosome 22, increases the risk of BAV and aortic aneurysm by sixteen-fold. The *TIMP* genes are of particular interest because they are well-known to regulate expression of extracellular matrix glycoproteins that are essential for maintaining the structural integrity of the aorta [17]. Other studies searching for gene dosage effects include RNA methylation and RNA or DNA expression profiling. These investigations have identified differential expression of a variety of genes when sex chromosome aneuploidies are compared to euploid sex chromosome complements [18–20]. One gene in particular, *KDM6A* (Xp11.2), a histone methylase, has been reported in most of these studies of differential expression and has also been implicated as a switch in the cardiac developmental program [21].

Environmental Factors

In addition to the influence of sex chromosome and autosomal genetic factors described above, the hemodynamic environment of the developing heart and subsequent postnatal conditions, particularly the marked increased risk for systemic hypertension [22], are likely to play a role in the origin of heart disease in TS, particularly the increased risk of aortic dissection and rupture. In this situation, intraluminal pressure conspires with a genetically vulnerable aortic wall. Another possible trigger for left heart disease in TS relates to the potential for abnormal development of the lymphatic vasculature as an epiphenomenon. It has been proposed that a fundamental mechanism of the TS phenotype altogether is developmental failure of the lymphatic system. Indeed, fetal and neonatal lymphedema are a hallmark of TS. Clark [23], initially, and others [24], more recently, reported that left heart obstructive diseases in TS are highly correlated with fetal lymphedema (hygroma coli or neck webbing). In this theory, impaired lymph return to the embryonic/fetal blood vasculature could produce under filling of the heart which has been postulated to contribute to underdevelopment of the left ventricle. In addition, distended lymphatic vessels could compress the aorta leading to coarctation or impede development of the pulmonary veins leading to anomalous pulmonary vein connections. This perhaps explains why the otherwise rare, left upper lobe anomalous pulmonary vein connections are frequently observed in TS. It is noteworthy that in TS, fetal demise before the end of the first trimester occurs in 99% of those affected [25], and left heart hypoplasia is typically found [26]. In support of a potential connection between lymphatic hypoplasia and left heart disease, knockout mice lacking the Vegfr3 receptor, an essential mediator of lymphatic vascular development, die at stage E9.5 from heart failure [27].

Congenital Heart Disease

Congenital heart disease is prevalent in TS, occurring in up to 50% of affected individuals and contributing significantly to early mortality [4]. Although the incidence is highest in 45,X karyotype, cardiac abnormalities may also be associated with X mosaicism or other X structural abnormalities [28]. Left-sided obstructive lesions are most common with the spectrum of cardiac involvement ranging from trivial with no associated symptoms to severe, requiring surgery in the neonatal period. For this reason, if TS is suspected or confirmed prenatally, a thorough fetal cardiac assessment should be performed so that appropriate parental counseling, delivery planning, and postnatal management can be provided in the event that significant heart disease is present.

Bicuspid Aortic Valve

Bicuspid aortic valve (BAV) has a prevalence of 15–30% in girls and women with TS, compared to 1–2% in the general population [29, 30]. Severe aortic valve abnormalities, such as critical aortic stenosis or aortic atresia, present as ductal-dependent lesions requiring intervention in the newborn period. More often, however, aortic valve dysfunction is minimal and may go undiagnosed unless a screening echocardiogram is performed. Aortic stenosis and insufficiency may develop and progress over time. Therefore, early diagnosis and regular follow-up are essential for optimizing long-term outcomes.

Aortic Arch Anomalies

Abnormalities of the aortic arch are also common in TS. Coarctation of the aorta occurs in up to 20% of affected individuals and may occur in isolation or in association with a BAV. Approximately 5–12% of identified cases of coarctation require repair during childhood. Another 5–8% of cases are found incidentally on cross-sectional imaging in otherwise asymptomatic adults with TS [31]. Perhaps because of the generalized vasculopathy in TS, even well-repaired coarctation can predispose to overt or exercise-induced hypertension. Ambulatory blood pressure monitoring may be useful in this setting. Elongation of the transverse arch, defined as a relative increase in vertical distance from the top of the aortic arch to the origin of the innominate artery, has also been described in close to 50% of individuals and has been associated with a higher risk of aortic dilation and hypertension [32]. Additional anatomic variants include an aberrant right subclavian artery (8%), bovine aorta (8%), and isolated cases of cervical aortic arch [31].

Pulmonary and Systemic Vascular Anomalies

An increased incidence of pulmonary and systemic vascular anomalies has been identified by cross-sectional imaging modalities that might not otherwise have been detected by echocardiography. There is a marked increase in the prevalence of partial anomalous pulmonary vein connection (13–15%), particularly involving the left upper lobe pulmonary vein [33, 34]. Other venous anomalies include left superior vena cava (8–13%), interrupted inferior vena cava with azygous continuation, and dilation of the head and neck arteries. Neck webbing and an increased anterior-posterior thoracic diameter have been shown to be strong predictors of arterial and venous anomalies in TS [35, 36].

Congenital coronary arterial anomalies are prevalent (20%) and most often affect the left coronary artery. Absence of the left main coronary artery, single coronary ostium, anomalous origins of the coronary arteries, coronary artery dilation, and coronary artery-to-pulmonary artery fistulae have also been reported. Most of these abnormalities are benign, but their identification is important prior to any cardiovascular surgical intervention as their presence may require modifications in operative approach [37, 38].

Associated Lesions

Additional, but less frequently seen, cardiac anomalies include Shone's complex, isolated mitral valve anomalies, dextroposition of the cardiac apex, atrial and ventricular septal defects, pulmonary valve abnormalities, and patent ductus arteriosus. Hypoplastic left heart syndrome is rare postnatally but is the most common cause of fetal demise in TS. This is important because it is estimated that 99% of all TS conceptions fail to reach term [39], and it is thought that up to 2% of *all* conceptions are due to the TS sex chromosome aneuploidy.

Surveillance and Management

Because of the preponderance of left heart disease in TS compared to 46, XX females (30–60-fold), it has been suggested that left heart disease is an independent marker for TS. Accordingly, it has been suggested that all females born with a bicuspid aortic valve or other structural left heart abnormalities, even those without additional features, should prompt genetic assessment for TS [9]. Despite the predilection for left heart malformations in TS, the operative and interventional catheterization outcomes are essentially no different in TS when compared to the general population with the notable exception of hypoplastic left heart syndrome where the results are dismal [40–42]. Therefore, it is reasonable that diagnosis and management of cardiac malformations in those with TS follow the standards of care and the published guidelines established for the general population. A critical exception relates to those with aortic enlargement where the presence or absence of BAV greatly modifies the risk for aortic dissection (discussed below) [43].

Aortic Enlargement and Risk for Dissection

Turner syndrome alone is an independent risk factor for aortic enlargement [44] suggesting that that there is a fundamental connection between X chromosome deficiency and aortopathy [45]. Enlargement of the mid-ascending aorta is common in TS and may be progressive, leading to aneurysm formation and a propensity for dissection and rupture. Aortic dissection typical occurs in young adult women (mean ~31 years) in contrast to euploid females in whom it occurs more rarely and later in life (mean age ~68 years) [46]. Dilation may also occur in the aortic root, proximal head and neck vessels, and descending aorta [31, 35, 36]. The risk for aortic dissection is significantly increased in TS, occurring in approximately 40 per 100,000 person-years compared with 6 per 100,000 years in the general population [6]. A more recent analysis from Sweden suggests a much higher risk, 354 per 100,000 per person-years, which is 12-fold higher than the general female population [47]. Aortic dissection occurs at a younger age than in the general population and at smaller dimensions than with other genetically triggered aortic conditions [48]. Additional risk factors common to TS include BAV, coarctation of the aorta, and hypertension [46, 49]. Pregnancy and assisted reproductive therapies are also of concern [50]. Growth hormone does not appear to promote aortic enlargement [46, 51]. There is also evidence that growth hormone may be protective [47], possibly through favorable effects on aortic wall distensibility [52].

Assessment of Aortic Dimensions

Short stature in Turner syndrome complicates decision-making because the usual tools available to clinicians to normalize aortic dimensions rely on formulae that employ body surface area or height. Consequently, for those of equivalent body size, Z-score calculations referenced to the larger body size of the general population produce higher values than Z-scores referenced to a healthy TS population [53]. Using the general population-based Z-score formulae carries the risk of stigmatizing children with TS, restricting them from sports participation, or subjecting them to potentially unnecessary medical or operative treatments. For these reasons, the use of Turner-specific Z-score formulae (TSZ) [54] have been recommended by both the American Heart Association [9] and the recently published Clinical Practice Guidelines for the Care of Girls and Women with Turner syndrome [55]. An online calculator is available (http://www.parameterz.com/refs/quezada-ajmg-2015). Because of the rarity of aortic dissection in the pediatric population, employing TSZ for risk stratification is based on extrapolation from the adult experience. In adults, an ascending aortic size index [56] (aortic dimensions at the level of the right pulmonary artery divided by body surface area) greater than 2.5 cm/m^2 appears to be a sensitive and specific marker of aortic dissection risk (see Fig. 6.1).

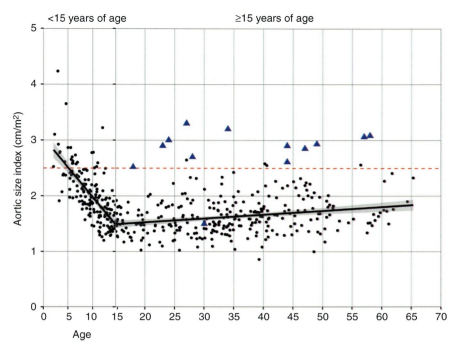

Fig. 6.1 Relationship between ascending aortic size index (ascending ASI) and age in individuals with TS with or without aortic dissection (AoD) modified from three studies [43, 49, 53]. Dots represent measurements determined by transthoracic echocardiography performed at study entry to the "Healthy Heart Project" during the annual meeting of the TS Society of the US between 2003 and 2015 ($n = 458$). For those who were ≥15 years of age ($n = 212$): the mean BSA was 1.62 m^2 and the mean absolute aortic size 2.6 ± 0.4 cm. At the time the study was performed, none of these individuals had either a history of AoD or an elective operation for an aortic aneurysm. Note that subjects <15 years of age with a negative history for AoD frequently have ascending ASI >2.5 cm/m^2 making ASI unreliable as a predictor of AoD in this age group [53]. Triangles represent echocardiographically determined ascending aorta ASI obtained prior to presentation with AoD in 13 individuals with TS reported in two studies [43, 49] (absolute aortic size 4.6 ± 0.7 cm, mean ascending ASI 2.8 ± 0.5 cm/m^2). Dashed line represents an absolute ascending aortic diameter of 4.1 cm, ascending ASI = 2.5 cm/m^2, Turner-specific Z-score [54] = 4 based on the average BSA of 1.62 m^2 for the 212 women ≥15 years of age without aortic dissection (dots). (Modified from Corbitt et al. [53] with permission from Copyright© 2017, John Wiley and Sons)

Medical and Operative Management

There is no published experience of Turner syndrome-specific medical or operative management of aortic aneurysm or dissection. However, there is limited data suggesting that deleterious TGF-β signaling pathways that are known to be active in Marfan syndrome may also play a role in the aortopathy of Turner syndrome [11]. Furthermore, the histologic appearance of the aorta in connective tissue diseases, cystic medial necrosis, is routinely found in TS aorta [6]. Therefore, it is reasonable to consider the use of standard therapies such as beta blocker and/or angiotensin receptor blockers as they have been shown to be beneficial in Marfan syndrome [57]. Decision-making regarding participation in sports must be determined on a case-by-case basis and largely depends on the likelihood that the patient and family will comply with the necessity for those with a significantly enlarged aorta to avoid isometric exercise such as heavy weightlifting and exercise to exhaustion. Detailed suggestions for appropriate sports participation in TS have been published by the American Heart Association [37]. With regard to the operative management for those with significant aortic enlargement, in general, the standards of care set for the non-TS population are appropriate. It is important to remember that, as with all genetically triggered aortopathies, proximal repair may result in extending aneurysmal disease distally. Conversely, placement of non-compliant conduits distal to preserved proximal structures, as in the so-called aortic valve-sparing operations that include the aortic root, can lead to severe sinus enlargement.

Surveillance

As for most genetically triggered aortopathies, Marfan syndrome being the best example, the degree of aortic dilation and aortic growth rate are the key predictors of risk. However, stable aortic diameters are not necessarily reassuring [3]. The risk for aortic dissection and rupture in all cases depends on the interplay of the intrinsic strength of the aortic wall, on the one hand, and the distending forces exerted by the blood flow on the other [58]. Therefore, surveillance and treatment of high blood pressure are critical. The hallmark of TS aortic size surveillance algorithms for TS suggested by the American Heart Association (see Figs. 6.2 and 6.3 below) is making the initial distinction between those with risk factors (BAV, coarctation, and/or hypertension) and those without [9]. For those who are under 15 years of age, TSZ normalization is preferred, and for those equal to or greater than 15 years of age, ascending aortic size index is preferable.

Electrocardiography

Electrocardiographic changes are prevalent in TS, occurring in approximately 50% of affected girls and women [59]. These differences can be classified into waveform changes (i.e., bundle branch block, T-wave or P-wave changes) or variable conduction intervals (i.e., PR shortening or QTc prolongation). Some of these changes may be related to excess sympathetic drive, resulting in an increased heart rate at baseline and accelerated atrioventricular conduction [60]. Others, such as right axis deviation, may signify the presence of underlying structural heart disease (i.e., partial anomalous pulmonary venous return) and should alert the clinician to obtain additional testing.

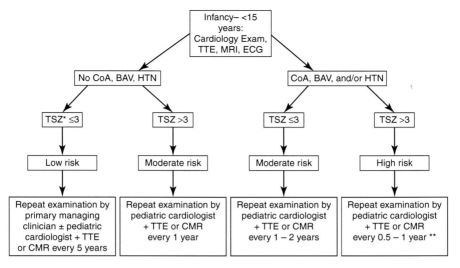

Fig. 6.2 Suggested monitoring protocol for girls with Turner syndrome from infancy to 15 years of age. BAV indicates bicuspid aortic valve, CMR cardiac magnetic resonance, CoA coarctation of the aorta, HTN hypertension, MRI magnetic resonance imaging, TSZ Turner-specific Z-score, and TTE transthoracic echocardiography. *Ascending aorta TSZ [54]. **It is important to remember that surveillance frequency may change with worse disease severity in terms of obstruction, regurgitation, or left ventricular hypertrophy. (Modified from Gravholt et al. [55] with permission from Bioscientifica Limited)

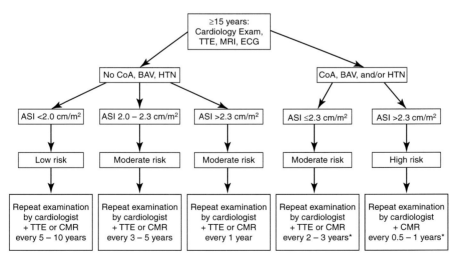

Fig. 6.3 Suggested monitoring protocol for girls and women with Turner syndrome who are ≥15 years of age. ASI indicates aortic size index, BAV bicuspid aortic valve, CMR cardiac magnetic resonance, CoA coarctation of the aorta, HTN hypertension, MRI magnetic resonance imaging, and TTE transthoracic echocardiography. *It is important to remember that surveillance frequency may change with worse disease severity in terms of obstruction, regurgitation, or left ventricular hypertrophy. (Modified from Gravholt et al. [55] with permission from Bioscientifica Limited)

Prolongation of the QT interval is a common phenomenon in TS [61]. Although this finding can be associated with arrhythmias and even sudden death in the general population, there have been no studies to date confirming this occurrence in individuals with TS. According to one study, QTc prolongation was shown to return to normal in up to 40% of ambulatory electrocardiograms and with exercise testing, suggesting that prolonged QTc does not carry an increased risk in TS [62]. Nevertheless, caution should be used when prescribing QTc-prolonging medications in women with TS, and counseling regarding the risks and benefits of such medication should be provided. It may be reasonable to avoid drugs that prolong the QTc altogether. However, if necessary a careful assessment of the QTc interval should be performed before and after initiation of any QTc-prolonging medications, as well as with any increase in dosing. A comprehensive list of QTc-prolonging medications may be found at www.crediblemeds.org.

Hypertension

Hypertension has been reported to occur in 20–40% of children and up to 60% of adult women with TS. Elevated blood pressure may be related to underlying renal anomalies which are common in this cohort or may be idiopathic [22]. Several factors may contribute to hypertension in this population, including the intrinsic shape of the aorta [63] and an underlying arteriopathy characterized by increased arterial stiffness and medial thickness which may result in abnormal vascular compliance and distensibility [64, 65]. Other related causes may include a propensity toward obesity, lack of estrogen, and abnormalities of the renin-angiotensin system.

Abnormal diurnal variation and increased vascular stiffness may result in masked hypertension (i.e., normal blood pressure in clinic but high on ambulatory blood pressure monitoring) [66]. This may contribute to increased left ventricular mass and diastolic dysfunction [67]. Hypertension is also a known risk factor for aortic dissection in TS, and therefore regular blood pressure surveillance should be part of the management plan for all individuals with TS [68]. Ambulatory blood pressure should be considered in children and adults with normal resting blood pressure, especially if there is unexplained left ventricular hypertrophy.

When present, hypertension should be treated promptly. Management is similar to the general population and should include adherence to a healthy diet and incorporation of physical activity into one's daily routine. Identification and treatment of secondary underlying causes such as renal issues abnormalities or coarctation should be pursued. Medical therapy with antihypertensive agents may be needed. Use of β-blockers and/or angiotensin receptor blockers may be preferred as they are effective in slowing aortic growth in other genetically triggered aortopathies [57].

Dyslipidemia and Thrombosis

Ischemic heart disease and stroke are more prevalent in adults with TS than in the general population [1, 2]. Contributing factors include an increase in type 2 diabetes, obesity, and lack of estrogen [69, 70]. Some of these risks are modifiable by following a healthy diet, incorporating regular exercise into one's daily routine, and maintenance of normal body weight. Identification and treatment of hypertension are also of key importance. The predisposition to dyslipidemia may also add to the risk for developing heart disease, and therefore lipids should be assessed in early adulthood. Treatment of dyslipidemia should follow current guidelines in the general population.

An increased risk for thrombus formation in adult women with TS has been suggested [71]. Fibrinogen has been reported to be elevated in 65% of women with TS, and proteins C and S are decreased [72]. However, other studies have found these factors to be within normal range [73], although high-normal procoagulant factors have been reported [74]. Mutations associated with thrombus formation are more frequently reported in TS. For example, Factor V Leiden G1691A gen polymorphism heterozygosity is more prevalent in individuals with TS (13%) than in the general population (2%). These findings do not appear to relate to estrogen replacement, since doses prescribed are within physiologic range [75].

Conclusions

Cardiovascular abnormalities pose a major threat to the lives of girl and women with Turner syndrome. Unfortunately, the responsible disease mechanisms are barely understood. In addition, the suggestions for surveillance and medical and operative management presented here are largely based on extrapolation from what is known about similar but fundamentally different disorders or on general consensus. There are a variety of reasons for the lack of TS clinical and basic evidence: (1) Turner syndrome is rare, making studies at a single site problematic. (2) TS is not inherited (except in rare circumstances), making the identification of research participants difficult because affected individuals do not segregate into families. (3) Overall, those affected do not fit into a single disease state precluding interest within one specific field of research.

One solution to the lack of TS research is the establishment of the Turner Syndrome Research Registry (TSRR) by the Turner Syndrome Society of the USA. This participant-powered registry is recruiting a large cohort from throughout the USA and soon will be making potentially identifiable data available to approved researchers for longitudinal studies [76]. An operating principle of the Registry is that after a period of embargo, new data will be returned to the Registry allowing it to be shared with other investigators. The hope is that this will create a "virtuous cycle" that increases the value of the registry to new investigators and, in turn, make it self-sustaining. While the evidence-based data is currently limited (the ideas and suggestions present in this chapter are limited), it should serve as the beginning of a process that will create quality indicators, structures for implementing standards of care, all leading to definitive outcome studies.

References

1. Stochholm K, Juul S, Juel K, Naeraa RW, Gravholt CH. Prevalence, incidence, diagnostic delay, and mortality in Turner syndrome. J Clin Endocrinol Metab. 2006;91:3897–902.
2. Schoemaker MJ, Swerdlow AJ, Higgins CD, Wright AF, Jacobs PA. Mortality in women with Turner syndrome in Great Britain: a national cohort study. J Clin Endocrinol Metab. 2008;93:4735–42.
3. Fuchs MM, Attenhofer Jost C, Babovic-Vuksanovic D, Connolly HM, Egbe A. Long-term outcomes in patients with Turner syndrome: a 68-year follow-up. J Am Heart Assoc. 2019;8:e011501.
4. Sybert VP. Cardiovascular malformations and complications in Turner syndrome. Pediatrics. 1998;101:E11.
5. Lin AE, Lippe BM, Geffner ME, Gomes A, Lois JF, Barton CW, Rosenthal A, Friedman WF. Aortic dilation, dissection, and rupture in patients with Turner syndrome. J Pediatr. 1986;109:820–6.
6. Gravholt CH, Landin-Wilhelmsen K, Stochholm K, Hjerrild BE, Ledet T, Djurhuus CB, Sylven L, Baandrup U, Kristensen BO, Christiansen JS. Clinical and epidemiological description of aortic dissection in Turner's syndrome. Cardiol Young. 2006;16:430–6.
7. Mortensen KH, Andersen NH, Gravholt CH. Cardiovascular phenotype in Turner syndrome—integrating cardiology, genetics, and endocrinology. Endocr Rev. 2012;33:677–714.
8. Gravholt CH, Juul S, Naeraa RW, Hansen J. Morbidity in Turner syndrome. J Clin Epidemiol. 1998;51:147–58.
9. Silberbach M, Roos-Hesselink JW, Anderson NH, Braverman A, Brown N, Collins RT, De Backer J, Eagle KA, Hirata K, Johnson WHJ, Kadian-Dodov D, Lopez L, Mortensen KH, Prakash SK, Ratchford EV, Saidi A, van Hagen IM, Young LT. Cardiovascular health in Turner syndrome: a scientific statement of the American Heart Association. Circ Genom Precis Med. 2018;11(10):e000048.
10. Sybert VP, McCauley E. Turner's syndrome. N Engl J Med. 2004;351:1227–38.
11. Corbitt H, Gutierrez J, Silberbach M, Maslen CL. The genetic basis of Turner syndrome aortopathy. Am J Med Genet C Semin Med Genet. 2019;181:117–25.
12. Wang L, Ming Wang L, Chen W, Chen X. Bicuspid aortic valve: a review of its genetics and clinical significance. J Heart Valve Dis. 2016;25:568–73.
13. Bondy CA, Matura LA, Wooten N, Troendle J, Zinn AR, Bakalov VK. The physical phenotype of girls and women with Turner syndrome is not X-imprinted. Hum Genet. 2007;121:469–74.
14. Bondy C, Bakalov VK, Cheng C, Olivieri L, Rosing DR, Arai AE. Bicuspid aortic valve and aortic coarctation are linked to deletion of the X chromosome short arm in Turner syndrome. J Med Genet. 2013;50:662–5.
15. Prakash S, Guo D, Maslen CL, Silberbach M, Milewicz D, Bondy CA. Single-nucleotide polymorphism array genotyping is equivalent to metaphase cytogenetics for diagnosis of Turner syndrome. Genet Med. 2014;16:53–9.
16. Corbitt H, Morris SA, Gravholt CH, Mortensen KH, Tippner-Hedges R, Silberbach M, Maslen CL, Gen TACRI. TIMP3 and TIMP1 are risk genes for bicuspid aortic valve and aortopathy in Turner syndrome. PLoS Genet. 2018;14:e1007692.

17. Ikonomidis JS, Gibson WC, Butler JE, McClister DM, Sweterlitsch SE, Thompson RP, Mukherjee R, Spinale FG. Effects of deletion of the tissue inhibitor of matrix metallo-proteinases-1 gene on the progression of murine thoracic aortic aneurysms. Circulation. 2004;110:II268–73.
18. Raznahan A, Parikshak NN, Chandran V, Blumenthal JD, Clasen LS, Alexander-Bloch AF, Zinn AR, Wangsa D, Wise J, Murphy DGM, Bolton PF, Ried T, Ross J, Giedd JN, Geschwind DH. Sex-chromosome dosage effects on gene expression in humans. Proc Natl Acad Sci U S A. 2018;115:7398–403.
19. San Roman AK, Page DC. A strategic research alliance: Turner syndrome and sex differences. Am J Med Genet C Semin Med Genet. 2019;181:59–67.
20. Trolle C, Nielsen MM, Skakkebaek A, Lamy P, Vang S, Hedegaard J, Nordentoft I, Orntoft TF, Pedersen JS, Gravholt CH. Widespread DNA hypomethylation and differential gene expression in Turner syndrome. Sci Rep. 2016;6:34220.
21. Lee S, Lee JW, Lee SK. UTX, a histone H3-lysine 27 demethylase, acts as a critical switch to activate the cardiac developmental program. Dev Cell. 2012;22:25–37.
22. Los E, Quezada E, Chen Z, Lapidus J, Silberbach M. Pilot study of blood pressure in girls with Turner syndrome: an awareness gap, clinical associations, and new hypotheses. Hypertension. 2016;68:133–6.
23. Clark EB. Neck web and congenital heart defects: a pathogenic association in 45 X-O Turner syndrome? Teratology. 1984;29:355–61.
24. Loscalzo ML, Van PL, Ho VB, Bakalov VK, Rosing DR, Malone CA, Dietz HC, Bondy CA. Association between fetal lymphedema and congenital cardiovascular defects in Turner syndrome. Pediatrics. 2005;115:732–5.
25. Hook EB, Warburton D. The distribution of chromosomal genotypes associated with Turner's syndrome: livebirth prevalence rates and evidence for diminished fetal mortality and severity in genotypes associated with structural X abnormalities or mosaicism. Hum Genet. 1983;64:24–7.
26. von Kaisenberg CS, Wilting J, Dörk T, Nicolaides KH, Meinhold-Heerlein I, Hillemanns P, Brand-Saberi B. Lymphatic capillary hypoplasia in the skin of fetuses with increased nuchal translucency and Turner's syndrome: comparison with trisomies and controls. Mol Hum Reprod. 2010;16:778–89.
27. Dumont DJ, Jussila L, Taipale J, Lymboussaki A, Mustonen T, Pajusola K, Breitman M, Alitalo K. Cardiovascular failure in mouse embryos deficient in VEGF receptor-3. Science. 1998;282:946–9.
28. Gotzsche CO, Krag-Olesn B, Nielsen J, Sorensen KE, Kristensen BO. Prevalence of cardiovascular malformations and association with karyotypes in Turner's syndrome. Arch Dis Child. 1994;71:433–6.
29. Sachdev V, Matura LA, Sidenko S, Ho VB, Arai AE, Rosing DR, Bondy CA. Aortic valve disease in Turner syndrome. J Am Coll Cardiol. 2008;51:1904–9.
30. Siu SC, Silversides CK. Bicuspid aortic valve disease. J Am Coll Cardiol. 2010;55:2789–800.
31. Mortensen KH, Hjerrild BE, Andersen NH, et al. Abnormalities of the major intrathoracic arteries in Turner syndrome as revealed by magnetic resonance imaging. Cardiol Young. 2010;20:191–200.
32. De Groote K, Devos D, Van Herck K, et al. Abnormal aortic arch morphology in Turner syndrome patients is a risk factor for hypertension. Heart Vessel. 2015;30:618–25.
33. Gutmark-Little I, Hor KN, Cnota J, Gottliebson WM, Backeljauw PF. Partial anomalous pulmonary venous return is common in Turner syndrome. J Pediatr Endocrinol Metab. 2012;25:435–40.
34. van den Hoven AT, Chelu RG, Duijnhouwer AL, Demulier L, Devos D, Nieman K, Witsenburg M, van den Bosch AE, Loeys BL, van Hagen IM, Roos-Hesselink JW. Partial anomalous pulmonary venous return in Turner syndrome. Eur J Radiol. 2017;95:141–6.
35. Kim HK, Gottliebsen W, Lor K, et al. Cardiovascular anomalies in Turner syndrome: spectrum, prevalence, and cardiac MRI findings in a pediatric and young adult population. AJR. 2011;196:454–60.

36. Ho VB, Bakalov VK, Cooley M, et al. Major vascular anomalies in Turner syndrome: prevalence and magnetic resonance angiographic features. Circulation. 2004;110:1694–700.
37. Viuff MH, Rolle C, Wen J, et al. Coronary artery anomalies in Turner syndrome. J Cardiovasc Comput Tomogr. 2016;10:480–4.
38. Oohara K, Yamazake I, Sakaguchi K, et al. Acute aortic dissection, aortic insufficiency and a single coronary artery in a patient with Turner's syndrome. J Cardiovasc Surg. 1995;36:273–5.
39. Hook EB, Warburton D. Turner syndrome revisited: review of new data supports the hypothesis that all viable 45,X cases are cryptic mosaics with a rescue cell line, implying an origin by mitotic loss. Hum Genet. 2014;133:417–24.
40. Madriago E, Nguyen T, McFerson M, Larson EV, Airhart N, Moller JH, Silberbach M. Frequency and outcomes of cardiac operations and catheter interventions in Turner syndrome. Am J Cardiol. 2012;110:580–5.
41. Chew JD, Soslow JH, Thurm C, Hall M, Dodd DA, Feingold B, Simmons J, Godown J. Heart transplantation in children with Turner syndrome: analysis of a linked dataset. Pediatr Cardiol. 2018;39:610.
42. Lara DA, Ethen MK, Canfield MA, Nembhard WN, Morris SA. A population-based analysis of mortality in patients with Turner syndrome and hypoplastic left heart syndrome using the Texas Birth Defects Registry. Congenit Heart Dis. 2017;12:105–12.
43. Carlson M, Airhart N, Lopez L, Silberbach M. Moderate aortic enlargement and bicuspid aortic valve are associated with aortic dissection in Turner syndrome: report of the international Turner syndrome aortic dissection registry. Circulation. 2012;126:2220–6.
44. Lopez L, Arheart KL, Colan SD, Stein NS, Lopez-Mitnik G, Lin AE, Reller MD, Ventura R, Silberbach M. Turner syndrome is an independent risk factor for aortic dilation in the young. Pediatrics. 2008;121:e1622–7.
45. Ostberg JE, Donald AE, Halcox JP, Storry C, McCarthy C, Conway GS. Vasculopathy in Turner syndrome: arterial dilatation and intimal thickening without endothelial dysfunction. J Clin Endocrinol Metab. 2005;90:5161–6.
46. Carlson M, Silberbach M. Dissection of the aorta in Turner syndrome: two cases and review of 85 cases in the literature. J Med Genet. 2007;44:745–9.
47. Thunstrom S, Krantz E, Thunstrom E, Hanson C, Bryman I, Landin-Wilhelmsen K. Incidence of aortic dissection in Turner syndrome. Circulation. 2019;139:2802–4.
48. Carlson M, Airhart N, Lopez L, Silberbach M. Moderate aortic enlargement and bicuspid aortic valve are associated with aortic dissection in Turner syndrome: report of the International Turner syndrome Aortic Dissection Registry. Circulation. 2012;126:2220–6.
49. Matura LA, Ho VB, Rosing DR, Bondy CA. Aortic dilatation and dissection in Turner syndrome. Circulation. 2007;116:1663–70.
50. Hadnott TN, Gould HN, Garib AM, Bondy CA. Outcomes of spontaneous and assisted pregnancies in Turner syndrome: the U.S. National Institutes of Health experience. Fertil Steril. 2011;95:2251–6.
51. Bondy CA, Van PL, Bakalov VK, Ho VB. Growth hormone treatment and aortic dimensions in Turner syndrome. J Clin Endocrinol Metab. 2006;91:1785–8.
52. van den Berg J, Bannink EM, Wielopolski PA, Pattynama PM, de Muinck Keizer-Schrama SM, Helbing WA. Aortic distensibility and dimensions and the effects of growth hormone treatment in the Turner syndrome. Am J Cardiol. 2006;97:1644–9.
53. Corbitt H, Maslen C, Prakash S, Morris SA, Silberbach M. Allometric considerations when assessing aortic aneurysms in Turner syndrome: implications for activity recommendations and medical decision-making. Am J Med Genet A. 2018;176:277–82.
54. Quezada E, Lapidus J, Shaughnessy R, Chen Z, Silberbach M. Aortic dimensions in Turner syndrome. Am J Med Genet A. 2015;167:2527.
55. Gravholt CH, Andersen NH, Conway GS, Dekkers OM, Geffner ME, Klein KO, Lin AE, Mauras N, Quigley CA, Rubin K, Sandberg DE, Sas TCJ, Silberbach M, Soderstrom-Anttila V, Stochholm K, van Alfen-van der Velden JA, Woelfle J, Backeljauw PF, International Turner Syndrome Consensus Group. Clinical practice guidelines for the care of girls and women

with Turner syndrome: proceedings from the 2016 Cincinnati International Turner Syndrome Meeting. Eur J Endocrinol. 2017;177:G1–G70.

56. Davies RR, Gallo A, Coady MA, Tellides G, Botta DM, Burke B, Coe MP, Kopf GS, Elefteriades JA. Novel measurement of relative aortic size predicts rupture of thoracic aortic aneurysms. Ann Thorac Surg. 2006;81:169–77.

57. Lacro RV, Dietz HC, Sleeper LA, Yetman AT, Bradley TJ, Colan SD, Pearson GD, Selamet Tierney ES, Levine JC, Atz AM, Benson DW, Braverman AC, Chen S, De Backer J, Gelb BD, Grossfeld PD, Klein GL, Lai WW, Liou A, Loeys BL, Markham LW, Olson AK, Paridon SM, Pemberton VL, Pierpont ME, Pyeritz RE, Radojewski E, Roman MJ, Sharkey AM, Stylianou MP, Wechsler SB, Young LT, Mahony L, for the Pediatric Heart Network Investigators. Atenolol versus losartan in children and young adults with Marfan syndrome. N Engl J Med. 2014;371:2061–71.

58. Edwards WD, Leaf DS, Edwards JE. Dissecting aortic aneurysm associated with congenital bicuspid aortic valve. Circulation. 1978;57:1022–5.

59. Bondy CA, Ceniceros I, Van PL, Bakalov VK, Rosing DR. Prolonged rate-corrected QT interval and other electrocardiogram abnormalities in girls with Turner syndrome. Pediatrics. 2006;118:e1220–5.

60. Sozen AB, Cefle K, Kudat H, Ozturk S, Oflaz H, Pamukcu B, Akkaya V, Isguven P, Palanduz S, Ozcan M, Goren T, Guven O. Atrial and ventricular arrhythmogenic potential in Turner syndrome. Pacing Clin Electrophysiol. 2008;31:1140–5.

61. Bondy CA, Van PL, Bakalov VK, Sachdeve V, Malone CA, Ho VB, Rosin DR. Prolongation of the cardiac QTc interval in Turner syndrome. Medicine (Baltimore). 2006;85:75–81.

62. Dalla Pozza R, Bechtold S, Urschel S, Netz H, Schwarz HP. QTc interval prolongation in children with Turner syndrome: the results of exercise testing and 24-h ECG. Eur J Pediatr. 2009;168:59–64.

63. De Groote K, Devos D, Van Herck K, Demulier L, Buysse W, De Schepper J, De Wolf D. Abnormal aortic arch morphology in Turner syndrome patients is a risk factor for hypertension. Heart Vessel. 2015;30:618–25.

64. Fox DA, Kang KT, Potts JE, Bradley TJ, Stewart LL, Dionne JM, Sandor GGS. Non-invasive assessment of aortic stiffness and blood pressure in young Turner syndrome patients. J Pediatr Endocrinol Metab. 2019;32:489–98.

65. Lawson SA, Urbina EM, Gutmark-Little I, Khoury PR, Gao Z, Backeljauw PF. Vasculopathy in the young Turner syndrome population. J Clin Endocrinol Metab. 2014;99:E2039–45.

66. Narayan O, Cameron JD. Ambulatory blood pressure monitoring and dipping status in predicting left ventricular hypertrophy. J Hypertens. 2014;32:1962–3.

67. Mortensen KH, Andersen NH, Hjerrild BE, Horlyck A, Stockhholm K, Hojbjerg Gravholt C. Carotid intima-media thickness is increased in Turner syndrome: multifactorial pathogenesis depending on age, blood pressure, cholesterol and oestrogen treatment. Clin Endocrinol (Oxf). 2012;77:844–51.

68. Flynn JT, Kaelber DC, Baker-Smith CM, Blowey D, Carroll AE, Daniels SR, De Ferranti SD, Dionne JM, Falkner B, Flinn SK, Gidding SS, Goodwin C, Leu MG, Powers ME, Rea C, Samuels J, Simasek M, Thaker VV, Urbina EM, Subcommittee on Screening and Management of High Blood Pressure in Children. Clinical practice guidelines for screening and management of high blood pressure in children and adolescents. Pediatrics. 2017;140:e2017–3035.

69. Van PL, Bakalov VK, Bondy CA. Monosomy for the X- chromosome is associated with an atherogenic lipid profile. J Clin Endocrinol Metab. 2006;91:2867–70.

70. Gravholt CH, Christian Klausen I, Weeke J, Sandahl Christiansen J. Lp(a) and lipids in adult Turner's syndrome: impact of treatment with 17-betaestradiol and norethisterone. Atherosclerosis. 2000;150:201–8.

71. Mortensen KH, Andersen NH, Gravholt CH. Cardiovascular phenotype in Turner syndrome: integrating cardiology, genetics, and endocrinology. Endocr Rev. 2012;33:667–714.

72. Calcaterra V, Gamba G, Montani N, de Silvestri A, Terulla V, Lanati G, Larizza D. Thrombophilic screening in Turner syndrome. J Endocrinol Investig. 2011;34:676–9.

73. Lanes R, Gunczler P, Palacios A, Villareal O. Serum lipids, lipoprotein lp(a) and plasminogen activator inhibitor-1 in patients with Turner's syndrome before and during growth hormone and estrogen therapy. Fertil Steril. 1997;68(4):473–7.
74. Gravholt CH, Mortensen KH, Andersen NH, Ibsen L, Ingergley J, Hjerrid BE. Coagulation and fibrinolytic disturbances are related to carotid intima thickness and arterial blood pressure in Turner syndrome. Clin Endocrinol (Oxf). 2012;76:649–56.
75. Cintron D, Rodriguez-Gutierrez R, Serrano V, Latortue-Albino P, Erwin PJ, Murad MH. Effect of estrogen replacement therapy on bone and cardiovascular outcomes in women with Turner syndrome: a systematic review and meta-analysis. Endocrine. 2017;55:366–75.
76. Prakash SK, Lugo-Ruiz S, Rivera-Davila M, Rubio N Jr, Shah AN, Knickmeyer RC, Scurlock C, Crenshaw M, Davis SM, Lorigan GA, Dorfman AT, Rubin K, Maslen C, Bamba V, Kruszka P, Silberbach M, Scientific Advisory Board of the TSRR. The Turner syndrome research registry: creating equipoise between investigators and participants. Am J Med Genet C Semin Med Genet. 2019;181:135–40.

Chapter 7
Renal Disorders and Systemic Hypertension

Yosuke Miyashita and Joseph T. Flynn

Abbreviations

TS	Turner syndrome
UT	Urinary tract
HTN	Hypertension
VUR	Vesicoureteral reflux
UPJ	Ureteropelvic junction
UVJ	Ureterovesical junction
UTI	Urinary tract infection
VCUG	Voiding cystourethrogram
DMSA	Dimercaptosuccinic acid
MAG3	Mercaptotriglycylglycine
DTPA	Diethylenetriaminepentacetate
CKD	Chronic kidney disease
ESRD	End-stage renal disease
CT	Computed tomography
BP	Blood pressure
ABPM	Ambulatory blood pressure monitoring
LVH	Left ventricular hypertrophy

Y. Miyashita
University of Pittsburgh School of Medicine, Pittsburgh, PA, USA
e-mail: yosuke.miyashita@chp.edu

J. T. Flynn (✉)
University of Washington School of Medicine, Seattle, WA, USA

Division of Nephrology, Seattle Children's Hospital, Seattle, WA, USA
e-mail: joseph.flynn@seattlechildrens.org

© Springer Nature Switzerland AG 2020
P. Y. Fechner (ed.), *Turner Syndrome*,
https://doi.org/10.1007/978-3-030-34150-3_7

Renal Disorders

Prevalence

There have been a number of published single-center retrospective studies from around the world (the United States, Ireland, Turkey, and Brazil) that provide prevalence data about renal malformations in TS females. Based on these studies, a sizeable percentage of TS females have anatomical malformation in the kidney and/or UT. Table 7.1 summarizes these prevalence studies [2–5]. Due to different methodologies and the small numbers of most anomalies, assessing the exact prevalence of individual anomalies is difficult. However, the broad categories of renal anomalies associated with TS can be divided into:

(a) Positional or rotational anomalies such as horseshoe kidney
(b) Collecting system anomalies such as duplicated collecting system and UT dilation

These broad categories will be discussed in detail below.

Three of these prevalence studies [3–5] and one additional study using renal scintigraphy [6] analyzed the rates of renal disorders categorized by monosomy TS versus mosaic/structural X chromosome TS. Table 7.2 summarizes the prevalence of renal/UT anomalies classified by the cytogenetics: 45, X versus mosaic/structural abnormalities. Although no association between specific renal/UT anomalies and karyotypes has been reported, monosomy TS girls and women appear to have more frequent anomalies compared to mosaic/structural X TS.

Anatomic Renal Anomalies

Human kidney development begins as early as the third week of embryonic development and involves a number of complex signaling pathways and transcription factors that coordinate cell differentiation, migration, and proliferation [7]. These signaling pathways and transcription factors may play distinct and different roles depending on the spatial and temporal relationships within the developmental sequence. The most common renal/UT malformations in TS – horseshoe kidney, ectopic kidney which includes malrotated kidney, and renal agenesis – are believed to be caused by one or more abnormal steps in the embryologic sequence.

Horseshoe kidney occurs when the lower poles of the contralateral kidneys are fused either with renal parenchymal tissue or, less commonly, with a fibrous isthmus [8]. Horseshoe kidney with parenchymal isthmus (Fig. 7.1) is thought to occur when there is migration of nephrogenic cells across the primitive streak before the fifth gestational week. In contrast, horseshoe kidney with fibrous isthmus is believed to occur when there is mechanical fusion of the two kidneys at or after the fifth week of gestation before the ascent of kidneys [9]. The horseshoe kidney is usually located

Table 7.1 Prevalence of renal anomalies in TS patients[a]

Study location, publication year	United States, 1988	Ireland, 1996	Turkey, 2000	Brazil, 2010
Number of subjects	141	43	82	123
Imaging technique	IVP (92) Renal ultrasonogram [1] Cardiac catheterization [2]	Renal ultrasonogram (all)	Renal ultrasonogram (all) IVP, DMSA scan, DTPA scan, and VCUG scan if clinically indicated	Renal ultrasonogram (all)
Renal anomalies	Overall prevalence – 33% Duplicated collecting system – 11 Horseshoe kidney – 10 Malrotation – 8 Absent kidney – 2 Crossed ectopia – 3 UPJ obstruction – 3 UVJ obstruction – 2 Aberrant vessels – 2 Pelvic kidney – 1 Multiple renal arteries – 1 Dilated calyx – 1 Extrarenal pelvis – 1	Overall prevalence – 24% Horseshoe kidney – 6 Duplicated collection system – 2 Absent kidney – 1 Renal cysts – 1	Overall prevalence – 38% Horseshoe kidney – 9 Malrotation-positional abnormalities – 5 Duplicated collecting system – 8 Mild hydronephrosis – 6 UPJ obstruction – 2 Megaureter – 1	Overall prevalence – 29% Horseshoe kidney – 11 Abnormal collecting system – 17 Nephrolithiasis – 4 Calcification – 1 Malrotation – 1 Multicystic kidney – 1 VUR – 1

[a]Information adapted from references [2–5]
Abbreviations used in table: *IVP* intravenous pyelogram, *DMSA* dimercaptosuccinic acid, *DTPA* diethylenetriamine penta-acetic acid, *VCUG* voiding cystourethrography, *UPJ* ureteropelvic junction, *UVJ* ureterovesical junction, *VUR* vesicoureteral reflux

in the pelvis or in the lower lumbar region, as it is unable to ascend further above the junction of the aorta and inferior mesenteric artery. The majority of patients with horseshoe kidneys are asymptomatic and have no clinically significant problems, but horseshoe kidneys can be associated with other genitourinary anomalies, including vesicoureteral reflux (VUR) and ureteropelvic junction (UPJ) obstruction, and

Table 7.2 Frequency of renal anomalies according to cytogenetic analysis[a]

Study location, publication year	United States, 1988	Ireland, 1996	Turkey, 2000	Egypt, 2015
45, X	45%	53%	51%	56%
Mosaic/structural X abnormalities	18%	7%	22%	44%

[a]Information adapted from references [3–6]

Fig. 7.1 Horseshoe kidney on three-dimensional reconstruction image from computed tomography urography in excretory phase, courtesy of Judy Squires, MD

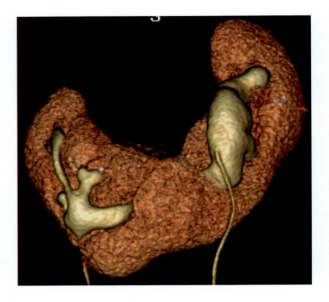

carry a higher risk of nephrolithiasis and infection. Although rarely seen in the pediatric age group, horseshoe kidney has an increased risk of renal tumors compared to normal kidneys, with renal cell carcinoma being the most common in adult case series [10]. A recent adult study with median follow-up period of 9 years reports horseshoe kidney complications of obstruction, kidney stones, urinary tract infection, and urogenital cancer rates of 26, 25, 19, and 4%, respectively [11]. The same report also indicates nearly an eightfold increased risk of developing end-stage renal disease compared to the matched controlled group, suggestive of the need for long-term regular monitoring of horseshoe kidney complications and renal function.

Ectopic kidney and malrotated kidney derive from abnormal ascent from the pelvis and can be either unilateral or bilateral. Fused kidney may occur due to fused ureteric buds or metanephric blastema during embryogenesis. Crossed ectopia occurs when an ectopic kidney's ureter crosses the midline. Often times, the ectopic kidney may be fused with the contralateral kidney resulting in crossed fused ectopic kidney. An ectopic kidney is often hypoplastic and malrotated, with anomalous small blood vessels and ureteric anomalies. Similar to horseshoe kidney, the majority of patients with ectopic kidneys have no clinically significant problems, but they are at slightly higher risk to develop infection and nephrolithiasis due to urinary stasis although no clear data has been reported [12], and ureteral obstruction from either UPJ or ureterovesical junction (UVJ) obstruction has been reported in the 52% of ectopic kidneys with UT dilatation [13].

Ureteral Anomalies

Ureteral duplication may be incomplete or complete. Complete ureteral duplication occurs when there are two separate ureters that continue and enter the bladder separately. Incomplete ureteral duplication is when the ureters join below the UPJ. If the two separate pyelocalyceal systems join at the UPJ, it is considered a bifid pelvis [14]. Individuals with duplicated collecting systems are at increased risk of urinary infection, but the majority of patients are asymptomatic.

UT dilation may occur with both single collecting systems and duplicated collecting systems. Among all neonates with UT dilatation, approximately 90% are due to physiological dilation, UPJ obstruction, VUR, and UVJ obstruction/megaureter with physiological dilatation being the most common [15]. In the typical clinical scenario of TS when diagnosis is made during the second decade of life or later, the latter three etiologies should be strongly considered. UVJ obstruction/megaureter should also show a dilated ureter in addition to collecting system dilation on ultrasonography, while ureters with VUR may or may not be visible on ultrasonography. In general, VUR and ureteral obstructive lesions may be associated with decreased renal mass either due to associated congenital renal dysplasia or due to previous pyelonephritis resulting in renal scarring.

Suggested Approach to Diagnosis and Management of Renal Disorders

Renal Malformations

When the diagnosis of TS occurs later in life, obtaining a detailed renal history will aid in the choice of diagnostic testing and formulation of management plans. (Fig. 7.2)summarizes a suggested approach to follow for evaluation of renal anomalies after making a confirmed diagnosis of TS. Specific history to be ascertained should include any knowledge of prenatal anatomic anomalies of the kidneys and UT, prior diagnosis of urinary tract infection (UTI) especially febrile UTI, unexplained febrile illnesses (could represent undiagnosed UTI), gross hematuria, nephrolithiasis, flank and/or abdominal pain, and history of abnormal blood urea nitrogen or serum creatinine level (if known). Physical exam must include accurate measurement of blood pressure including the use of proper equipment and technique (see

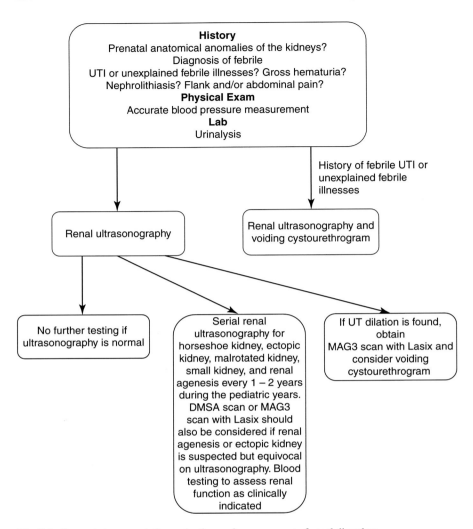

Fig. 7.2 Suggested approach for evaluation and management of renal disorders

following discussion of systemic HTN). Urinalysis should be obtained during this initial evaluation. Given that approximately 1/3 of TS females have renal anomalies, all newly diagnosed TS females should have screening renal ultrasonography, including the bladder. In addition, if they have had febrile UTI or unexplained febrile illnesses that could have been UTI, a voiding cystourethrogram (VCUG) should be considered in addition to ultrasonography to evaluate for VUR. In TS females with a negative renal history, normal blood pressure measurements, normal urinalysis, and normal renal ultrasonography, no further routine imaging or laboratory testing is recommended.

If anatomical anomalies such as horseshoe kidney, ectopic kidney, malrotated kidney, small kidney, and renal agenesis are found on ultrasonography but with no UT dilation and no history of UTI, these patients can be followed by serial ultrasonography mainly for assessment of kidney growth. These anatomical anomalies do have a higher risk of other associated anomalies such as VUR, but if these TS females are in their second decade of their life or older and have been infection free, the authors do not endorse routine VCUG (see below for further discussion). In some suspected cases with ectopic kidney, small kidney, or renal agenesis, renal ultrasonography images may be equivocal, especially in determining whether the renal moiety contains normal functioning parenchyma. In these cases, radionuclide scans such as 99mTc-dimercaptosuccinic acid (DMSA) scan or 99mTc-mercaptotriglycylglycine (MAG3) offer more definitive evaluation. The DMSA scan is a static scan to assess function of kidneys including differential function of the two kidneys and/or detection of decreased renal mass from congenital malformation or from acquired scarring due to pyelonephritis. In contrast, the MAG3 scan, often performed with IV furosemide, is a dynamic scan where ureteral obstructive lesions (see below) can be diagnosed in addition to what DMSA assesses. Blood testing, including electrolytes, blood urea nitrogen, and creatinine may be clinically useful at the time of initial evaluation and in follow-up evaluations especially if there is reduction in renal mass noted on ultrasonography or radionuclide scans. Another suggested time to obtain blood testing is after completion of physical growth, as the estimation of glomerular filtration rate using serum creatinine should not be confounded by changing muscle mass at that point. A recent publication compared renal ultrasonography with another radionuclide scan, 99mTc-diethylenetriaminepentacetate (DTPA) scan, in TS patients, and the study showed ultrasonography being superior in detecting anatomical anomalies where DTPA scan may be more reliable in detecting mild reduction in glomerular filtration rate [6].

Historically, many pediatric nephrologists have recommended barring otherwise healthy children with solitary kidneys from participating in competitive contact sports in attempt to reduce the risk of kidney loss from traumatic injury [16]. However, available data consistently show that the risk of lost kidney due to sports-related trauma is minimal especially when compared to some of the other organ systems, and no catastrophic or surgery-requiring injury occurred out of 23,666 injuries in 4.4 million athlete exposures [16, 17]. Especially when weighing in the health and social benefits of regular exercising, the authors do not endorse the practice of barring children from athletics because of their solitary kidney.

Ureteral Dilatation

UT dilation can be caused by VUR or obstructive lesions such as UPJ obstruction or UVJ obstruction. UPJ obstruction may be asymptomatic or cause intermittent flank pain and/or hematuria. MAG3 scan with IV furosemide will diagnose these ureteral obstructive lesions and can help determine whether urologic surgery is indicated. If MAG3 scan with IV furosemide does not show an obstructive lesion, the decision to obtain VCUG carries some clinical dilemma. Traditionally, children with confirmed VUR were placed on prophylactic antibiotics until they either "grew out" of their VUR or they underwent surgical intervention to repair VUR. The traditional paradigm was that VUR increased the risk of renal scarring from pyelonephritis resulting in reflux nephropathy manifested by hypertension and chronic kidney disease (CKD), including end-stage renal disease (ESRD). By using prophylaxis, the aim was to prevent pyelonephritis and thus reflux nephropathy.

However, more recent randomized trials have demonstrated conflicting results in prophylaxis reducing infection or renal scarring [18–21]. A recent large pediatric randomized, double-blinded, placebo-controlled trial with VUR diagnosed after a first or second febrile or symptomatic UTI showed reduction of infection risk by 50% with prophylactic antibiotics, but there was no difference in incidence of renal scarring, severe scars, or new scars compared to the baseline scan between the prophylaxis group and the placebo group [22]. Given these results, the decision to obtain a VCUG should be made based on individual patient clinical factors such as age (prevalence of VUR decreases with increasing age; VCUG is partially invasive and is easier to perform in infants), UTI history, other UTI risk factors such as constipation and dysfunctional voiding, and open communication with patients and their families about the benefits and risks of VCUG and prophylactic antibiotics.

Nephrolithiasis

One of the major risk factors for nephrolithiasis, particularly in children, is congenital or acquired structural abnormalities that lead to urinary stasis, eventually causing crystallization and stone formation [23]. Given this, there is a theoretical increased risk of nephrolithiasis in TS females, although only case has been reported in the literature [24]. Thus, TS females with known kidney or UT anatomical anomalies presenting with flank and/or abdominal pain, gross hematuria, dysuria, or urgency should be promptly evaluated for nephrolithiasis and infection. Imaging options for diagnosis of nephrolithiasis are mainly ultrasonography and non-contrast helical computed tomography (CT). Ultrasonography can detect radiolucent stones such as uric acid, and it can also diagnose UT obstruction. However, it can sometimes miss stones <5 mm, or ureteral stones. Helical CT has much better sensitivity to detect small nephrolithiasis and is considered the gold standard for nephrolithiasis diagnosis. However, one should weigh the risk of radiation exposure with CT, especially in younger patients. A recent large randomized adult trial in the emergency department showed a higher 6-month cumulative radiation exposure in the initial CT group compared to the initial ultrasonography group while showing no difference in incidence of high-risk diagnoses with complications, serious adverse events, pain scores, return to emergency department visits, or hospitalization [25]. Especially in children, ultrasonography should be used as the first-line imaging modality in nephrolithiasis evaluation for this reason. If obstructive nephrolithiasis is diagnosed, urology should be involved for consideration of surgical management, and nephrology evaluation for metabolic risk factors for stone formation should be obtained.

Neonatal Evaluation

In rare occasions of prenatal diagnosis of TS, renal ultrasonography should be obtained after day of life two or three because UT dilation may not be detected due to extracellular fluid shifts in neonates that may underestimate the degree of dilation. If any renal or UT anomalies are found on ultrasonography, pediatric nephrology or urology should be involved for consideration of further imaging evaluation such as VCUG and MAG3 scan with IV furosemide and biochemical evaluation.

Chronic Kidney Disease

Although the aforementioned anatomical anomalies of the kidney and UT in TS females are well-known, the prevalence of CKD and ESRD is unknown including whether if TS females have higher rates of CKD compared to the general population. Certainly, if TS females are born with reduced nephron mass, they are at increased risk of progression to CKD later in life [26, 27]. In addition, anatomical anomalies such as UPJ obstruction can result in decreased nephron mass even if surgically repaired early in life. Lastly, TS females have higher rates of HTN which can also lead to progression to CKD. Thus, TS patients with the above risk factors for CKD should have monitoring of renal mass with renal ultrasonography and biochemical assessment of renal function every 1 to 2 years. If they have evidence of CKD, they should be routinely followed by a nephrologist and be treated for known contributors to CKD such as HTN and be monitored for other manifestations of CKD, including metabolic acidosis, metabolic bone disease, anemia, and cardiovascular disease.

When CKD progresses to ESRD, dialysis and/or renal transplantation may be needed. At present, there is no consensus on a preferred dialysis modality specific to TS patients. One report suggests peritoneal dialysis as the first-line modality due to theoretical difficulty in creating vascular access either by arteriovenous fistula or placement of cuffed hemodialysis catheter [28]. This is due to higher risk of failure for fistula maturation in post-ductal extremity with coarctation of aorta and generalized dilation of vessels seen in TS females [29]. In contrast, successful peritoneal dialysis management requires well-trained caregivers and appropriate living environment, and infectious peritonitis is a significant risk factor for mortality and morbidity. Thus, the authors advocate an individualized approach for the choice of dialysis modality.

Systemic Hypertension

Diagnosis and Classification of Blood Pressure

A comprehensive discussion of the approach to patients with elevated blood pressure (BP) is beyond the scope of this chapter; however, some basic points regarding diagnosis are important to mention. First, the diagnosis of HTN depends on accurate BP measurement, which has been described in detail elsewhere [30, 31]. Ideally, BP should be measured in the right arm in the seated position after several minutes of rest. In children and adolescents, auscultation is the preferred method of BP measurement, but automated devices may be used for screening [31]. The diagnosis of HTN in children requires documentation of elevated office BPs on three occasions in order to avoid overdiagnosis of HTN [31], but in adults, the diagnosis is made after documented high office BP readings on two occasions [32]. Cuff size is important in both children and adults, as too small of a cuff will result in falsely high BP readings. The high prevalence of obesity in both children and adults means that larger cuffs may need to be used to obtain accurate BP readings given obese patients' increased arm circumferences [33, 34].

Thresholds for identification of elevated BP differ between children and adults; in children, the thresholds vary according to age, gender, and height, whereas in adults, any reading >120/80 is considered elevated, with readings of ≥130/80 considered hypertensive [31, 32]. Once a patient has been confirmed to have elevated BP, the severity of HTN should be staged for both children and adults, according to the classification summarized in Table 7.3. Detailed tables of normal values for BP in children have been published by the American Academy of Pediatrics [31].

Ambulatory blood pressure monitoring (ABPM), a procedure in which the patient's BP is recorded by a wearable device for 24 hours or longer, is becoming increasingly used in both adults and children to confirm the diagnosis of HTN made using office BP measurements [35, 36]. In addition to confirming the diagnosis of

Table 7.3 Approach to classification of blood pressure in TS patients by age

Blood pressure classification	Children aged 1 to 12 years[a]	Adolescents aged ≥13 years and adults[b]
Normal	SBP and DBP < 90th percentile	SBP <120 mmHg and DBP <80 mmHg
Elevated blood pressure	SBP or DBP ≥ 90th percentile to <95th percentile or 120/80 mm Hg to <95th percentile (whichever is lower)	120 to 129/<80 mm Hg
Stage 1 hypertension	SBP or DBP ≥ 95th percentile to <95th percentile +12 mm Hg or 130–139/80–89 mm Hg whichever is lower	130–139/80–89 mm Hg
Stage 2 hypertension	SBP or DBP ≥ 95th percentile +12 mm Hg or ≥ 140/90 mm Hg (whichever is lower)	≥140/90 mm Hg

[a]Adapted from reference [31]
[b]Adapted from reference [32]

HTN based on office measurements, ABPM can identify patients with white coat HTN (elevated office BP but normal BP on ABPM) and masked HTN (normal office BP but elevated BP on ABPM), which have significantly different prognostic implications. In TS patients who have undergone repair of coarctation of the aorta, ABPM should be performed no matter what the office BP level, as they may have a high rate of masked HTN and nocturnal HTN [36, 37].

Prevalence

Adult TS Women

HTN is well-known to be a major risk factor for cardiovascular disease in adult women with TS, although exact prevalence data are difficult to come by [38]. One recent study using office BP measurement only found that 41% of adult TS women were hypertensive [39], while an older study focusing on risk factors for aortic root dilatation found a prevalence of 50% [40]. Cross-sectional studies using ABPM have demonstrated prevalences between 17 and 58% [41, 42]. ABPM in adult TS women consistently demonstrates abnormalities of circadian BP regulation, most notably blunted nocturnal BP dipping [10, 41, 42]. This phenomenon is a well-known risk factor for cardiovascular disease in the general population of adults with HTN [38], so its frequency in women with TS is certainly alarming.

Indeed, HTN in adult women with TS is felt to be a risk factor for aortic root dilatation and also for aortic dissection. Aortic root diameter was significantly associated with systolic BP in the study of Elsheikh et al. [40] and with ambulatory BP in the study of Hjerrild et al., which found that 23% of women studied had dilated aortic roots [21]. HTN has been reported to be present in up to 50% of adult TS patients with aortic dissection [10], although other authors feel that the link between HTN and aortic dissection in TS is not as clear [43]. Despite this uncertainty, HTN is clearly a risk factor for other cardiovascular disease, so appropriate detection and treatment is definitely warranted in the adult TS patient.

Pediatric TS Patients

Fewer data are available on the prevalence of HTN in pediatric TS patients. Mainly this is either because available studies contain a mixture of both pediatric and adult TS patients or because of a lack of sufficient BP measurements to fulfill pediatric criteria for HTN. In an early study of HTN in TS patients aged 2–22 years, elevated BP was found in up to 47% of subjects, with many exhibiting high BP values since childhood [44]. A study of 75 TS girls by Nathwani and colleagues found that over 30% had elevated manual BP readings, and in another study conducted at the Hospital for Sick Children in Toronto, Canada, TS girls were found to have higher office BP than controls; criteria for HTN were not met, however, as BP was measured on just one occasion in both studies [41, 45]. On the other end of the spectrum, no patient was found to be hypertensive in a small group of asymptomatic Korean girls with TS [1].

ABPM has been increasingly applied to the study of BP in pediatric TS and has helped to clarify the extent of abnormal BP. In the study of 75 girls with TS previously mentioned [41], mean BP levels on ABPM were higher than in age-matched normal controls, and approximately 50% had abnormal circadian BP regulation, especially blunted BP dipping. More recently, other investigators have demonstrated that ABPM was superior to manual BP measurements for detection of TS patients with HTN [46, 47] and that abnormal BP dipping in TS is correlated with metabolic indicators of insulin resistance and other markers of subclinical cardiovascular disease [48]. Given these data, the authors recommend that ABPM be obtained as part of the routine cardiovascular evaluation of both pediatric and adult TS patients. At our center, all girls with TS undergo an initial ABPM study and then have periodic repeat ABPM depending on the results of the initial study (Fig. 7.3).

The frequency of aortic root dilatation appears to be lower in pediatric TS patients than in adult TS women, and strong correlations with BP have not been seen. Early work by Lin et al. using echocardiography found that 8.8% of a cohort of TS patients

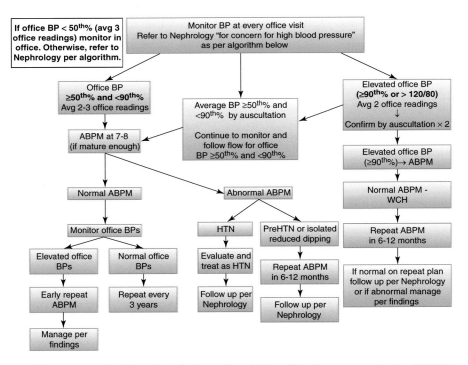

Fig. 7.3 Suggested algorithm for evaluation with ambulatory blood pressure monitoring (ABPM) in females with Turner syndrome/males with 45,X cell line with either normal or elevated office blood pressure, courtesy of Coral Hanevold, MD, Seattle Children's Hospital

had dilated aortic roots, most of whom had other structural heart defects such as bicuspid aortic valve [49]. More recently, Cleemann et al. found that only 12% of a carefully studied population of pediatric and young adult TS patients (mean age 17 ± 3 years) had dilated aortic roots and that aortic root dilatation was best correlated with a history of aortic coarctation [50]. Aortic dissection in the pediatric TS patient appears to be a rare event, with only a few case reports in the literature [49]. However, in a recent age-matched prospective cohort study of young women aged 8–25 years, Fox et al. found 16 out of 21 TS patients to have abnormal ABPM, dilated proximal aortas when scaled for height, and stiffer aortas by pulse wave velocity when compared to age-matched controls [47]. Therefore, careful screening for HTN should clearly be part of the routine care of pediatric TS patients, as early identification and treatment may prevent complications later in life.

Pathophysiology

Aside from those with unrepaired aortic coarctation and advanced CKD, HTN in TS patients appears to occur independently of cardiac and renal abnormalities [41]. Obesity is common in both TS and non-TS females, and similar mechanisms are probably operative in obese TS females as in obese females without TS [38]. Other factors that have been cited as contributing to HTN in TS include use of estrogen and growth hormone, yet the data on the effects of these hormonal therapies are not clear. Studies of hormonal replacement therapy in TS have tended to show adverse effects on glucose metabolism, but the effects on BP and other parameters of cardiovascular risk have not been consistent [51, 52]. Growth hormone may have an effect of increasing systolic BP in TS girls [53], but this effect has not been universally seen, and no adverse effects on left ventricular hypertrophy have been observed [54].

What is more likely is that HTN in TS is the result of a diffuse vasculopathy, which may lead to HTN in the absence of other pathogenic mechanisms. In addition to enlargement of the aortic root (see above), a variety of other abnormalities of vascular structure and function have been demonstrated in TS patients, including impaired flow-mediated dilatation and increased intimal-medial thickness [55, 56]. The increased occurrence of HTN years after repair of coarctation in TS is further indirect evidence of this concept.

Evaluation and Management

A comprehensive discussion of the evaluation and management of HTN is beyond the scope of this chapter. However, some points pertinent to HTN in TS are worth emphasizing.

Patient Evaluation

BP should be measured according to the guidelines previously discussed [30, 31]. In addition to carefully measured office BP, ABPM should be performed at least in TS patients who have a history of repaired aortic coarctation, bicuspid aortic valve, or other known cardiac abnormalities. TS patients with obesity should also undergo ABPM, as should those with a history of a renal anomaly. ABPM should be interpreted according to age-appropriate criteria [48, 57].

Basic laboratory studies including urinalysis and electrolytes/BUN/creatinine should be obtained in all patients; additional studies to further delineate cardiovascular risk include lipid profile, serum uric acid, and fasting glucose, especially in the obese. Renal ultrasonography should be obtained in those with no known history of a renal malformation but with abnormal urinalysis or renal function and in hypertensive TS patients ≤6 years of age. Echocardiography, if not recently done, should be ordered to evaluate for target organ effects of hypertension such as left ventricular hypertrophy (LVH) and/or aortic root dilatation. Cardiac MRI has emerged as a potentially superior modality for identification of aortic root dilatation [10, 42] and can also be used to assess for LVH.

Treatment of Hypertension

Once a diagnosis of HTN has been confirmed, lifestyle changes including dietary sodium restriction, weight loss when appropriate, and increased physical activity should be instituted, no matter what age the patient may be and no matter whether antihypertensive medications are prescribed. Although specific studies in patients with TS are lacking, all of these measures have robust evidence bases in the general HTN population and are logical to include in the management of HTN in TS.

Antihypertensive medications are generally prescribed in hypertensive adults once the diagnosis of HTN has been made and lifestyle changes have proven ineffective. In TS women, the case has been made that antihypertensive medications should be initiated at a lower BP level than in the general population if there is a history of any cardiac abnormality and that lower BP targets are reasonable in such individuals [14]. Clearly if there is any evidence of CKD, a lower threshold for initiating treatment and lower BP goal should be followed in TS as in any adult with CKD [58]. Prior recommendations for the use of hydrochlorothiazide as the preferred initial agent in most hypertensive adults have been recently revised, and other classes of antihypertensive medications are now recommended [59].

In children specific criteria are usually required for the initiation of antihypertensive medications. These have been reviewed in detail elsewhere [31, 60]. Choice of medication is generally left up to the individual clinician in children and adolescents, but care must be taken to prescribe agents with FDA-approved pediatric labeling and to consider specific side effect profiles that may differ from those seen in adults [60]. As in adult patients with TS, the presence of cardiac complications or CKD in a pediatric TS patient would warrant initiation of medication treatment at a lower BP and use of a lower BP target during therapy. At our center we have also been treating masked HTN found on ABPM for the reasons outlined earlier.

References

1. Lee SH, Jung JM, Song MS, Choi S, Chung WY. Evaluation of cardiovascular anomalies in patients with asymptomatic turner syndrome using multidetector computed tomography. J Korean Med Sci. 2013;28(8):1169–73.
2. Carvalho AB, Guerra Junior G, Baptista MT, de Faria AP, Marini SH, Guerra AT. Cardiovascular and renal anomalies in Turner syndrome. Rev Assoc Med Bras. 2010;56(6):655–9.
3. Lippe B, Geffner ME, Dietrich RB, Boechat MI, Kangarloo H. Renal malformations in patients with Turner syndrome: imaging in 141 patients. Pediatrics. 1988;82(6):852–6.
4. Flynn MT, Ekstrom L, De Arce M, Costigan C, Hoey HM. Prevalence of renal malformation in Turner syndrome. Pediatr Nephrol. 1996;10(4):498–500.
5. Bilge I, Kayserili H, Emre S, Nayir A, Sirin A, Tukel T, et al. Frequency of renal malformations in Turner syndrome: analysis of 82 Turkish children. Pediatr Nephrol. 2000;14(12):1111–4.
6. Hamza RT, Shalaby MH, Hamed LS, Abdulla DB, Elfekky SM, Sultan OM. Renal anomalies in patients with turner syndrome: is scintigraphy superior to ultrasound? Am J Med Genet A. 2016;170(2):355–62.
7. Reidy KJ, Rosenblum ND. Cell and molecular biology of kidney development. Semin Nephrol. 2009;29(4):321–37.
8. Limwongse C. Developmental syndromes and malformations of the urinary tract. In: Avner ED, Harmon WE, Niaudet P, Yoshikawa N, Emma F, Goldstein SL, editors. Pediatric nephrology. 7th ed. Berlin: Springer; 2014.
9. Domenech-Mateu JM, Gonzalez-Compta X. Horseshoe kidney: a new theory on its embryogenesis based on the study of a 16-mm human embryo. Anat Rec. 1988;222(4):408–17.
10. Stimac G, Dimanovski J, Ruzic B, Spajic B, Kraus O. Tumors in kidney fusion anomalies–report of five cases and review of the literature. Scand J Urol Nephrol. 2004;38(6):485–9.
11. Kang M, Kim YC, Lee H, Kim DK, Oh KH, Joo KW, et al. Renal outcomes in adult patients with horseshoe kidney. Nephrol Dial Transplant. 2019. https://doi.org/10.1093/ndt/gfz217.
12. Cinman NM, Okeke Z, Smith AD. Pelvic kidney: associated diseases and treatment. J Endourol. 2007;21(8):836–42.
13. Gleason PE, Kelalis PP, Husmann DA, Kramer SA. Hydronephrosis in renal ectopia: incidence, etiology and significance. J Urol. 1994;151(6):1660–1.
14. Rodriguez MM. Congenital anomalies of the kidney and the urinary tract (CAKUT). Fetal Pediatr Pathol. 2014;33(5–6):293–320.
15. Nguyen HT, Benson CB, Bromley B, Campbell JB, Chow J, Coleman B, et al. Multidisciplinary consensus on the classification of prenatal and postnatal urinary tract dilation (UTD classification system). J Pediatr Urol. 2014;10(6):982–98.
16. Grinsell MM, Showalter S, Gordon KA, Norwood VF. Single kidney and sports participation: perception versus reality. Pediatrics. 2006;118(3):1019–27.
17. Grinsell MM, Butz K, Gurka MJ, Gurka KK, Norwood V. Sport-related kidney injury among high school athletes. Pediatrics. 2012;130(1):e40–5.
18. Garin EH, Olavarria F, Garcia Nieto V, Valenciano B, Campos A, Young L. Clinical significance of primary vesicoureteral reflux and urinary antibiotic prophylaxis after acute pyelonephritis: a multicenter, randomized, controlled study. Pediatrics. 2006;117(3):626–32.
19. Pennesi M, Travan L, Peratoner L, Bordugo A, Cattaneo A, Ronfani L, et al. Is antibiotic prophylaxis in children with vesicoureteral reflux effective in preventing pyelonephritis and renal scars? A randomized, controlled trial. Pediatrics. 2008;121(6):e1489–94.
20. Montini G, Rigon L, Zucchetta P, Fregonese F, Toffolo A, Gobber D, et al. Prophylaxis after first febrile urinary tract infection in children? A multicenter, randomized, controlled, noninferiority trial. Pediatrics. 2008;122(5):1064–71.
21. Craig JC, Simpson JM, Williams GJ, Lowe A, Reynolds GJ, McTaggart SJ, et al. Antibiotic prophylaxis and recurrent urinary tract infection in children. N Engl J Med. 2009;361(18):1748–59.
22. Hoberman A, Chesney RW. Antimicrobial prophylaxis for children with vesicoureteral reflux. N Engl J Med. 2014;371(11):1072–3.
23. Milliner DS, Murphy ME. Urolithiasis in pediatric patients. Mayo Clin Proc. 1993;68(3):241–8.

24. Francois I, Proesmans W, de Zegher F. Case of the month: a girl with Ullrich-Turner syndrome, nephrolithiasis and hypercalcaemia. Eur J Pediatr. 1996;155(7):615–6.
25. Smith-Bindman R, Aubin C, Bailitz J, Bengiamin RN, Camargo CA Jr, Corbo J, et al. Ultrasonography versus computed tomography for suspected nephrolithiasis. N Engl J Med. 2014;371(12):1100–10.
26. Brenner BM, Garcia DL, Anderson S. Glomeruli and blood pressure. Less of one, more the other? Am J Hypertens. 1988;1(4 Pt 1):335–47.
27. Brenner BM, Chertow GM. Congenital oligonephropathy and the etiology of adult hypertension and progressive renal injury. Am J Kidney Dis. 1994;23(2):171–5.
28. Liu WS, Li SY, Yang WC, Chen TW, Lin CC. Dialysis modality for patients with Turner syndrome and renal failure. Perit Dial Int. 2012;32(2):230–2.
29. Bondy CA. Care of girls and women with Turner syndrome: a guideline of the Turner Syndrome Study Group. J Clin Endocrinol Metab. 2007;92(1):10–25.
30. Pickering TG, Hall JE, Appel LJ, Falkner BE, Graves J, Hill MN, et al. Recommendations for blood pressure measurement in humans and experimental animals: part 1: blood pressure measurement in humans: a statement for professionals from the Subcommittee of Professional and Public Education of the American Heart Association Council on High Blood Pressure Research. Hypertension. 2005;45(1):142–61.
31. Flynn JT, Kaelber DC, Baker-Smith CM, Blowey D, Carroll AE, Daniels SR, et al. Clinical practice guideline for screening and management of high blood pressure in children and adolescents. Pediatrics. 2017;140(3):e20171904.
32. Chobanian AV, Bakris GL, Black HR, Cushman WC, Green LA, Izzo JL Jr, et al. The seventh report of the joint national committee on prevention, detection, evaluation, and treatment of high blood pressure: the JNC 7 report. JAMA. 2003;289(19):2560–72.
33. Ostchega Y, Hughes JP, Prineas RJ, Zhang G, Nwankwo T, Chiappa MM. Mid-arm circumference and recommended blood pressure cuffs for children and adolescents aged between 3 and 19 years: data from the National Health and Nutrition Examination Survey, 1999–2010. Blood Press Monit. 2014;19(1):26–31.
34. Ostchega Y, Hughes JP, Zhang G, Nwankwo T, Chiappa MM. Mean mid-arm circumference and blood pressure cuff sizes for U.S. adults: National Health and Nutrition Examination Survey, 1999-2010. Blood Press Monit. 2013;18(3):138–43.
35. Pickering TG, Shimbo D, Haas D. Ambulatory blood-pressure monitoring. N Engl J Med. 2006;354(22):2368–74.
36. Flynn JT, Urbina EM. Pediatric ambulatory blood pressure monitoring: indications and interpretations. J Clin Hypertens (Greenwich). 2012;14(6):372–82.
37. O'Sullivan J. Late hypertension in patients with repaired aortic coarctation. Curr Hypertens Rep. 2014;16(3):421.
38. De Groote K, Demulier L, De Backer J, De Wolf D, De Schepper J, T'Sjoen G, et al. Arterial hypertension in Turner syndrome: a review of the literature and a practical approach for diagnosis and treatment. J Hypertens. 2015;33(7):1342–51.
39. De Groote K, Cools M, De Schepper J, Craen M, Francois I, Devos D, et al. Cardiovascular pathology in males and females with 45,X/46,XY mosaicism. PLoS One. 2013;8(2):e54977.
40. Elsheikh M, Casadei B, Conway GS, Wass JA. Hypertension is a major risk factor for aortic root dilatation in women with Turner's syndrome. Clin Endocrinol. 2001;54(1):69–73.
41. Nathwani NC, Unwin R, Brook CG, Hindmarsh PC. The influence of renal and cardiovascular abnormalities on blood pressure in Turner syndrome. Clin Endocrinol. 2000;52(3):371–7.
42. Hjerrild BE, Mortensen KH, Sorensen KE, Pedersen EM, Andersen NH, Lundorf E, et al. Thoracic aortopathy in Turner syndrome and the influence of bicuspid aortic valves and blood pressure: a CMR study. J Cardiovasc Magn Reson. 2010;12:12.
43. Bondy CA. Aortic dissection in Turner syndrome. Curr Opin Cardiol. 2008;23(6):519–26.
44. Virdis R, Cantu MC, Ghizzoni L, Ammenti A, Nori G, Volta C, et al. Blood pressure behaviour and control in Turner syndrome. Clin Exp Hypertens A. 1986;8(4–5):787–91.

45. O'Gorman CS, Syme C, Lang J, Bradley TJ, Wells GD, Hamilton JK. An evaluation of early cardiometabolic risk factors in children and adolescents with Turner syndrome. Clin Endocrinol. 2013;78(6):907–13.
46. Fudge EB, Constantacos C, Fudge JC, Davenport M. Improving detection of hypertension in girls with turner syndrome using ambulatory blood pressure monitoring. Horm Res Paediatr. 2014;81(1):25–31.
47. Fox DA, Kang KT, Potts JE, Bradley TJ, Stewart LL, Dionne JM, et al. Non-invasive assessment of aortic stiffness and blood pressure in young Turner syndrome patients. J Pediatr Endocrinol Metab. 2019;32(5):489–98.
48. Akyurek N, Atabek ME, Eklioglu BS, Alp H. Ambulatory blood pressure and subclinical cardiovascular disease in children with turner syndrome. Pediatr Cardiol. 2014;35(1):57–62.
49. Lin AE, Lippe BM, Geffner ME, Gomes A, Lois JF, Barton CW, et al. Aortic dilation, dissection, and rupture in patients with Turner syndrome. J Pediatr. 1986;109(5):820–6.
50. Cleemann L, Mortensen KH, Holm K, Smedegaard H, Skouby SO, Wieslander SB, et al. Aortic dimensions in girls and young women with turner syndrome: a magnetic resonance imaging study. Pediatr Cardiol. 2010;31(4):497–504.
51. Gravholt CH, Naeraa RW, Nyholm B, Gerdes LU, Christiansen E, Schmitz O, et al. Glucose metabolism, lipid metabolism, and cardiovascular risk factors in adult Turner's syndrome. The impact of sex hormone replacement. Diabetes Care. 1998;21(7):1062–70.
52. Giordano R, Forno D, Lanfranco F, Manieri C, Ghizzoni L, Ghigo E. Metabolic and cardiovascular outcomes in a group of adult patients with Turner's syndrome under hormonal replacement therapy. Eur J Endocrinol. 2011;164(5):819–26.
53. Radetti G, Crepaz R, Milanesi O, Paganini C, Cesaro A, Rigon F, et al. Cardiac performance in Turner's syndrome patients on growth hormone therapy. Horm Res. 2001;55(5):240–4.
54. Sas TC, Cromme-Dijkhuis AH, de Muinck Keizer-Schrama SM, Stijnen T, van Teunenbroek A, Drop SL. The effects of long-term growth hormone treatment on cardiac left ventricular dimensions and blood pressure in girls with Turner's syndrome. Dutch Working Group on Growth Hormone. J Pediatr. 1999;135(4):470–6.
55. Ostberg JE, Donald AE, Halcox JP, Storry C, McCarthy C, Conway GS. Vasculopathy in Turner syndrome: arterial dilatation and intimal thickening without endothelial dysfunction. J Clin Endocrinol Metab. 2005;90(9):5161–6.
56. Radetti G, Mazzanti L, Di Somma C, Salerno M, Gottardi E, Capalbo D, et al. Evaluation of function and structure of arterial wall in girls and young women with Turner syndrome. J Endocrinol Investig. 2015;38(9):963–70.
57. Flynn JT, Daniels SR, Hayman LL, Maahs DM, McCrindle BW, Mitsnefes M, et al. Update: ambulatory blood pressure monitoring in children and adolescents: a scientific statement from the American Heart Association. Hypertension. 2014;63(5):1116–35.
58. KDIGO. Clinical practice guideline for the management of blood pressure in chronic kidney disease. Kidney Int Suppl. 2012;2(5):343.
59. Weber MA, Schiffrin EL, White WB, Mann S, Lindholm LH, Kenerson JG, et al. Clinical practice guidelines for the management of hypertension in the community: a statement by the American Society of Hypertension and the International Society of Hypertension. J Clin Hypertens (Greenwich). 2014;16(1):14–26.
60. Ferguson MA, Flynn JT. Rational use of antihypertensive medications in children. Pediatr Nephrol. 2014;29(6):979–88.

Chapter 8
Endocrine and Metabolic Consequences of Turner Syndrome

Mette H. Viuff and Claus H. Gravholt

Introduction

Women with Turner syndrome (TS) have a considerable decrease in life expectancy with a standardized mortality ratio of 2.86 (95% CI, 2.18–3.55) [1]. This is caused by the several comorbidities seen in Turner syndrome of which endocrine disorders are a substantial part. The overall relative risk of developing endocrine diseases in TS is 4.87 (95% CI, 3.63–6.41) [2]. The endocrine conditions range from metabolic syndrome, diabetes, altered lipid metabolism, and impaired bone metabolism, including osteoporosis, to autoimmune diseases including thyroid disorders, celiac disease, and inflammatory bowel disease.

Turner syndrome is a complex condition and several issues have to be considered when taking care of these girls and women. In the clinical practice of Turner syndrome, a careful monitoring of glucose and bone metabolism, weight, thyroid function, bone mineral density, and blood pressure should be performed.

In the following we will discuss the endocrine issues that girls and women with TS are at increased risk of developing. Through a review of literature we will aim at

M. H. Viuff
Department of Endocrinology and Medical Research Laboratories, Aarhus University Hospital, Aarhus, Denmark
e-mail: metteviuff@clin.au.dk

C. H. Gravholt (✉)
Department of Endocrinology and Internal Medicine, Aarhus University Hospital, Aarhus, Denmark

Department of Molecular Medicine, Aarhus University Hospital, Aarhus, Denmark

Department of Endocrinology and Internal Medicine and Medical Research Laboratories, Aarhus University Hospital, Aarhus, Denmark
e-mail: ch.gravholt@dadlnet.dk

© Springer Nature Switzerland AG 2020
P. Y. Fechner (ed.), *Turner Syndrome*,
https://doi.org/10.1007/978-3-030-34150-3_8

elucidating the pathophysiology behind each condition and present estimates of prevalence and incidence. Furthermore we will attempt to provide information on diagnosis and treatment of these disorders, thus ensuring that caregivers will be properly informed and prepared to handle the screening and treatment of Turner syndrome in regard to endocrine and metabolic issues.

Thyroid Disease – Epidemiology and Clinical Aspects

Thyroid dysfunction is common in Turner syndrome. The main etiology behind is autoimmune hypothyroidism [3–6], with a prevalence of Hashimoto's disease between 30% and 50% [4, 7, 8] and increasing with advancing age, such that about 50% of a given Turner syndrome population will have clinical or subclinical hypothyroidism by the age of 50 years [4]. The presence of TPO antibodies is even more frequent, with 40–45% of women with Turner syndrome having TPO antibodies in their bloodstream [3, 8].

Especially those with an isochromosome X karyotype (i(Xq)) are particular at risk of thyroid dysfunction [3], although other studies have presented data showing no correlation between percentage of cells with a 45,X karyotype and the number of patients with hypothyroidism [4]. Hence the risk of developing hypothyroidism appears to be present in all Turner karyotypes including mosaicisms.

It is well-known that hypothyroidism increases with advanced age, female karyotype, and a positive family history of hypothyroidism. Furthermore it is associated with other autoimmune conditions such as type 1 diabetes and coeliac disease. But when matching all these risk factors, the incidence of thyroid dysfunction is still drastically higher in Turner syndrome compared to 46,XX women. It remains a scientifically enigma why autoimmune diseases and especially hypothyroidism is more common in women with Turner syndrome.

Several hypotheses have been proposed. One correlated to the ovarian dysfunction and lack of estrogen and/or androgen synthesis [7]. Interestingly, premature ovarian failure in general, especially due to endometriosis, is also associated with thyroid disorders and elevated TPO antibody concentrations [9]. In one study, Hashimoto's thyroiditis was prevalent in respectively 37% of patients with Turner syndrome and 15% of 46,XX women suffering from primary ovarian insufficiency [7]. This implies that ovarian dysgenesis somehow may promote thyroid autoimmunity, but is not the sole reason.

Another hypothesis proposes that the absence of a second X-chromosome may contribute to increased autoimmunity in TS – called the haploinsufficiency hypothesis. The haploinsufficiency hypothesis is based on the fact that the development of autoimmune disorders, such as autoimmune thyroid disease, is characterized by a higher X-chromosome monosomy rate in peripheral B and T cells [10, 11].

The isochromosome Xq is a relatively common rearrangement in which long arm (Xq) duplicates are fused together head to head, with deletion of the short arm.

This creates a karyotype that is monosomic for Xp and trisomic for Xq. Women with isochromosome X are more prone to develop autoimmune disorders along with thyroid diseases [12].

The cause of the thyroid dysfunction in women with Turner syndrome thus seems to be multifactorial and probably not explained alone by lack of genes, estrogen/androgen deficit, or age.

Viewing the clinical aspect, levels of TSH, free T3, and free T4 were in one study significantly higher in Turner syndrome patients, with levels of total T4 and T3 being comparable to 46,XX women [13]. This was partly supported by research finding a significantly higher level of TSH, while free T4 was comparable to controls [4]. Turner syndrome women seem often to suffer from compensated hypothyreosis, before progressing into overt hypothyreosis. Therefore monitoring of the thyroid function is recommended on a yearly basis.

Other Autoimmune Diseases – Epidemiology and Clinical Aspects

As mentioned, women with TS are at increased risk of developing a wide range of autoimmune diseases (AID) [2, 4, 14–17]. The overall risk of autoimmune disease among women with Turner syndrome was twice that among Danish women in general (SIR 2.1 [95% CI 1.6–2.7]) [18]. For autoimmune diseases with a female predominance, the SIR among women with Turner syndrome was 1.7 (95% CI 1.2–2.4), whereas the SIR for autoimmune diseases with a male predominance among these women was 3.9 (95% CI 2.5–5.8). Women with Turner's syndrome are at excess risk of autoimmune diseases, notably autoimmune diseases characterized by male predominance [18].

The most common are autoimmune thyroid diseases [2, 3, 19], diabetes mellitus [2, 18, 20], inflammatory bowel disease [15, 21] like ulcerative colitis [18, 20], and Crohn's disease [2, 18, 20, 22] along with coeliac disease [18, 20, 23–25]. Also rheumatoid arthritis [2, 18, 20, 26, 27], psoriasis, vitiligo, and alopecia areata [2, 14, 16, 18, 20, 28, 29] are seen in TS.

Haploinsufficiency for X-chromosome-related genes likely plays a prominent role in pathogenesis of autoimmune conditions [10]. A Danish study found a 2–3-fold increased risk of autoimmune disease development independent of karyotype (X monosomy, isochromosome Xq, and 45,X/46,XX mosaicism) and in spite of different phenotypic expression [18]. However isochromosome Xq seems to be related to a higher frequence of thyroid autoimmunity and inflammatory bowel disease compared to other karyotypes [3, 15, 17].

Another study compared TS women to 46,XX women with primary ovarian insufficiency (POI). 50% of women with TS and 20% of women with idiopathic POI was affected by at least one autoimmune disease, suggesting that karyotype plays a role independent of gonadal functioning [7].

One of the genes located on the X-chromosome with possible immune regulatory functions is FOXP3. This gene encodes a transcription factor critical for the function of natural regulatory T cells that suppress autoreactive T cell in the periphery [30].

Autoantibodies (against gliadin, transglutaminase, adrenal cortex, intrinsic factor, antithyroid peroxidase (anti-TPO), and glutamic acid decarboxylase 65 (GAD-65)) have been found in 58% of TS women investigated [8]. TS patients with autoantibodies were significantly older than those without. 18% presented with coeliac disease autoantibodies, of which 26% had coeliac disease. Among four patients with anti-GAD-65 none had T1DM, but two were classified as having T2DM. One patient had adrenocortical autoantibodies but not adrenal failure. Anti-GAD-65 was increased in isochromosomal karyotypes with no other association found between autoantibodies and karyotype [8].

MHC (major histocompatibility complex) alleles play a significant role in the pathogeneses of AID [31].

One of these MHC paralogues is located in the long arm of the X-chromosome, so that people defective in this region, like TS, are less efficient in controlling immune adaptions during the life span [32]. Hence, women with TS are more likely to develop immune-mediated disorders. The following HLA alleles in TS have an association with underlying AID: HLA-B14 is associated with 21-hydroxylase mutation [33]. HLA-Cw6-positive subjects are likely to present with halo nevi and vitiligo [34]. HLA-DRB1*0301 is associated with autoimmune thyroid disease after infection with *Helicobacter pylori* [35]. A positive association exists between the presence of autoantibodies and HLA-DR7;DQ2 and HLA-DR7;DQ9 haplotypes in Turner patients and fathers [36].

TS women represent a unique immunological population, different from matched 46,XX women. The most significant immune abnormalities are low levels of immunoglobulin G and M subclasses [37], weak chemotaxis of polymorphonucleates [38], low CD4/CD8 ratio [38], high CD16+ natural killer cell count [39], and impaired T-cell response to mitogens [39]. Serum levels of pro-inflammatory cytokines IL6 and TGF β1 are approximately twofold higher in TS compared to POI and normal 46,XX women, while serum levels of anti-inflammatory cytokines TGF β2 and IL10 are decreased [7].

Inflammatory bowel diseases (IBD) like ulcerative colitis and Crohn's disease are more frequent in Turner syndrome with a pooled relative risk of 2.25 (0.61–5.75) [2]. A relative risk of 3.9 (2.3–6.1) [20] has been reported for ulcerative colitis and a SIR of 2.5 (1.2–4.7) [18]. Crohn's disease has a SIR of 1.5 (0.4–3.9) [18] and a RR between 2.25 and 5.3 (0.61–7.8) [2, 20]. There are a few details that distinguish inflammatory bowel diseases in TS to that of non-TS population. Crohn's disease usually involves the colon and appears to be twice as common as ulcerative colitis; they develop at younger age, are often severe and complicated with fistulae, and require colectomy [32]. Inflammatory bowel diseases seem to be more related to the presence of an abnormal X-chromosome than to its absence. Among TS women with isochromosome Xq karyotype, one study found an almost 11.6-fold increased risk of ulcerative colitis [18]. IBD should be suspected in girls and women with TS in case of unexplained weight loss, diarrhea, anemia, abdominal pain, or gastrointestinal bleeding.

The relative risk of developing celiac disease in Turner syndrome in comparison with the background population has found to be 14.0 (10.2–18.8) [20] and an incidence ratio of 2.7 (0.2–11.7) has been reported [18]. A recent study demonstrated that the risk of CD in females with TS increases substantially with age. Odds ratio ranged from twofold in the first 5 years of life to a fivefold increase in females aged >10 years at CD diagnosis [25]. Celiac disease may deteriorate the short stature, hypogonadism, and osteoporosis, already seen in TS [32]. An Italian study found a prevalence of 6.4% in TS patients, however in 60% of these cases presented with a subclinical picture, either completely asymptomatic or with atypical symptoms, which suggests that routine screening is necessary to avoid the diagnostic delay [40].

The relation between Turner syndrome and dermatological diseases has been poorly investigated. Psoriasis has been found to have a RR between 2.3 and 5.4 (0.06–12.51)) [2, 20] and a SIR of 1.6 (0.4–4.2) [18].

In a recent epidemiological study based on 2459 women with TS, alopecia areata was reported to have RR of 20.4 (2.5–75.0) in comparison to the control cohort; however this finding was only based on two cases [20]. Vitiligo has been reported in several cases of TS; however a report of 72 cases of TS found a prevalence of 2.77%, but this finding was insignificant [34]. Karyotype is not likely to have effect on described skin abnormalities. Vulvar lichen sclerosis is also more frequent among females with TS and in a recent study 17% were reported to suffer from the condition and an association with autoimmune thyroiditis and hepatitis was found [41]. The diagnosis is confirmed by a skin biopsy and treatment is initiated with highly potent topical corticosteroids applied locally and followed prospectively [42]. Vulvar lichen sclerosis is associated with later development of vulvar cancer [43] and as such increased vigilance is necessary when performing gynecological examination.

Rheumatoid arthritis has a relative risk between 1.8 and 3.18 (0.87–8.15) [2, 20] and SIR of 4.4 (0.7–13.6) [18]. In pediatric populations of TS, juvenile rheumatoid arthritis has a RR of 3.18 (0.87–8.15)) [2] and a SIR 0.9 (0.2–2.4) [18]. Especially the oligoarticular form seems to be frequent in Turner syndrome girls [27]. Other studies, though inconclusive, report a possible association with Addison disease [20, 44] and primary biliary cirrhosis [45].

Type 1 Diabetes – Epidemiology and Clinical Aspects

Type 1 diabetes is, along with thyroid disorders, one of the most common autoimmune disorders in Turner syndrome. An incidence ratio of 4.1 (95% CI 2.5–6.3) has been reported [18], and epidemiological studies have found the relative risk between 8.2 and 11.6 (95% CI 5.3–21.9) of having type 1 diabetes [2, 20]. These results, however, are based on registers and a risk of coding misclassification exists. Very few clinical studies have been performed on Turner syndrome women with type 1 diabetes and most published data are in case reports [46, 47]. On balance, it is evident that the risk type 1 diabetes is increased in Turner syndrome, and similar to thyroid disease, the pathophysiological background, this increase is not thoroughly understood and may well be multifactorial and may well include interesting genes or genetic backgrounds.

Type 2 Diabetes and the Metabolic Syndrome – Epidemiology and Clinical Aspects

Impaired glucose tolerance (IGT) is present in approximately 25–78% of adult Turner syndrome populations [12, 48–51] and contributes to about 25% of the death causes in Turner syndrome [2]. It seems to be more prevalent in TS compared to both healthy controls and women with primary ovarian failure [49]. This difference is apparent in all women with TS, even nonobese young girls with normal insulin sensitivity [49, 50, 52, 53]. Early reports showed IGT in girls and women with TS [54, 55], and since then epidemiological studies have shown an increased risk of developing both type 1 diabetes (T1DM) (relative risk, 11.6) and type 2 diabetes (T2DM) (relative risk, 4.38 (2.40–7.72)) [2], in addition to increased mortality due to diabetes [1, 56] (Table 8.1).

The pathophysiology of impaired glucose tolerance in TS still remains unsolved, but several hypotheses have been proposed and studied over the years. Early studies showed that TS have reduced insulin sensitivity compared to age-matched controls

Table 8.1 Increased risks of endocrine diseases based on epidemiological studies

Diagnosis	Relative risk (95% CI)
Thyroid diseases, overall	2.00 (0.96–3.69) [2]
Thyrotoxicosis	2.01 (0.41–5.86) [2]
Hypothyreosis	5.80 (1.20–16.94) [2]
Thyroiditis	16.60 (3.42–48.50) [2]
Type 1 diabetes	8.2–11.6 (95% CI 5.3–21.9) [2, 20]
Type 2 diabetes	4.38 (2.40–7.72) [2]
Inflammatory bowel	2.25 (0.61–5.75) [2]
Ulcerative colitis	3.9 (2.3–6.1) [20]
Crohn's disease	2.25–5.3 (0.61–7.8) [2, 20]
Celiac disease	14.0 (10.2–18.8) [20]
Psoriasis	2.3–5.4 (0.06–12.51)) [2, 20]
Alopecia areata	20.4 (2.5–75.0) [20]
Rheumatoid arthritis	1.8–3.18 (0.87–8.15) [2, 20]
Fracture risk, overall	2.16–1.25 (1.005–3.0) [2, 86]
Vitiligo	Unknown [34]
Vulvar lichen sclerosis	Unknown [41]
Vitamin D deficiency	Unknown, but frequent in clinical studies [88, 94]

[57, 58]. However, when the same hypothesis was tested later using both age- and body mass index-matched controls, insulin sensitivity was similar in TS and controls [48–50, 59]. Deficits in glucose metabolism seem to be present after glucose stimulation, and it has been demonstrated that especially the first-phase insulin secretion in response to both OGTT and IVGTT is insufficient in TS [48, 49, 51]. Insulin secretion seems to be comparable to controls, but not sufficient in response to the glucose load resulting in reduced insulin-to-glucose ratio in TS [48]. Insufficient first-phase insulin response may postpone a suppression of hepatic gluconeogenesis which may contribute to IGT [60]. Furthermore, the first-phase insulin response, hence beta-cell function, appears to decrease significantly with advanced age in TS, meaning that with time IGT progress into overt T2DM [49].

The frequency of impaired glucose metabolism varies with karyotype, with mosaic TS patients having normal glucose tolerance compared to monosomy X [61]. One study reported that TS with delXq had a T2DM rate of 9%, 45,X a rate of 18%, delXp a rate of 23%, and individuals with isochromosome Xq a remarkable rate of 43% [62]. These data suggest that haploinsufficiency for genes on Xp makes TS more susceptibility for T2DM and that excessive copies of Xq greatly increase the likelihood of developing T2DM [63, 64]. Bakalov et al. investigated the gene expression profiles in 45,X vs. 46,Xi(Xq) individuals, to clarify whether the Xq genes escape inactivation and promote the diabetic phenotype. The most distinct difference (>16-fold) between these two groups was in the level of XIST (X inactivation specific transcript; Xq13.2) expression. XIST is a noncoding RNA involved in X-chromosome inactivation. XIST and several other Xq transcription factors were overexpressed in 46,Xi(Xq) along with other autosomal gene expressions involved in the functioning of the pancreatic islets and beta-cells [62].

Metabolic syndrome is a condition that includes a combination of visceral adiposity, abnormalities in glucose metabolism, hypertension, and dyslipidemia. All of which are present in Turner syndrome. Furthermore TS have decreased physical fitness by 25% compared to controls [50], and VO_{2max} is significantly lower in TS [65]. A recent Italian study investigated the prevalence of metabolic syndrome in Turner syndrome and surprisingly found a lower prevalence (4.7%) in comparison to the incidence of the background population (10–18%) [66]. Furthermore metabolic syndrome in TS was not correlated to BMI; hence BMI does not seem a good predictor of metabolic risk in subjects with TS. Instead visceral fat was linked to metabolic syndrome [66]. A novel study found no differences in mean fasting, and post-load glucose, or insulin levels when comparing TS girls treated with growth hormone with obese age-matched 46,XX girls, but overall metabolic risk factor was lower in TS [67].

Estrogen replacement treatment seems to be important for glucose homeostasis even though the findings in TS diverge. Fasting insulin and glucose concentrations are found to be lower during estrogen therapy [68], and fat-free mass and physical fitness seem to increase during treatment in TS [50]. All factors have a beneficial effect on the impaired glucose tolerance. However, more studies are needed to determine the efficiency of exogenous estrogen treatment.

GH treatment in girls with Turner syndrome does not negatively influence glucose levels and HbA1c remains unchanged or even decreases during GH therapy [69–71]. Insulin levels increase during GH treatment, indicating relative insulin resistance, but decrease after termination of treatment [69–71]. Interestingly, when considering the high prevalence of myocardial disease in Turner syndrome, the myocardial glucose uptake is reduced in these women; however GH treatment does not alter this fact [72]. Further studies are needed to investigate the long-term effects of hyperinsulinism during GH treatment.

Lipid Disorders – Epidemiology and Clinical Aspects

Body composition is altered in Turner syndrome compared to age-matched controls. They are about 20 cm shorter [73], but often have similar weight, resulting in an increased body mass index [66, 73–75]. Alterations in fat distribution are evident with increased waist-hip ratio, total fat mass, visceral fat mass, and decreased truncal lean body mass [50, 65, 76].

Hypercholesterolemia has been reported in approximately 50% of adolescents with TS and was found to be independent of BMI and unrelated to the karyotype [77, 78]. Overall TS have elevated serum triglyceride and LDL cholesterol concentrations, both when comparing with normal 46,XX women and women with primary ovarian failure [76, 78, 79], and a positive correlation exists between total cholesterol and LDL levels and age [77, 79]. Some authors have found that higher triglyceride levels may be a direct consequence of their body mass index [58, 59, 76, 78]. Low levels of high-density lipoprotein cholesterol occur in about 25% of adult TS women [76].

Lipid particle size is an important predictor of coronary disease independent of absolute lipid levels, with larger particle size being more salutary. Interestingly LDL and HDL particle size is significantly smaller in 45,X women compared to POF [79].

Theories attempting to explain these aberrations in in TS are inconclusive, but gene dosage may be important. Women with 45,X exhibit a more atherogenic (higher LDL cholesterol and triglyceride levels) lipid profile than 46,XX women with ovarian failure, suggesting that the second X-chromosome contributes to a more beneficial lipid profile in normal women, independent of sex steroid effects [79]. A novel study compared TS girls with a paternally inherited X-chromosome with TS girls having a maternal X-chromosome, showing that TS with a paternally inherited X-chromosome was associated with higher total and low-density lipoprotein cholesterol and lower body mass index than the maternal group [80].

Growth hormone treatment in girls with TS has a beneficial effect on body composition and lipid profile (lower BMI, decreased body fat percentage, less visceral fat, increase in muscle mass, and more salutary serum lipid profile) [81–83]. Sex hormone administration increases fat-free mass and physical fitness, while the lipid profile remains unchanged [50].

It is important to realize that in TS a disadvantageous lipid profile will often be superimposed on a number of congenital malformations of the heart and acquired conditions, like atherosclerosis and hypertension [84], and therefore may be more serious than when seen in isolation and actually aggravate the preexisting conditions. Whether this should lead to more aggressive treatment with statins and other lipid lowering drugs has yet to be shown.

Metabolic Bone Disease – Epidemiology and Clinical Aspects

Women with Turner syndrome have approximately 25% increased risk of bone fractures [85]. Estimations of fracture risks in TS are primarily based on retrospective epidemiological studies [2, 86, 87]. Gravholt et al. found a relative risk of 2.16 (95% CI, 1.5–3.0) of fractures in relation to hospital admissions [2]. Later a questionnaire-based study confirmed the presence of increased fracture risk in TS, but to a lesser degree with a relative risk of 1.25 (95% CI, 1.005–1.54) [86]. Studies investigating fracture risk in TS women with mean age 31–33 (16–71) found an increased fracture risk of 16–32% [87, 88]. In a prepubertal population of young TS girls (<13 years old), Ross et al. did not find an increase in total fracture incidence [89], but did find a higher number of wrist fractures.

Fractures have been reported in the cortical and trabecular bones. Patients with TS experience fractures at the arm [88], forearm [85–87], wrist [2, 89], appendicular skeleton [90], vertebra [88, 91], and femur neck [2, 88]. In summary, the risk seems to be higher during childhood (wrist fractures) and after age 45 years. In this older age-group fractures are related to osteoporosis and can be prevented by estrogen replacement therapy [88].

Bone metabolism depends on genetic background, nutrition, physical activity, local growth factors, and a spectrum of hormones. The pathophysiology behind this increase in bone fractures in TS has been investigated throughout the years and several mechanisms have been proposed.

The haploinsufficiency of the homeobox gene (SHOX) is causing short stature in TS [92, 93]. This gene might also be responsible for altered mechanical strength of the skeleton in Turner syndrome. There is no correlation between the TS karyotypes and the risk of fractures or osteoporosis [88, 94, 95]. However, individuals who have cell mosaicism (45,X/46,XX) tend to have better and close to normal spine BMD compared to individuals with only 45,X cells [96].

Speculations regarding skeletal dysmorphogenesis have been proposed, since one study found an altered hip geometry; however this could not explain the increased risk of hip fracture in TS [97]. Others have considered if a primary bone defect exists in TS [90, 94]. An increased bone resorption was present, with normal or reduced bone formation, suggesting imbalance in bone remodeling. Skeletal changes may be induced by chromosome abnormalities or secondary related to a relative estrogen deficiency and other endocrine deficiencies [94].

A number of studies have shown decreased bone mineral density (BMD) in girls and women with TS [88, 94, 98–101]. However, BMD measured by DXA scan can be affected by body size, due to the two-dimensional nature of this method (measures grams per square centimeter) [102]. Hence short individuals are likely to be misdiagnosed with osteoporosis and osteopenia unless volumetric BMD (vBMD) is used (grams per cubic centimeter) [90]. Using volumetric BMD, studies have shown similar results in TS and controls [94, 103]. We have recently studied BMD using high-resolution pQCT (hr-pQCT) and found that patients had compromised trabecular microarchitecture and lower bone strength at both skeletal sites (radius and tibia), which may partly account for the increased risk of fracture observed in these patients (Fig. 8.1) [104]. Thus, the use of hr-pQCT has extended our understanding of the physiology of bone in TS.

Cortical bone constitutes the outer part of all skeletal structures, whereas trabecular bone is found in the end of long bones, throughout the vertebral bodies, and in the inner portions of the pelvis. Low BMD at the cortical bone had been reported in individuals with TS [98, 105]. This differential affection of cortical and trabecular BMD may predispose to fracture. Bakalov et al. compared women with TS to women with premature ovarian failure and found a selective reduction in cortical BMD suggesting that the deficiency in BMD of the cortical bone in TS could be related to X-chromosome haploinsufficiency [98].

Data, however, are conflicting, since low BMD can occur in the trabecular bone with or without cortical bone [94, 106–108]. Some studies found low BMD at the lumbar spine, proximal femur [105–107], and hip [107]. Another study using volumetric BMD found reduced density at the lumbar spine, but not at the femoral neck or forearm [94].

Plasma levels of calcium and 25-hydroxyvitamin-D are often reduced in Turner syndrome; levels of PTH are increased [88, 94]. One study found an altered renal vitamin D metabolism in response to low calcium diet in TS compared to controls [109].

Proper hormone replacement therapy can maintain BMD in Turner syndrome [107]. Growth hormone treatment in TS is also associated with an increased height and larger bones, while no significant increase in DXA-derived BMD or bone strength has been detected [103, 110]. Estrogen therapy has a protective effect on the development of osteoporosis and bone fractures [88, 90, 91] and exerts an anabolic effect in the skeleton of young women with TS [106]. The impact of proper gonadal functioning was demonstrated by a study showing that adolescent TS girls who had induced puberty all had BMD in the osteopenic range, while TS girls with spontaneous puberty had normal range BMD [100]. Young TS does not attain peak BMD despite proper HRT started in adolescence [90].

Gonadal dysfunction in TS leads to almost non-existing levels of estrogens; however this may also explain the lower level of androgens seen among TS. A reduction of 25–40% of circulating androstenedione, testosterone, free testosterone, and dihydrotestosterone was reported [111]. Adrenarche is an early sexual maturation. During adrenarche the adrenal cortex secretes increased levels of androgens. Hence, the early increase of androgen secretion is independent of gonadal hormone

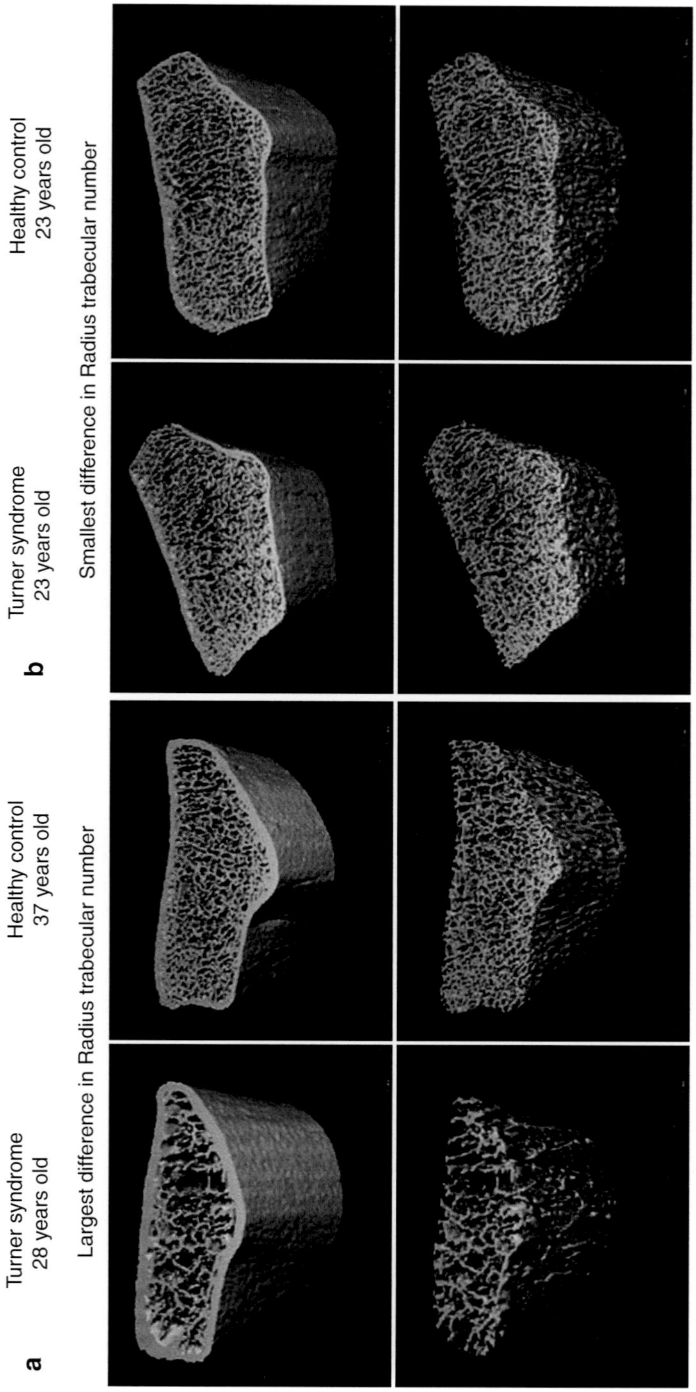

Fig. 8.1 Pictures from hr-pQCT illustrating the microarchitecture of patients with Turner syndrome and controls. (**a**) Illustrates the difference in microarchitecture between the matched pair with the largest differences. (**b**) Illustrates the difference in microarchitecture between the matched pair with the smallest differences. (Adapted from Hansen et al. [104])

secretion contrary to the pubertal increase in androgens where the ovaries are the principal source [112].

There have been suggestions that androgen replacement therapy should become standard treatment in TS girls. The beneficial effects might be increased bone mineral density and final height [113, 114], reduced sexual problems [115], and decrease in frequency of severe arithmetic learning disabilities [116]. A small study of young adults with TS, treated for a year with 1.5 mg of methyltestosterone or placebo, showed improvements in body composition and bone mineral density, along with positive effects on attention, verbal memory, and reaction time. Interestingly, total cholesterol and triglycerides decreased along with a slight decrease in HDL cholesterol, while LDL cholesterol was unaffected [117]. However, so far this area, albeit interesting, has only been sparingly investigated and there is a clear need for more studies.

Patient-Oriented Management

At transition from pediatric to adult care it is important to emphasize that the long-term goal is manifold and includes optimized hormonal replacement therapy, early diagnosis of additional medical diseases and appropriate treatment thereof, monitoring of weight and exercise habits, and encouragement of a healthy lifestyle. It is therefore necessary to discuss these issues and attempt a consensus with the patient to achieve these goals.

A yearly consultation and clinical examination is recommended; this should include measurement of blood pressure, thyroid function, and glycated hemoglobin (HbA1c). In order to obtain proper management of bone density and prevent fractures, it is recommended to perform DEXA scans at first encounter. Transglutaminase should be monitored every third year, to observe an eventual development of coeliac disease. Increased vigilance in relation to other rarer autoimmune condition is advised and appropriate testing should be put in place.

Treatment should follow clinical guidelines for the specific diseases.

We recommend a healthy lifestyle with appropriate intervention with regard to diet, exercise, and weight. We put much emphasis on keeping weight within normal limits and vigorously encourage exercise fitted to the individual patient.

Conclusion

Endocrine diseases are frequently seen in TS, necessitating a systematic approach in the clinical setting. Strikingly, the pathophysiology behind this increase in especially autoimmune disease proneness is not clear and remains an enigma. Likely, genes or genetic mechanisms are involved, but these have yet to be elucidated. Most endocrine diseases within the realm of TS should be treated according to international guidelines concerning the specific disease.

References

1. Stochholm K, Juul S, Juel K, Naeraa RW, Gravholt CH. Prevalence, incidence, diagnostic delay, and mortality in Turner syndrome. J Clin Endocrinol Metab. 2006;91(10):3897–902.
2. Gravholt CH, Juul S, Naeraa RW, Hansen J. Morbidity in Turner syndrome. J Clin Epidemiol. 1998;51(2):147–58.
3. Elsheikh M, Wass JA, Conway GS. Autoimmune thyroid syndrome in women with Turner's syndrome–the association with karyotype. Clin Endocrinol. 2001;55(2):223–6.
4. El-Mansoury M, Bryman I, Berntorp K, Hanson C, Wilhelmsen L, Landin-Wilhelmsen K. Hypothyroidism is common in Turner syndrome: results of a five-year follow-up. J Clin Endocrinol Metab. 2005;90(4):2131–5.
5. Wilson R, Chu CE, Donaldson MD, Thomson JA, McKillop JH, Connor JM. An increased incidence of thyroid antibodies in patients with Turner's syndrome and their first degree relatives. Autoimmunity. 1996;25(1):47–52.
6. Pai GS, Leach DC, Weiss L, Wolf C, Van Dyke DL. Thyroid abnormalities in 20 children with Turner syndrome. J Pediatr. 1977;91(2):267–9.
7. Bakalov VK, Gutin L, Cheng CM, et al. Autoimmune disorders in women with Turner syndrome and women with karyotypically normal primary ovarian insufficiency. J Autoimmun. 2013;38(4):315–21.
8. Mortensen KH, Cleemann L, Hjerrild BE, et al. Increased prevalence of autoimmunity in Turner syndrome – influence of age. Clin Exp Immunol. 2009;156(2):205–10.
9. Poppe K, Velkeniers B. Thyroid disorders in infertile women. Ann Endocrinol (Paris). 2003;64(1):45–50.
10. Invernizzi P, Miozzo M, Selmi C, et al. X chromosome monosomy: a common mechanism for autoimmune diseases. J Immunol. 2005;175(1):575–8.
11. Invernizzi P, Miozzo M, Oertelt-Prigione S, et al. X monosomy in female systemic lupus erythematosus. Ann N Y Acad Sci. 2007;1110:84–91.
12. Libert C, Dejager L, Pinheiro I. The X chromosome in immune functions: when a chromosome makes the difference. Nat Rev Immunol. 2010;10(8):594–604.
13. Højbjerg Gravholt C, Christian Klausen I, Weeke J, Sandahl Christiansen J. Lp(a) and lipids in adult Turner's syndrome: impact of treatment with 17beta-estradiol and norethisterone. Atherosclerosis. 2000;150(1):201–8.
14. Lowenstein EJ, Kim KH, Glick SA. Turner's syndrome in dermatology. J Am Acad Dermatol. 2004;50(5):767–76.
15. Hayward PA, Satsangi J, Jewell DP. Inflammatory bowel disease and the X chromosome. QJM. 1996;89(9):713–8.
16. Wihlborg CE, Babyn PS, Schneider R, Canada MG. The association between Turner's syndrome and juvenile rheumatoid arthritis. Pediatr Radiol. 1999;29(9):676–81.
17. Grossi A, Crinò A, Luciano R, Lombardo A, Cappa M, Fierabracci A. Endocrine autoimmunity in Turner syndrome. Ital J Pediatr. 2013;39:79.
18. Jørgensen KT, Rostgaard K, Bache I, et al. Autoimmune diseases in women with Turner's syndrome. Arthritis Rheum. 2010;62(3):658–66.
19. Germain EL, Plotnick LP. Age-related anti-thyroid antibodies and thyroid abnormalities in Turner syndrome. Acta Paediatr Scand. 1986;75(5):750–5.
20. Goldacre MJ, Seminog OO. Turner syndrome and autoimmune diseases: record-linkage study. Arch Dis Child. 2014;99(1):71–3.

21. Price WH. A high incidence of chronic inflammatory bowel disease in patients with Turner's syndrome. J Med Genet. 1979;16(4):263–6.
22. Kohler J, Grant D. Crohn's disease in Turner's syndrome. Br Med J. 1981;282:950.
23. Arslan D, Kuyucu T, Kendirci M, Kurtoglu S. Celiac disease and Turner's syndrome: patient report. J Pediatr Endocrinol Metab. 2000;13(9):1629–31.
24. Rujner J, Wisniewski A, Gregorek H, Wozniewicz B, Młynarski W, Witas HW. Coeliac disease and HLA-DQ 2 (DQA1∗ 0501 and DQB1∗ 0201) in patients with Turner syndrome. J Pediatr Gastroenterol Nutr. 2001;32(1):114–5.
25. Mårild K, Størdal K, Hagman A, Ludvigsson JF. Turner syndrome and celiac disease: a case-control study. Pediatrics. 2016;137(2):1–8.
26. Scarpa R, Lubrano E, Castiglione F, Morace F, Ames PR, Oriente P. Juvenile rheumatoid arthritis, Crohn's disease and Turner's syndrome: a novel association. Clin Exp Rheumatol. 1996;14(4):449–50.
27. Zulian F, Schumacher HR, Calore A, Goldsmith DP, Athreya BH. Juvenile arthritis in Turner's syndrome: a multicenter study. Clin Exp Rheumatol. 1998;16(4):489–94.
28. Rosina P, Segalla G, Magnanini M, Chieregato C, Barba A. Turner's syndrome associated with psoriasis and alopecia areata. J Eur Acad Dermatol Venereol. 2003;17(1):50–2.
29. Oiso N, Ota T, Kawara S, Kawada A. Pustular psoriasis and vitiligo in a patient with Turner syndrome. J Dermatol. 2007;34(10):727–9.
30. Pessach IM, Notarangelo LD. X-linked primary immunodeficiencies as a bridge to better understanding X-chromosome related autoimmunity. J Autoimmun. 2009;33(1):17–24.
31. Lessard CJ, Ice JA, Adrianto I, et al. The genomics of autoimmune disease in the era of genome-wide association studies and beyond. Autoimmun Rev. 2012;11(4):267–75.
32. Larizza D, Calcaterra V, Martinetti M. Autoimmune stigmata in Turner syndrome: when lacks an X chromosome. J Autoimmun. 2009;33(1):25–30.
33. Larizza D, Cuccia M, Martinetti M, et al. Adrenocorticotrophin stimulation and HLA polymorphisms suggest a high frequency of heterozygosity for steroid 21-hydroxylase deficiency in patients with Turner's syndrome and their families. Clin Endocrinol. 1994;40(1):39–45.
34. Brazzelli V, Larizza D, Martinetti M, et al. Halo nevus, rather than vitiligo, is a typical dermatologic finding of Turner's syndrome: clinical, genetic, and immunogenetic study in 72 patients. J Am Acad Dermatol. 2004;51(3):354–8.
35. Larizza D, Calcaterra V, Martinetti M, et al. Helicobacter pylori infection and autoimmune thyroid disease in young patients: the disadvantage of carrying the human leukocyte antigen-DRB1∗0301 allele. J Clin Endocrinol Metab. 2006;91(1):176–9.
36. Larizza D, Martinetti M, Lorini R, et al. Parental segregation of autoimmunity in patients with Turner's syndrome: preferential paternal transmission? J Autoimmun. 1999;12(1):65–72.
37. Jensen K, Petersen PH, Nielsen EL, Dahl G, Nielsen J. Serum immunoglobulin M, G, and A concentration levels in Turner's syndrome compared with normal women and men. Hum Genet. 1976;31(3):329–34.
38. Rongen-Westerlaken C, Rijkers GT, Scholtens EJ, et al. Immunologic studies in Turner syndrome before and during treatment with growth hormone. The Dutch Growth Hormone Working Group. J Pediatr. 1991;119(2):268–72.
39. Lorini R, Ugazio AG, Cammareri V, et al. Immunoglobulin levels, T-cell markers, mitogen responsiveness and thymic hormone activity in Turner's syndrome. Thymus. 1983;5(2):61–6.
40. Bonamico M, Pasquino AM, Mariani P, et al. Prevalence and clinical picture of celiac disease in Turner syndrome. J Clin Endocrinol Metab. 2002;87(12):5495–8.
41. Chakhtoura Z, Vigoureux S, Courtillot C, Tejedor I, Touraine P. Vulvar lichen sclerosus is very frequent in women with Turner syndrome. J Clin Endocrinol Metab. 2014;99(4):1103–4.
42. Neill SM, Lewis FM, Tatnall FM, Cox NH. British association of dermatologists' guidelines for the management of lichen sclerosus 2010. Br J Dermatol. 2010;163(4):672–82.
43. Haidopoulos D, Bakolas G, Michala L. Turner syndrome: don't forget the vulva. Endocrinol Diabetes Metab Case Rep. 2016;2016:160016.

44. Irvine WJ, Chan MMW, Scarth L, et al. Immunological aspects of premature ovarian failure associated with idiopathic Addison's disease. Lancet. 1968;2(7574):883–7.
45. Sokol L, Stueben ET, Jaikishen JP, Lamarche MB. Turner syndrome associated with acquired von Willebrand disease, primary biliary cirrhosis, and inflammatory bowel disease. Am J Hematol. 2002;70(3):257–9.
46. Obara-Moszynska M, Banaszak M, Niedziela M. Growth hormone therapy in a girl with Turner syndrome and diabetes type 1 – case report. Pediatr Endocrinol Diabetes Metab. 2015;20(2):75–81.
47. Gonc EN, Ozon A, Alikasifoglu A, Kandemir N. Type 1 diabetes mellitus in a 3 1/2 year-old girl with Turner's syndrome. J Pediatr Endocrinol Metab. 2002;15(8):1203–6.
48. Hjerrild BE, Holst JJ, Juhl CB, Christiansen JS, Schmitz O, Gravholt CH. Delayed β-cell response and glucose intolerance in young women with Turner syndrome. BMC Endocr Disord. 2011;11:6.
49. Bakalov VK, Cooley MM, Quon MJ, et al. Impaired insulin secretion in the Turner metabolic syndrome. J Clin Endocrinol Metab. 2004;89(7):3516–20.
50. Højbjerg Gravholt C, Naeraa RW, Nyholm B, et al. Glucose metabolism, lipid metabolism, and cardiovascular risk factors in adult Turner's syndrome. Diabetes Care. 1998;21(7):1062–70.
51. Holl RW, Kunze D, Etzrodt H, Teller W, Heinze E. Turner syndrome: final height, glucose tolerance, bone density and psychosocial status in 25 adult patients. Eur J Pediatr. 1994;153(1):11–6.
52. Polychronakos C, Letarte J, Collu R, Ducharme JR. Carbohydrate intolerance in children and adolescents with Turner syndrome. J Pediatr. 1980;96(6):1009–14.
53. AvRuskin TW, Crigler JF, Soeldner JS. Turner's syndrome and carbohydrate metabolism. I. Impaired insulin secretion after tolbutamide and glucagon stimulation tests: evidence of insulin deficiency. Am J Med Sci. 1979;277(2):145–52.
54. Nielsen J, Johansen K, Yde H. The frequency of diabetes mellitus in patients with Turner's syndrome and pure gonadal dysgenesis. Blood glucose, plasma insulin and growth hormone level during an oral glucose tolerance test. Acta Endocrinol. 1969;62(2):251–69.
55. Forbes AP, Engel E. The high incidence of diabetes mellitus in 41 patients with gonadal dysgenesis, and their close relatives. Metabolism. 1963;12:428–39.
56. Schoemaker MJ, Swerdlow AJ, Higgins CD, Wright AF, Jacobs PA. Mortality in women with Turner syndrome in Great Britain: a national cohort study. J Clin Endocrinol Metab. 2008;93(12):4735–42.
57. Caprio S, Boulware S, Diamond M, et al. Insulin resistance: an early metabolic defect of Turner's syndrome. J Clin Endocrinol Metab. 1991;72(4):832–6.
58. Salgin B, Amin R, Yuen K, Williams RM, Murgatroyd P, Dunger DB. Insulin resistance is an intrinsic defect independent of fat mass in women with Turner's syndrome. Horm Res. 2006;65(2):69–75.
59. Ostberg JE, Attar MJH, Mohamed-Ali V, Conway GS. Adipokine dysregulation in Turner syndrome: comparison of circulating interleukin-6 and leptin concentrations with measures of adiposity and C-reactive protein. J Clin Endocrinol Metab. 2005;90(5):2948–53.
60. Gravholt CH. Epidemiological, endocrine and metabolic features in Turner syndrome. Eur J Endocrinol. 2004;151(6):657–87.
61. Cicognani A, Mazzanti L, Tassinari D, et al. Differences in carbohydrate tolerance in Turner syndrome depending on age and karyotype. Eur J Pediatr. 1988;148:64–8.
62. Bakalov VK, Cheng C, Zhou J, Bondy CA. X-chromosome gene dosage and the risk of diabetes in Turner syndrome. J Clin Endocrinol Metab. 2009;94(9):3289–96.
63. Menzinger G, Fallucca F, Andreani D, Wais S. Klinefelter's syndrome and diabetes mellitus. Lancet. 1966;288(7466):747–8.
64. Bojesen A, Kristensen K, Birkebaek NH, et al. The metabolic syndrome is frequent in Klinefelter's syndrome and is associated with abdominal obesity and hypogonadism. Diabetes Care. 2006;29(7):1591–8.

65. Gravholt CH, Hjerrild BE, Mosekilde L, et al. Body composition is distinctly altered in Turner syndrome: relations to glucose metabolism, circulating adipokines, and endothelial adhesion molecules. Eur J Endocrinol. 2006;155(4):583–92.
66. Calcaterra V, Brambilla P, Carnevale Maffe G, et al. Metabolic syndrome in Turner syndrome and relation between body composition and clinical, genetic, and ultrasonographic characteristics. Metab Syndr Relat Disord. 2014;12(3):159–64.
67. Wojcik M, Janus D, Zygmunt-Gorska A, Starzyk JB. Insulin resistance in adolescents with Turner syndrome is comparable to obese peers, but the overall metabolic risk is lower due to unknown mechanism. J Endocrinol Investig. 2015;38(3):345–9.
68. Elsheikh M, Bird R, Casadei B, Conway GS, Wass JA. The effect of hormone replacement therapy on cardiovascular hemodynamics in women with Turner's syndrome. J Clin Endocrinol Metab. 2000;85(2):614–8.
69. Sas T, de Muinck Keizer-Schrama S, Aanstoot HJ, Stijnen T, Drop S. Carbohydrate metabolism during growth hormone treatment and after discontinuation of growth hormone treatment in girls with Turner syndrome treated with once or twice daily growth hormone injections. Clin Endocrinol. 2000;52(6):741–7.
70. Radetti G, Pasquino B, Gottardi E, Boscolo Contadin I, Aimaretti G, Rigon F. Insulin sensitivity in Turner's syndrome: influence of GH treatment. Eur J Endocrinol. 2004;151(3):351–4.
71. Sas TCJ, De Muinck Keizer-Schrama SMPF, Stijnen T, Aanstoot HJ, Drop SLS. Carbohydrate metabolism during long-term growth hormone (GH) treatment and after discontinuation of GH treatment in girls with Turner syndrome participating in a randomized dose-response. J Clin Endocrinol Metab. 2000;141(2):769–75.
72. Christian T, Britta H, Kristian Havmand M, et al. Low myocardial glucose uptake in Turner syndrome is unaffected by growth hormone: a randomized, placebo-controlled FDG-PET study. Clin Endocrinol. 2015;83(1):133–40.
73. Gravholt CH, Naeraa RW. Reference values for body proportions and body composition in adult women with Ullrich-Turner syndrome. Am J Med Genet. 1997;72(4):403–8.
74. Bondy CA. Care of girls and women with Turner syndrome: a guideline of the Turner Syndrome Study Group. J Clin Endocrinol Metab. 2007;92(1):10–25.
75. Giordano R, Forno D, Lanfranco F, Manieri C, Ghizzoni L, Ghigo E. Metabolic and cardiovascular outcomes in a group of adult patients with Turner's syndrome under hormonal replacement therapy. Eur J Endocrinol. 2011;164(5):819–26.
76. Elsheikh M, Conway GS. The impact of obesity on cardiovascular risk factors in Turner's syndrome. Clin Endocrinol. 1998;49(4):447–50.
77. Garden AS, Diver MJ, Fraser WD. Undiagnosed morbidity in adult women with Turner's syndrome. Clin Endocrinol. 1996;45(5):589–93.
78. Ross JL, Feuillan P, Long LM, Kowal K, Kushner H, Cutler GB. Lipid abnormalities in Turner syndrome. J Pediatr. 1995;126(2):242–5.
79. Van PL, Bakalov VK, Bondy CA. Monosomy for the X-chromosome is associated with an atherogenic lipid profile. J Clin Endocrinol Metab. 2006;91(8):2867–70.
80. Sagi L, Zuckerman-Levin N, Gawlik A, et al. Clinical significance of the parental origin of the X chromosome in Turner syndrome. J Clin Endocrinol Metab. 2007;92(3):846–52.
81. Wooten N, Bakalov VK, Hill S, Bondy CA. Reduced abdominal adiposity and improved glucose tolerance in growth hormone-treated girls with Turner syndrome. J Clin Endocrinol Metab. 2008;93(6):2109–14.
82. Gravholt CH, Naeraa RW, Brixen K, et al. Short-term growth hormone treatment in girls with turner syndrome decreases fat mass and insulin sensitivity: a randomized, double-blind, placebo-controlled, crossover study. Pediatrics. 2002;110(5):889–96.
83. Bannink EMN, Van Der Palen RLF, Mulder PGH, De Muinck Keizer-Schrama SMPF. Long-term follow-up of GH-treated girls with turner syndrome: metabolic consequences. Horm Res. 2009;71(6):343–9.
84. Mortensen KH, Andersen NH, Gravholt CH. Cardiovascular phenotype in Turner syndrome—integrating cardiology, genetics, and endocrinology. Endocr Rev. 2012;33(5):677–714.

85. Bakalov VK, Bondy CA. Fracture risk and bone mineral density in Turner syndrome. Rev Endocr Metab Disord. 2008;9(2):145–51.
86. Gravholt CH, Vestergaard P, Hermann AP, Mosekilde L, Brixen K, Christiansen JS. Increased fracture rates in Turner's syndrome: a nationwide questionnaire survey. Clin Endocrinol. 2003;59(1):89–96.
87. Han TS, Cadge B, Conway GS. Hearing impairment and low bone mineral density increase the risk of bone fractures in women with Turner's syndrome. Clin Endocrinol. 2006;65(5):643–7.
88. Landin-Wilhelmsen K, Bryman I, Windh M, Wilhelmsen L. Osteoporosis and fractures in Turner syndrome-importance of growth promoting and oestrogen therapy. Clin Endocrinol. 1999;51(4):497–502.
89. Ross JL, Long LM, Feuillan P, Cassorla F, Cutler GB. Normal bone density of the wrist and spine and increased wrist fractures in girls with Turner's syndrome. J Clin Endocrinol Metab. 1991;73(2):355–9.
90. Bakalov VK, Chen ML, Baron J, et al. Bone mineral density and fractures in turner syndrome. Am J Med. 2003;115:259–64.
91. Hanton L, Axelrod L, Bakalov V, Bondy CA. The importance of estrogen replacement in young women with Turner syndrome. J Womens Health (Larchmt). 2003;12(10):971–7.
92. Rao E, Weiss B, Fukami M, et al. Pseudoautosomal deletions encompassing a novel homeobox gene cause growth failure in idiopathic short stature and Turner syndrome. Nat Genet. 1997;16(1):54–63.
93. Clement-Jones M, Schiller S, Rao E, et al. The short stature homeobox gene SHOX is involved in skeletal abnormalities in Turner syndrome. Hum Mol Genet. 2000;9(5):695–702.
94. Gravholt CH, Lauridsen AL, Brixen K, Mosekilde L, Heickendorff L, Christiansen JS. Marked disproportionality in bone size and mineral, and distinct abnormalities in bone markers and calcitropic hormones in adult Turner syndrome: a cross-sectional study. J Clin Endocrinol Metab. 2002;87(6):2798–808.
95. Bakalov VK, Van PL, Baron J, Reynolds JC, Bondy CA. Growth hormone therapy and bone mineral density in Turner syndrome. J Clin Endocrinol Metab. 2004;89(10):4886–9.
96. El-Mansoury M, Barrenäs M-L, Bryman I, et al. Chromosomal mosaicism mitigates stigmata and cardiovascular risk factors in Turner syndrome. Clin Endocrinol. 2007;66(5):744–51.
97. Nissen N, Gravholt CH, Abrahamsen B, et al. Disproportional geometry of the proximal femur in patients with Turner syndrome: a cross-sectional study. Clin Endocrinol. 2007;67(6):897–903.
98. Bakalov VK, Axelrod L, Baron J, et al. Selective reduction in cortical bone mineral density in turner syndrome independent of ovarian hormone deficiency. J Clin Endocrinol Metab. 2003;88(12):5717–22.
99. Stěpán JJ, Musilová J, Pacovský V. Bone demineralization, biochemical indices of bone remodeling, and estrogen replacement therapy in adults with Turner's syndrome. J Bone Miner Res. 1989;4(2):193–8.
100. Carrascosa A, Gussinyé M, Terradas P, Yeste D, Audí L, Vicens-Calvet E. Spontaneous, but not induced, puberty permits adequate bone mass acquisition in adolescent turner syndrome patients. J Bone Miner Res. 2000;15(10):2005–10.
101. Costa AMG, Lemos-Marini SHV, Baptista MTM, Morcillo AM, Maciel-Guerra AT, Guerra G. Bone mineralization in Turner syndrome: a transverse study of the determinant factors in 58 patients. J Bone Miner Metab. 2002;20(5):294–7.
102. Nielsen SP, Kolthoff N, Bärenholdt O, et al. Diagnosis of osteoporosis by planar bone densitometry: can body size be disregarded? Br J Radiol. 1998;71(849):934–43.
103. Bertelloni S, Cinquanta L, Baroncelli GI, Simi P, Rossi S, Saggese G. Volumetric bone mineral density in young women with Turner's syndrome treated with estrogens or estrogens plus growth hormone. Horm Res. 2000;53(2):72–6.
104. Hansen S, Brixen K, Gravholt CH. Compromised trabecular microarchitecture and lower finite element estimates of radius and tibia bone strength in adults with turner syndrome: a cross-sectional study using high-resolution-pQCT. J Bone Miner Res. 2012;27(8):1794–803.

105. Holroyd CR, Davies JH, Taylor P, et al. Reduced cortical bone density with normal trabecular bone density in girls with Turner syndrome. Osteoporos Int. 2010;21(12):2093–9.
106. Khastgir G, Studd JWW, Fox SW, Jones J, Alaghband-zadeh J, Chow JWM. A longitudinal study of the effects of subcutaneous estrogen replacement on bone in young women with Turner's syndrome. J Bone Miner Res. 2003;18(5):925–32.
107. Cleemann L, Hjerrild BE, Lauridsen AL, et al. Long-term hormone replacement therapy preserves bone mineral density in Turner syndrome. Eur J Endocrinol. 2009;161(2):251–7.
108. Hogler W, Briody J, Moore B, Garnett S, Lu PW, Cowell CT. Importance of estrogen on bone health in Turner syndrome: a cross-sectional and longitudinal study using dual-energy X-ray absorptiometry. J Clin Endocrinol Metab. 2004;89(1):193–9.
109. Saggese G, Federico G, Bertelloni S, Baroncelli GI. Mineral metabolism in Turner's syndrome: evidence for impaired renal vitamin D metabolism and normal osteoblast function. J Clin Endocrinol Metab. 1992;75(4):998–1001.
110. Nour MA, Burt LA, Perry RJ, Stephure DK, Hanley DA, Boyd SK. Impact of growth hormone on adult bone quality in turner syndrome: a HR-pQCT study. Calcif Tissue Int. 2016;98(1):49–59.
111. Gravholt CH, Svenstrup B, Bennett P, Christiansen JS. Reduced androgen levels in adult Turner syndrome: influence of female sex steroids and growth hormone status. Clin Endocrinol. 1999;50(6):791–800.
112. Apter D, Lenko HL, Perheentupa J, Söderholm A, Vihko R. Subnormal pubertal increases of serum androgens in Turner's syndrome. Horm Res. 1982;16(3):164–73.
113. Stahnke N, Keller E, Landy H, Serono Study Group. Favorable final height outcome in girls with Ullrich-Turner syndrome treated with low-dose growth hormone together with oxandrolone despite starting treatment after 10 years of age. J Pediatr Endocrinol Metab. 2002;15(2):129–38.
114. Zeger MPD, Shah K, Kowal K, Cutler GB, Kushner H, Ross JL. Prospective study confirms oxandrolone-associated improvement in height in growth hormone-treated adolescent girls with Turner syndrome. Horm Res pædiatrics. 2011;75(1):38–46.
115. Menke LA, Sas TCJ, Visser M, et al. The effect of the weak androgen oxandrolone on psychological and behavioral characteristics in growth hormone-treated girls with Turner syndrome. Horm Behav. 2010;57(3):297–305.
116. Ross JL, Mazzocco MMM, Kushner H, Kowal K, Cutler GB, Roeltgen D. Effects of treatment with oxandrolone for 4 years on the frequency of severe arithmetic learning disability in girls with Turner syndrome. J Pediatr. 2009;155(5):714–20.
117. Zuckerman-Levin N, Frolova-Bishara T, Militianu D, Levin M, Aharon-Peretz J, Hochberg Z. Androgen replacement therapy in Turner syndrome: a pilot study. J Clin Endocrinol Metab. 2009;94(12):4820–7.

Chapter 9
Care of Girls with Turner Syndrome: Beyond Growth and Hormones

Angel Siu Ying Nip and Darcy King

Turner syndrome (TS) is a relatively common genetic disorder, with associated neurocognitive differences, characterized by complete or partial monosomy X in a phenotypic female [1]. TS is associated with a cognitive profile that typically includes intact intellectual function and verbal abilities with relative weaknesses in visual-spatial, executive, and social domains. In this chapter, we provide a summary of cognitive, social, and executive challenges that girls with TS may encounter and measures used in the assessment of visual-spatial and executive skills.

Females with TS often demonstrate a unique cognitive profile characterized by relative strengths in verbal domains but weaknesses in visual-spatial and executive areas. There is also increasing evidence for deficits in the domain of social function and interpersonal relationship. While studies largely suggest that adult women with TS do not have increased incidence of psychiatric illnesses, there is some indication that global psychosocial functioning may be impaired. Several studies also suggest that girls with TS are at risk for social, cognitive, and emotion processing difficulties. Significant problems in academic achievement, especially in mathematics, and poor social interactions are evident and indicate a need for a multidisciplinary team whose members often include medical providers, educators, therapists, psychologists, and mental health providers [1]. Early identification of these issues and preventive interventions are warranted. We encourage clinicians to pay greater attention to areas of social, academic, and emotional functioning in girls with TS as potential targets in an overall treatment plan.

A. S. Y. Nip (✉) · D. King
University of Washington, Seattle, WA, USA

© Springer Nature Switzerland AG 2020
P. Y. Fechner (ed.), *Turner Syndrome*,
https://doi.org/10.1007/978-3-030-34150-3_9

Cognitive Profile

Verbal skills are relatively strong in girls with TS across all ages, with normal to above average scores generally reported [2]. Recent studies indicate a possible specific TS profile in language use abilities with increased vocabulary, initial verbal memory, reading comprehension, and understanding of rarely used words. Slow responding and weak performances in verbal fluency tasks have sometimes been reported but are thought to be less related to linguistic skills but rather reflect underlying deficits in executive functioning [3, 4].

Turner syndrome typically leads to a slight decrease in scores of overall intelligence, except in cases of intellectual disability associated with a ring chromosome karyotype, which is very infrequent [5]. Many early studies demonstrated that full-scale IQ is normal in girls with TS, but the subtest profile indicated that the performance intelligence quotient (PIQ) is low when compared with that of a normal or even above-average verbal IQ (VIQ) [6]. Studies also showed a consistent discrepancy in PIQ scores in girls with TS at the same level or below that of their mothers [7]. Although impairments in PIQ in girls with TS have been examined extensively and generally been attributed to problems with visual-spatial processing, visual memory, and executive function, there is also evidence that select components of verbal performance may additionally be affected [8].

Social Differences

Psychosocial difficulties and adaptive function are commonly reported problems in girls with TS. Studies found that girls with TS performed more poorly than their peers on several measures of social competence and recognition [9]. Girls with TS similarly placed in the mild-to-moderate range of clinical significance for the social cognition and autistic mannerisms SRS domains, which are designed to assess an individual's ability to interpret social cues and the presence of restricted interests or stereotypic behaviors [10]. Although there is no clear increase in incidence of psychiatric disorders when compared with general norms, numerous studies indicate increased self-report of anxiety, depression, low self-esteem, and impaired social competence when compared with peers [11, 12]. Girls with TS often have difficulties understanding subtle social cues that studies have described as atypical social cognition in TS. Facial recognition has been repeatedly shown to be an area of vulnerability as determined by tasks such as the Benton Facial Recognition Test [13–15] and delayed face-matching tests [16, 17]. Lawrence et al., (2003) noted poor facial recognition based on several tasks examining faces manipulated by several visual-spatial constructs, such as less accurate performance in recognizing halftone images of faces [18]. More recently, studies of individuals with TS have demonstrated aberrant face recognition abilities including affect recognition, specifically for fearful or angry faces [19].

Studies to date indicate that impaired social function in TS is not related to intelligence quotient (IQ) alone nor to overall stigmata of disease, such as short stature or delayed puberty [20]. However, both shyness and low self-esteem are frequently linked to self-consciousness over physical appearance in studies of individuals with TS. Data from studies of sex hormone replacement are similarly inconclusive but also suggest that while induction of puberty improves self-concept and other aspects of cognition such as working memory, difficulties in social competence continue to persist after sex hormone replacement [21, 22].

Psychosocial problems become more obvious between 6 and 12 years. Poorer social skills have consistently been described as affecting all aspects of social behavior and functioning [2, 23, 24]. The girls tend to have fewer close friends, spend less time with peers, and appear emotionally less mature than age-matched normally developing girls. Building up friendships and maintaining relationships are difficult for them, and parents report that their daughters with TS are less socially competent than their peers [25].

Visual-Spatial Differences

Visual-spatial processing weakness is one of the most commonly and consistently observed impairments among individuals with TS [19]. Visuoperception deficits are apparent on object identification and location identification tasks and yet appear associated with poor visual working memory. Others have also reported slower response times on visual-spatial tasks by girls with TS [26]. Neuroimaging studies suggest that spatial/executive difficulties are related to frontal-parietal structural, functional, and biochemical abnormalities [27–29]. It is likely that haploinsufficiency of several inactivation-escaping X chromosome genes interacts with other genetic and environmental factors to increase the risk for neurodevelopmental alterations and related cognitive impairments. The specific causal factors are likely highly complex and currently unknown.

One issue contributing to the complexity of determining specific genetic or other causes of visual-spatial in TS is the significant inconsistency across studies in terms of the specific visual-spatial deficits observed.

Executive Function

During adolescence, girls with TS increasingly fall behind in normal cognitive development. High cognitive tasks such as abstract reasoning, clustering, and arithmetic calculation are likely to become a challenge. The prevalence of mathematics learning disability among girls with TS is higher than the estimated prevalence in the general population (~6–10%) [30]. Rover et al. found that 55% of the 7- to 16-year-old girls with TS met criteria for mathematics learning disability, versus 7%

for comparison group [31]. Processing speed appears to play a significant role, as girls with TS are significantly slower [32] on arithmetic fact retrieval and on response times during calculations [33, 34]. Many everyday tasks require spatial skills, including reading maps, driving, and finding one's way around an unfamiliar place, are examples of skills that are difficult. Limitations in working memory and slower response times indicate deficits in executive functioning that commonly result in weak planning, self-organization, and self-regulation performances. In one study of working memory and executive function, girls with TS made more than twice as many errors as their peers on the naming tasks, when working memory demands increased [35]. Girls with TS were less accurate despite taking as much time to complete the timed tasks as their peers. More research is needed to determine the nature of these processing deficits. Studies showed both an increased incidence of ADHD (24%) and a higher frequency of the hyperactive/impulsive subtype of ADHD, in girls with TS when compared with children in the general population [36–39].

Motor Performance

In general, girls with TS had evidence of decreased motor coordination and motor learning. They have difficulty with motor function and tend to make more errors across aspects on motor skills including gross and fine motor skills [40]. They may appear clumsy and their hand-eye coordination is often very poor. Physical education (PE) and team games can be challenging for girls with TS, and they often prefer individual sports. Studies did not show a specific profile of motor impairment or correlation between intelligence scores and motor performance scores. However, girls with TS indeed experience a significant general motor impairment [41] in tasks requiring dexterity such as handwriting and drawing. Specifically, getting dressed for PE may be difficult if they cannot manage buttons or tie their shoes. Speed and neatness may be a problem in later school years. Proper physical and occupational evaluations during school age are necessary, and accommodation is important to ensure success at school.

Emotional Health

Though outcome studies of adult women with TS are not always consistent, the extent literature indicates that relative to age-matched peers, these individuals experience higher incidence of anxiety, depression, poor body image, low self-esteem, and self-perception of impaired social competence [11, 42]. Clinical reports have documented that girls with TS experience more social anxiety and shyness than matched controls [43]. In contrast, few studies have systematically evaluated the presence of mood and behavioral syndromes in patients with TS. Recent studies found that women with TS reported a higher rate of lifetime depression compared with rates observed in community-based studies [44]. Overall, 52% of the TS women met criteria for a current or a past depressive or anxiety disorder. McCauley et al. studied 30 women with TS and found high levels of major psychiatric difficulties and low self-esteem [45]. Lifetime major depression occurred in 36% of women, and lifetime affective disorders in 47% of women, compared with rates in the community of 20% and 24%, respectively. Lifetime histories of anxiety disorders were observed in 15% of women with TS and in 15–30% of women in community studies [43]. Thus, it should be recognized and addressed in a timely manner [24].

Transition to Adult Care

Unfortunately, many women with TS do not receive regular medical care and adequate health surveillance, which results in poor medical outcomes [46, 47]. Effective coordination and continuity of care during transition to adult care is critical for their medical, emotional, and psychological health in adulthood. Transition challenges such as poor self-advocacy or self-management, little family support, or unsatisfactory cooperation between healthcare professionals have been reported [48, 49]. Unfortunately, self-planning and organizational skills in girls with TS are impaired even more than in other chronic conditions due to the impairment in executive function. Taking over responsibilities from their parents is likely to be a major challenge for them. Thus, extra effort and proactive action are important from healthcare professionals at this stage of development to enhance smooth transition to adult care [50, 51]. Various transition models have been developed and those commonly recommend informing patients early about their health issues, building up a relationship with new healthcare providers, and having a social network as essential for a successful transition.

Assessment and Management

According to the clinical practice guideline for the care of girls and women with TS, the importance of neuropsychology and allied behavioral health services should be integrated into the care for girls and women with TS. It is also recommended that annual developmental and behavioral screenings be performed until adulthood with referrals as indicated. Conducting neuropsychological assessments at key transitional stages in schooling and aiming for on-time puberty and aggressive management of hearing impairment are recommended to facilitate positive psychosocial and psychosexual adaptation and accommodate learning and performance issues. It is suggested that evidence-based interventions for cognitive or psychosocial problems in other populations may be utilized or adapted to meet the needs of girls and women with TS.

Early diagnosis and treatment of comorbidities are known to enhance the overall health of adult patients with TS. Experienced clinicians have discussed inclusion of psychological testing and routinely screening of girls with TS for developmental progress, but evidence-based recommendations are rare. Consequently, intervention guidelines for the psychosocial aspects of TS are scarce. It is important to include supportive interventions encompassing the family system and caregivers. The overall aim is to empower patients with TS to keep up with their peers at school and in their working life and to improve their self-esteem and thus their quality of life. Counseling and treating girls with TS are complicated because although the karyotype differences may affect the phenotypes of TS, the karyotype is not a distinct predictor of the physical or psychological phenotypical outcome. Consequently, in TS we must acknowledge normal and healthy development while being attuned to the possible impairments.

When concerns are identified, evaluations are recommended to identify cognitive, emotional, and social deficits. Examples of standardized assessments that may be appropriate are as follows:

- *Bayley Scales* assess developmental levels of infants and young children in the domains of motor skills, cognition, language, and social-emotional and adaptive behavior [52].
- The *Wechsler Preschool and Primary Scale of Intelligence (WIPPSI)*, the *Wechsler Intelligence Scale for Children (WISC)*, and the *Wechsler Adult intelligence Scale (WAIS)* assess verbal and nonverbal abilities [53–55].
- The *Developmental NEuroPSYchological Assessment (NEPSY-II)* examines neuropsychological domains including social cognition and is useful in planning intervention for various childhood disorders [56].
- The *Social Skills Improvement System Rating Scale (SSIS)* locates social skills, competing behavior problems, and academic competence [57].
- The *Child Behavior Checklist (CBCL)* is a caregiver report form, whereas the *Youth Self Report Form (YSR)* is filled out by children and adolescents. The *Teacher Report Form (TRF)* may be of additional use for providing information in school matters.

Awareness of the psychological and psychosocial issues in TS is as important as the knowledge of medical treatments. Importantly, information on the aspects of cognitive development should not instill fear of intellectual disability, but stress the variability and strengths of cognitive development in TS. Developmental or neuropsychological screening should be initiated at an early age and remain an integral part of the patient's routine assessment.

Early intervention, 504 plans, and individualized education plans (IEPs) should be considered for school success. Many girls with TS thrive utilizing interventions for children with ADHD and nonverbal learning disabilities. Some girls may benefit from social skills classes or interventions for anxiety. It is important to know what resources are in your community. The Turner Syndrome Support Society (TSSS, TSS.org.UK) has published some tips for parents and schools in helping girls with TS [58].

Summary and Conclusions

Turner syndrome impacts girls and women across their lifespan. The phenotypes vary widely across individuals. Special attention should be given to the psychosocial sequelae of the syndrome, and appropriate interventions should be undertaken. Given the evidence of a specific cognitive and psychosocial phenotype in TS, pediatricians should be attuned to upcoming developmental differences and monitor their development closely. With the proper evaluations and interventions, we can optimize health and developmental outcomes for girls and women with TS.

References

1. Pinsker JE. Clinical review: Turner syndrome: updateing the paradigm of clinical care. J Clin Endocrinol Metab. 2012;97:994–1003.
2. Temple CM. Oral fluency and narrative production in children with Turner's syndrome. Neuropsychologia. 2002;40:1419–27.
3. Rovet J. Turner syndrome: a review of genetic and hormonal influences on neuropsychological functioning. Child Neuropsychol. 2004;10:262–79.
4. Sterling A, Abbeduto L. Language development in school-age females. J Intellect Disabil Res. 2012;56:974–83.
5. Van Dyke DL, Wiktor A, Palmer CG, Miller DA, Witt M, Babu VR, Worsham MJ, Roberson JR, Weiss L. Ullrich-Turner syndrome with a small ring X chromosome and presence of mental retardation. Am J Med Genet. 1992;43:996–1005.
6. Temple CM, Carney RA. Intellectual functioning of children with Turner syndrome: a comparison of behavioral phenotypes. Dev Med Child Neurol. 1993;35:691–8.
7. Wechsler D. Wechsler abbreviated scale of intelligence: WASI. San Antonio: The Psychological Corporation; 1999.
8. Silbert A, Wolff PH, Lilienthal J. Spatial and temporal processing in patients with Turner's syndrome. Behav Genet. 1977;7:11–21.
9. Lagrou K, Xhrouet-Heinrichs D, Heinrichs C, Craen M, Chanoine JP, Malvaux P, Bourguignon JP. Age-related perception of stature, acceptance of therapy, and psychosocial functioning in human growth hormone-treated girls with Turner's syndrome. J Clin Endocrinol Metab. 1998;83:1494–501.
10. Hong DS, Dunkin B, Reiss AL. Psychosocial functioning and social cognitive processing in girls with Turner syndrome. J Dev Behav Pediatr. 2011;32:512–20.
11. Boman UW, Bryman I, Halling K, Moller A. Women with Turner syndrome: psychological well-being, self-rated health and social life. J Psychosom Obstet Gynaecol. 2001;22:113–22.
12. Lagrou K, Froidecoeur C, Verlinde F, Craen M, De Schepper J, Francois I, Massa G, Belgian Study Group of Paediatric Endocrinology. Psychosocial functioning, self-perception and body image and their auxologic correlates in growth hormone and oestrogen-treated young adult women with Turner syndrome. Horm Res. 2006;66:277–84.
13. Reiss AL, Freund L, Plotnick L, Baumgardner T, Green K, Sozer AC, Reader M, Boehm C, Denckla MB. The effects of X monosomy on brain development: monozygotic twins discordant for Turner's syndrome. Ann Neurol. 1993;34:95–107.
14. Ross JL, Feuillan P, Kushner H, Roeltgen D, Cutler GB Jr. Absence of growth hormone effects on cognitive function in girls with Turner syndrome. J Clin Endocrinol Metab. 1997;82:1814–7.
15. Romans SM, Stefanatos G, Roeltgen DP, Kushner H, Ross JL. Transition to young adulthood in Ullrich-Turner syndrome: neurodevelopmental changes. Am J Med Genet. 1998;79:140–7.

16. Murphy DG, Allen G, Haxby JV, Largay KA, Daly E, White BJ, Powell CM, Schapiro MB. The effects of sex steroids, and the X chromosome, on female brain function: a study of the neuropsychology of adult Turner syndrome. Neuropsychologia. 1994;32:1309–23.
17. Buchanan L, Pavlovic J, Rovet J. The contribution of visuospatial working memory to impairments in facial processing and arithmetric in Turner syndrome. Brain Cogn. 1998;37:72–5.
18. Lawrence K, Kuntsi J, Coleman M, Campbell R, Skuse D. Face and emotion recognition deficits in Turner syndrome: a possible role for X-linked genes in amygdala development. Neuropsychology. 2003;17:39–49.
19. McCauley E, Kay T, Ito J, Treder R. The Turner syndrome: cognitive deficits, affective discrimination, and behavior problems. Child Dev. 1987;58:464–73.
20. Downey J, Ehrhardt AA, Gruen R, Bell JJ, Morishima A. Psychopathology and social functioning in women with Turner syndrome. J Nerv Ment Dis. 1989;177:191–201.
21. Hong DS, Reiss AL. Cognition and behavior in Turner syndrome: a brief review. Pediatr Endocrinol Rev. 2012;9:710–2.
22. Carel JC, Elie C, Ecosse E, Tauber M, Leger J, Cabrol S, Nicolino M, Brauner R, Chaussain JL, Coste J. Self-esteem and social adjustment in young women with Turner syndrome – influence of pubertal management and sexuality: population-based cohort study. J Clin Endocrinol Metab. 2006;91:2972–9.
23. Mazzocco MMM. The cognitive phenotype of Turner syndrome: specific learning disabilities. Int Congr Ser. 2006;1298:83–92.
24. Mccauley E, Feuillan P, Kushner H, Ross JL. Psychosocial development in adolescents with Turner syndrome. J Dev Behav Pediatr. 2001;22:360–5.
25. Lepage JF, Dunkin B, Hong DS, Reiss AL. Impact of cognitive profile on social functioning in prepubescent females with Turner syndrome. Child Neuropsychol. 2013;19:161–72.
26. Buchanan L, Pavlovic J, Rovet J. A reexamination of the visuospatial deficit in Turner syndrome: contributions of working memory. Dev Neuropsychol. 1998;14:341–67.
27. Brown WE, Kesler SR, Eliez S, Warsofsky IS, Haberecht M, Reiss AL. A volumetric study of parietal lobe subregions in Turner syndrome. Dev Med Child Neruol. 2004;46:607–9.
28. Kesler SR. Turner syndrome. Child Adolesc Psychiatr Clin N Am. 2007;16:709–22.
29. Cutter WJ, Daly EM, Robertson DM, Chitnis XA, van Amelsvoort TA, Simmons A, Ng VW, Williams BS, Shwa P, Conway GS, DH SK, Colier DA, Craig M, Murphy BG. Influence of X chromosome and hormones on human brain development: a magnetic resonance imaging and proton magnetic resonance spectroscopy study of Tuner syndrome. Biol Psychiatry. 2006;59:273–83.
30. Rovet JF. The psychoeducational characteristics of children with Turner syndrome. J Learn Disabil. 1993;26:333–41.
31. Mazzocco MMM. Math learning disability and math LD subtypes: evidence from studies of Turner syndrome, fragile X syndrome, and neurofibromatosis type 1. J Learn Disabil. 2001;34:520–33.
32. Nijhuis-Van der Sanden MW, Eling PA, Van Asseldonk EH, Van Galen GP. Decreased movement speed in girls with Turner syndrome: a problem in motor planning or muscle initiation? J Clin Exp Neuropsyhol. 2004;26:795–816.
33. Bruandet M, Molko N, Cohen L, Dehaene S. A cognitive characterization of dyscalculia in Turner syndrome. Neuropsychologia. 2004;42:288–98.
34. Temple CM, Marriott AJ. Arithmetical ability and disability in Turner's syndrome: a cognitive neuropsychological analysis. Dev Neuropsychol. 1998;14:47–67.
35. Kirk JW, Mazzocco MM, Kover ST. Assessing executive dysfunction in girls with fragile X or Turner syndrome using the Contingency Naming Test (CNT). Dev Neuropsychol. 2005;28:755–77.
36. Russlee HF, Wallis D, Mazzocco MM, Moshang T, Zackai E, Zinn AR, Ross JL, Muenke M. Increased prevalence of ADHD in Turner syndrome with no evidence of imprinting effects. J Pediatr Psychol. 2006;31:945–55.
37. Kilic BG, Erqur AT, Ocal G. Depression, levels of anxiety and self-concept in girls with Turner's syndrome. J Pediatr Endocrinol Metab. 2005;18:1111–7.

38. Russell HF, Wallis D, Mazzocco MM, Moshang T, Zackai E, Zinn AR, Ross JL, Muenke M. Increased prevalence of ADHD in Turner syndrome with no evidence of imprinting effects. J Pediatr Psychol. 2006;31:945–55.
39. Green T, Naylior PE, Davies W. Attention deficit hyperactivity disorder (ADHD) in phenotypically similar neurogenetic conditions: Turner syndrome and the RASopathies. J Neurodev Disord. 2017;9:25.
40. Nijhuis-van der Sanden RW, Smits-Engelsman BC, Eling PA. Motor performance in girls with Turner syndrome. Dev Med Child Neurol. 2000;42:685–90.
41. Ross JL, Kushner H, Roeltgen DP. Development changes in motor function in girls with Turner syndrome. Pediatr Neurol. 1996;15:317–22.
42. Lagrou K, Froidecoeur C, Verlinde F, Craen M, De Schepper J, Francois I, Massa G, Gelgian Study Group of Paediatric Endocrinology. Psychosocial functioning, self-perception and body image and their auxologic correlates in growth hormone and estrogen-treated young adult women with Turner syndrome. Horm Res. 2006;66:277–84.
43. Lesniak-Karpiak K, Mazzocco MM, Ross JL. Behavioral assessment of social anxiety in females with Turner syndrome or fragile X syndrome. J Autism Dev Disord. 2003;33:55–67.
44. Cardoso G, Daly R, Hag NA, Hanton L, Rubinow DR, Bondy CA, Schmidt P. Current and lifetime psychiatric illness in women with Turner syndrome. Gynecol Endocrinol. 2004;19:313–9.
45. McCauley E, Sybert VP, Ehrhardt AA. Psychosocial adjustment of adult women with Turner syndrome. Clin Genet. 1986;19:284–90.
46. Davies MC. Lost in transition: the needs of adolescents with Turner syndrome. BJOG. 2010;117:134–6.
47. Freriks K, Timmermans J, Beerendonk CCM, Verhaak CM, Netea-Maier RT, Otten BJ, Braat DD, Smeets DF, Kunst DH, Hermus AR, Timmers HJ. Standardized multidisciplinary evaluation yields significant previously undiagnosed morbidity in adult women with Turner syndrome. J Clin Endocrinol Metab. 2011;96:1517–26.
48. Viner RM. Transition of care from paediatric to adult services: one part of improved health services for adolescents. Arch Dis Child. 2008;93:160–3.
49. Gleeson H, Turner G. Transition to adult services. Arch Dis Child Educ Pract Ed. 2012;97:86–92.
50. Gleeson H. 'Part of the problem, part of the solution' – adult physicians' role in adolescent and young adult health. Clin Med. 2015;15:413–4.
51. Hokken-Koelega A, van der Lely AJ, Hauffa B, Hausler G, Johannsson G, Maghnie M, Argente J, DeSchepper J, Gleeson H, Gregory JW, Hoybye C, Kelestimur F, Luger A, Muller HL, Neggers S, Popovic-Brkic V, Porcu E, Savendahl L, Shalet S, Spiliotis B, Tauber M. Bridging the gap: metabolic and endocrine care of patients during transition. Endocr Connect. 2016;5:44–54.
52. Bayler N. Bayley scales of infant and toddler development. 3rd ed. San Antonio: Pearson; 2006.
53. Wechsler preschool and primary scale of intelligence (WPPSI-IV). 4th ed. San Antonio: Pearson; 2012.
54. Wechsler intelligence scale for children (WISC-V). 5th ed. Bloomington, MN: NCS Pearson; 2014.
55. Wechsler D. Wechsler adult intelligence scale – fourth edition (WAIS-IV). San Antonio: Pearson; 2008.
56. Korkman M, Kirk U, Kemp S. NEPSY – Second Edition (NEPSY – II). San Antonio: PsychCorp; 2007.
57. Gresham F, Elliott SN. Social skills improvement system (SSIS) rating scales. Minneapolis: NCS Pearson; 2008.
58. How to help your child survive and succeed at school – a guide for parents and teachers. Turner Syndrome Support Society, Clydebank, United Kingdom, TSSS.org; 2009.

Chapter 10
Ear and Hearing Problems in Turner Syndrome

Åsa Bonnard and Malou Hultcrantz

Abbreviation

Tfh cells   T follicular helper cells

Ear and hearing problems are frequent in women with Turner syndrome and have a negative effect on well-being and quality of life [1, 2]. Throughout life different periods of ear and hearing problems can be seen in girls and women with Turner syndrome. During childhood, there is a high incidence of otitis media resulting in a conductive hearing loss, frequent tympanostomy tube insertions, and antibiotic treatment [3–5]. Women with Turner syndrome also have a higher incidence of chronic otitis and cholesteatoma over time [6, 7]. Sensorineural hearing loss in the form of a mid-frequency dip can be present as early as age 5 and progresses over the years [8, 9]. A high-frequency sensorineural hearing loss that develops in early adulthood is often present, and this can have a devastating effect on the hearing situation for the individual. In such cases, hearing aids are often required earlier than in the normal population [10–13]. There is an increased risk for ear and hearing problems in all women with Turner syndrome, but it is more common in karyotype 45,X and 46,X,i(Xq) [3, 10, 14]. On an individual level, however, the phenotype penetration can vary which is why medical advice based on karyotype has to be carefully planned.

Å. Bonnard (✉) · M. Hultcrantz
Department of Clinical Science, Intervention and Technology, Division of Otorhinolaryngology, Karolinska Institutet, Stockholm, Sweden

Department of Otorhinolaryngology, Karolinska University Hospital, Stockholm, Sweden
e-mail: asa.bonnard@sll.se

P. Y. Fechner (ed.), *Turner Syndrome*,
https://doi.org/10.1007/978-3-030-34150-3_10

185

Anatomy and Function of the Ear

The purpose of the ear is to transform the soundwaves in the air into electrical signals and forward these to the auditory cortex in the brain via the auditory nerve and the auditory nuclei in the brain stem. The ear can be divided into three different sections where the first part, the auricle and the ear canal, will capture the soundwaves in the air and direct them toward the eardrum. The eardrum is the first part of the middle ear, a normally air-filled space containing the ossicles (malleus, incus, and stapes), the facial nerve, the taste nerve (chorda tympani), and the round and oval window, membrane-covered openings to the inner ear (Fig. 10.1a). The purpose of the middle ear is to transform the soundwaves in the air into a mechanical force transmitted to the liquid (perilymph) in the inner ear. The middle ear will also enhance the sound which is why a perforated eardrum or a discontinuation in the ossicular chain will have a negative effect on hearing accounting for a maximal loss of 60 dB. This hearing loss is called a *conductive hearing loss*. The ossicular chain is attached to the inner ear via the stapes footplate in the oval window.

The inner ear contains three liquid filled canals, the scala vestibuli, scala media, and scala tympani (Fig. 10.1b). The movement of the stapes footplate in the oval window will create a pressure wave in the perilymph in the scala vestibule. This pressure wave will travel the 2.5 turns up to the apex of the cochlea via the scala vestibuli and down again via the scala tympani. The organ of Corti is situated in

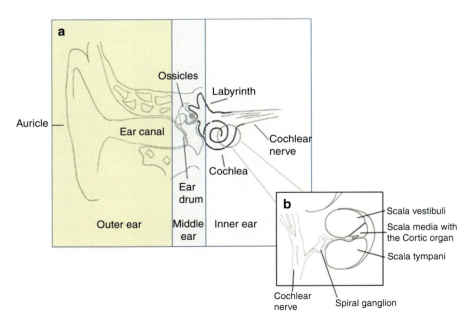

Fig. 10.1 Schematic figure of (**a**) the outer, middle, and inner ear with (**b**) a detail of the inner ear (Drawing by Mattias Krakau)

scala media and contains one row of inner hair cells and three rows of outer hair cells covered by the tectorial membrane, where the stereocilia (hairs) are embedded. When a pressure wave produces a movement in the basilar membrane where the hair cells are anchored, the stereocilia then bend, and the mechanical force is transformed into a release of nerve-stimulating neurotransmitters activating the cochlear nerve. The signal is then transmitted to the brain stem and further to the auditory cortex in the brain. The spiral ganglion nerve threads comprise the cochlear nerve which connects to the cochlear nuclei in the brain stem. Nerve fibers continue through the brain stem, mid-brain, and thalamus to the primary auditory cortex in the temporal region. If the hair cells or nerves are malfunctioning, the result would be a hearing loss called *sensorineural hearing loss*. The afferent system also crosses over in the brain stem; thus, the auditory input from one ear stimulates the cortex region on both sides of the brain.

Hearing Tests

Pure Tone Audiometry

In order to establish the hearing level of the quietest sound detectable for an individual, the normal "hearing test," pure tone audiometry, is performed in a sound-proof room. Adults and older children listen to a sound coming from headphones and push a button, while younger children may build a tower with building blocks when a sound is detected. For the youngest, a behavioral observation audiometry is performed when the audiologist detects a behavioral change in the child as a reaction to a given sound. Air conduction and bone conduction for the frequencies 0.125–8 kHz and 0.250–4 kHz, respectively, are usually performed, thus covering most of the spectrum for speech. The cochlea is tonotopic; i.e., the highest frequencies will activate the hair cells in the base of the cochlea and the lowest frequencies in the top, apex.

OAE

Oto-acoustic emissions, OAE, are generated in the outer hair cells in the cochlea in response to sound stimuli and are measured with a probe in the ear canal. The purpose of this test is to determine cochlear function, specifically the function of the inner hair cells, and is used in hearing screening programs for newborns in some countries. It can also be used as an objective measurement of normal hearing in individuals who cannot perform an audiogram, i.e., in a coma, young children, or handicapped, or in hearing loss to determine a cochlear or retrocochlear origin of the hearing impairment. A response is generated if the hearing is better than

25–35 dB. There are different types of optoacoustic emissions used where TEOAE and DPOAE are the most common. TEOAE, transient-evoked optoacoustic emissions, is the recording of the cochlear response to transient click sounds or sound bursts with a wide frequency range. In DPOAE, distortion product optoacoustic emissions, two tones are used simultaneously to provoke a response from the inner hair cells.

ABR

Auditory brain stem response is an objective measure of hearing threshold and the function of the retrocochlear auditory system from signals in the brain stem. The stimulation is usually rapid multifrequency clicks (*Michael I.G. Simpson∗, Garreth Prendergast, in Handbook of Clinical Neurophysiology, 2013*) that are recorded with scalp EEG electrodes. In adults, this measurement can be performed while the person sits relaxed in a dark room, while young children often need sedation or general anesthesia. The result is typically five different components in waveforms (wave I–V) where the first (I) is the auditory nerve response and the last is the superior olivary nucleus in the brain stem. An automatized version, eABR, is used as a hearing screening tool in some countries.

Speech Audiometry

Speech is harder to hear than the sound detection as is measured in pure tone audiometry. Speech audiometry is a way to measure a more complex form of hearing that better mimics the demands in normal listening environments. These tests can be single words or sentences with and without noise in the background. Hard-of-hearing children and adults usually have difficulty hearing in noisy environments (discrimination). Hearing in noise has a higher demand on the overall auditory system due to the activation of both primary auditory cortex and other auditory associated areas in the brain. Loss of function in the auditory-associated areas, e.g., in aging or hearing impairment, will hamper the hearing in noise [15].

Type, Grade, and Configuration of Hearing Loss

Hearing loss can be divided in different *types*, *grades*, and *configuration* in regard to the reason for the severity of and the aspect of the impairment. There are three main *types* of peripheral hearing loss: conductive, sensorineural, and mixed. Conductive hearing loss is due to a disturbed pathway for the sound from the ear canal through the middle ear and can be expected in acute and chronic otitis, in tympanic membrane perforations, and in disturbances in the ossicular chain. Problems interfering with the inner ear or nerve give rise to sensorineural hearing loss. A combination of these two is referred to as a mixed hearing loss.

Pure tone average (PTA4) is calculated as the mean of 0.500, 1, 2, and 4 (or 3) kHz and is used to determine the *grade of hearing loss*. Normal hearing is usually classified as a PTA4 at 25 dB or better according to WHO (http://www.who.int/pbd/deafness/hearing_impairment_grades/en/). Slight or mild hearing loss means having trouble hearing in background noise or at a distance and is diagnosed when the mean hearing loss (PTA) is between 26 and 40 dB. Between 41 and 60 dB, there is a moderate hearing loss with troubles hearing regular speech even at a normal distance. In severe hearing loss, 61–80 dB, it is difficult to hear normal conversational speech, and the person might only hear loud environmental sounds as fire sirens. Eighty dB is the limit for profound hearing loss, and with that level of hearing, a person might only perceive loud sounds as vibrations.

The *configuration of hearing loss* can be divided into five main types according to the modified classification by Hederstierna et al.: high-frequency hearing loss, high-frequency U-shaped, mid-frequency U-shaped, low-frequency rising, and flat loss [16, 17]. High-frequency U-shaped is not frequent in Turner syndrome and is not further discussed. An isolated high-frequency hearing loss, *high-frequency sloping*, is described as when a person hears the lower frequencies better than the higher. This can affect hearing even at the level of mild hearing loss due to a number of important phonemic sounds that demand a good high-frequency hearing as the f and s sound and the "th" sound in the English language. A *mid-frequency U-shaped* hearing loss, an audiogram shaped like a basin with worse hearing in 1.5 and 2 kHz, is less likely to be detected early due to a lesser demand for hearing in those frequencies. In the configuration *low-frequency rising* hearing loss, the person hears better in the higher frequencies than in the lower, something that might affect hearing in noise and difficulties with male voices. In *flat* hearing loss, all frequencies will be evenly affected with no frequency better than another (Fig. 10.2).

Ear and Hearing Problems in Turner Syndrome

Hearing: A Main Factor for Quality in Life

Girls and women with Turner syndrome are affected with ear and hearing problems to a greater extent than women in the general population [11]. There is an increased risk for recurrent otitis media in childhood as well as an augmented need of ear surgery throughout life [4, 7]. Hearing loss, both conductive and sensorineural, is more frequent and affects all aspects of communication, both in personal relations and at work or leisure-related activities. In surveys, women with Turner syndrome grade hearing as one of the most important medical problems [1]. Women in general have a quite stable hearing up until the age of menopause in comparison with men whose hearing start to decline already around the age of 30 [18, 19]. Studies have

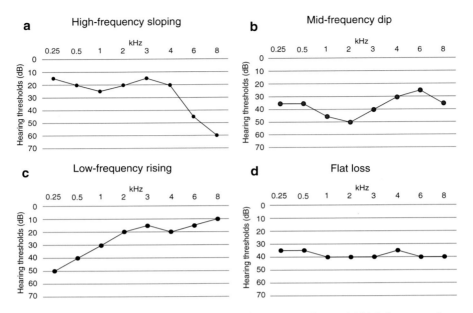

Fig. 10.2 Hearing configurations commonly seen in Turner syndrome: (**a**) high-frequency sloping, (**b**) mid-frequency U-shaped (or Turner dip), (**c**) low-frequency rising, and (**d**) flat loss. A combination of high-frequency sloping (**a**) and mid-frequency U-shaped (**b**) configurations is often seen and is devastating for speech understanding

shown that compared to women in the general population, the mean hearing in girls and women with Turner syndrome is worse at all ages in life [16] and mitigates the hearing decline in men in regard to the high-frequency loss. At the age of 40, the mean hearing level is comparable with women 20 years their age (60 years) in the general population (Fig. 10.3). The need for a good audiological surveillance and rehabilitation is crucial for maintaining the quality of life and to reduce hearing-related problems at work and in social situations.

Ear Infections: Otitis Media and Treatment

Girls and women with Turner syndrome are particularly prone to ear infections. In different studies, a prevalence between 24% and 88% of girls with Turner syndrome has had recurrent ear infections during childhood [1, 3–5, 20–22]. The prevalence of otitis media with effusion is also high, between 55% and 78% in different studies [6, 23]. This is more frequent in the general population. When having an acute otitis media or a period of otitis media with effusion, a conductive hearing loss will be present leading to a hearing loss of between 10 and 30 dB. About 40% of girls with Turner syndrome under the age of 16 have conductive hearing loss [6, 23]. This may interfere with language development and general learning in school [24]. Girls with karyotype 45,X are more prone to otitis media than other karyotypes [3, 4, 11, 22, 23, 25–27].

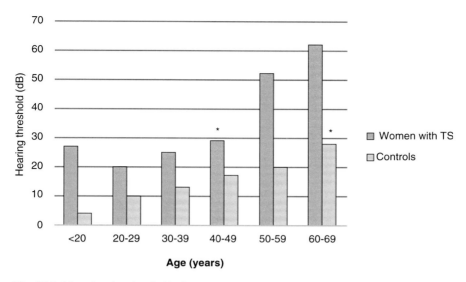

Fig. 10.3 Mean hearing thresholds for women with Turner syndrome (TS) and controls within different age spans. Women with Turner syndrome have a worse hearing in each category. The asterisk (∗) shows the comparable hearing thresholds for women with Turner syndrome aged 40–49 and controls aged 60–69

Background

The reason for the high incidence of otitis media in girls and women with Turner syndrome is not entirely known, but there are some anatomical and immunological differences that play a part. In Turner syndrome, a lack of the growth-promoting SHOX gene on the X chromosome is responsible for the short stature and also affects the development of the skull base [4, 5, 14, 23, 28, 29]. This results in a shortening of the skull base leading to a more horizontal projection of the Eustachian tube. This is associated with an increased risk for otitis media and a negative middle ear pressure [28]. Recent studies have also identified a deficiency of a specific immune cell, the *T* follicular helper (*T*fh) cells, in women with Turner syndrome [30]. The *T*fh cells are critical for antibody generation from the B cells, and an important step in the immunological response to infection. Further studies are needed to enhance the knowledge in this field.

Treatment

There is no medical treatment present today to prevent neither acute otitis media nor otitis media with effusion. An episode of acute otitis media can be treated with antibiotics and/or symptomatic treatment in regard to age and local treatment programs. For recurrent problems with both acute otitis media and otitis media with effusion, a surgical treatment with trans-tympanic tubes is common in girls with Turner syndrome [4]. The tubes ensure air to enter the middle ear, thus preventing effusion and a possible conductive hearing loss. The tubes are normally extruded within 6 months to 2 years after surgery why the procedure might need to be repeated surgery can be possible. In most cases, the perforation in the eardrum heals by itself, but in girls with Turner syndrome, about 10–20% have chronic persisting perforations [4, 8, 23]. A tympanoplasty can be performed to close the perforation. To ensure proper treatment and follow up, all girls and women with Turner syndrome with ear problems should be followed by an otorhinolaryngologist. According to the Clinical Practice Guidelines for the care of girls and women with Turner syndrome [31], the treatment for detected middle ear disease should be aggressive, and an audiogram should be performed every 5 years.

Chronic Otitis, Cholesteatoma, and Surgery

The frequency of tympanic membrane retraction and cholesteatoma formation is elevated in women with Turner syndrome with a prevalence of 19 and 3–15%, respectively, found in studies [6, 7, 22, 23]. A retracted tympanic membrane, with or without cholesteatoma formation (a sac formation of the eardrum filled with keratin debris), is thought to be due partly to a decreased pressure in the middle ear caused by the altered anatomy and function of the Eustachian tube [28]. Other contributing factors are the scarring and weakening of the eardrum due to recurrent infections. A retracted eardrum can negatively affect the underlying ossicles in the middle ear, leading to destruction of the bones with conductive hearing loss as a result. There is also an increased number of chronic otitis in women with Turner syndrome. It presents with discharging, sometimes smelly ears with hearing loss, and a perforated or retracted eardrum.

Treatment

The first step in treating these conditions is to establish a dry ear by local cleaning, using eardrops, and avoiding water in the ear while showering and bathing. An ear with a cholesteatoma formation can sometimes avoid surgical treatment by recurrent cleaning by an otolaryngologist, but surgery is usually needed at some point to prevent a negative effect on hearing and creating a waterproof ear. The literature presents a high recurrence rate of cholesteatoma after surgery in girls and women with Turner syndrome [6, 7].

Sensorineural Hearing Loss

Sensorineural hearing loss is common in women with Turner syndrome, and it usually presents in one of two ways: the mid-frequency dip or the high-frequency loss (high-frequency sloping configuration). The mid-frequency dip can be present as a mild hearing loss as early as the age of 5 and has a tendency to aggravate over the years [8, 9]. A hearing loss in these frequencies usually pass unnoticed for a longer time compared with a high-frequency loss due to a lower demand on hearing in the mid-frequencies. The high-frequency loss resembles presbycusis, a high-frequency loss in old age, but women with Turner syndrome are younger, and the progress is faster [11, 12, 16, 20]. The combination of the mid- and high-frequency loss has a devastating effect on hearing, and hearing aids are often needed. At the age of 40, only about 25% of women with Turner syndrome have a normal hearing [12]. The sensorineural hearing loss together with a conductive hearing loss, i.e., mixed hearing loss, is often present in women having had ear surgery or having chronic otitis.

Background

The reason for the sensorineural hearing loss is still debated, but genetic and hormonal causes have been discussed. Estrogen has neuroprotective effects in the brain and is crucial for the hearing process in the inner ear. Mice lacking one of two estrogen receptors in the inner ear become deaf within a year and show an increased sensitivity for acoustic trauma [32, 33]. Studies have shown presence of estrogen receptors in the inner ear in Turner syndrome, but the function of the receptors is still unknown [34]. There are associated neurocognitive problems in Turner syndrome including impaired visual-spatial abilities, attention, working memory, and spatially dependent executive functions [35] which is why a central origin to the hearing loss could be possible. Studies using OAE, ABR, and speech recognition tests have shown that the hearing loss seems to be connected to the inner ear and not central auditory pathways [13]. The lack of endogenous estrogen could be implicated in the cochlear malfunction, but no studies have been able to show this.

Women with karyotype 45,X or karyotypes with a loss of the short, p-arm of the X-chromosome appear to be more prone to ear and hearing problems [10, 14], while women with mosaic karyotype are less affected. This has led to a search for a gene affecting ear and hearing in this part of the genome, but none has been identified yet. Recent advances in the genetic field have revealed that many genes on the X chromosome, rather than having a proper effect on its own, affect other genes in the genome. This opens up a new range of possible genes or combination of genes and other interacting agents responsible for the ear and hearing problems in Turner syndrome, and a lot of work remains before certain answers can be given.

Treatment

The hearing loss in middle-aged women with Turner syndrome (age 41–61) is most commonly in the moderate range [12] which is why a normal hearing aid is usually enough. Severe to profound hearing loss ir rare but if present a wider hearing rehabilitation might be needed, somtimes including a cochlear implant can be needed. For conductive or mixed hearing loss, a bone-anchored hearing aid system (BAHS) can be beneficial if a normal hearing aid cannot be worn due to discharge. It is important with regular audiological follow-up every 3–5 years to ensure an optimal treatment [31].

Hearing Rehabilitation

An adult onset of hearing loss affects social interactions at all levels. It might induce social uncertainty, anxiety, and reluctance to interact with others due to fear of misunderstandings which can lead to social withdrawal and isolation [36]. Hearing loss is associated with decreased health-related quality of life and depression [37]. There are different types of treatment for hearing loss depending on the type and degree. Surgery with ossiculoplasty or middle ear implants can be efficient for mild to moderate conductive or mixed hearing loss. In other cases, a hearing aid is a better solution. For severe to profound hearing loss, a cochlear implant is the treatment of choice.

Audiologic Rehabilitation

The importance of contact with and counseling from an experienced audiology team cannot be stressed enough. Besides discussions regarding hearing aid solutions for hearing loss, the individual might be in need of acquiring knowledge in speech reading, communication strategies, psychosocial exercises, additional assistive devices, and lectures aiming to give an understanding of the reason for hearing loss and the effects on the daily life. Performing audiologic rehabilitation in a group setting improves the possibility to face the problems with the help of others facing the same problem but are effective on an individual basis as well [38].

Hearing Aids

The most common treatment for hearing loss today is hearing aids. It is used in mild to severe hearing loss and works as a sound amplifier, resembling the function of the middle ear. It collects the sound with an external microphone, enhances the signal, and projects it into the ear canal. In bone-anchored hearing systems, BAHS, the vibrations are created and transmitted from a percutaneous titanium screw or a subcutaneous floating mass transducer in the bone, where it will be conducted directly to the inner ear. For these systems to work, the ear must have enough hair cells remaining in the inner ear in order to create an electric signal to the brain. When there is a lack of hair cells, the possibility to hear will decrease in general, but a lack of hair cells can also affect the quality of the sound making it harder to interpret words. For people with severe to profound hearing loss, a cochlear implant might be the treatment of choice.

Cochlear Implants

In severe to profound hearing loss, a cochlear implant is usually the hearing aid most appropriate. A cochlear implant has two parts, an outer part with microphone and processor that transfers the sound as an electric signal to the inner part via a magnet. Under the skin, an inner part receives the signals that will reach the auditory nerve via an electrode inserted in the inner ear. This hearing aid is not dependent on existing hair cells but affects the nerve endings directly. Due to limitations in the spectral and temporal resolution, an individual with a cochlear implant will be needing a certain amount of training before reaching a satisfying hearing result.

Surgery

A conductive hearing loss might be due to a perforated eardrum or a fixed or disconnected ossicular chain. This can most often be treated with surgery if no contraindications are present. Middle ear surgery are routine procedures with a high chance of positive hearing results but have a small risk of affecting the function in the taste nerve (the chorda tympani) and the facial nerve. Other side effects can include deterioration of hearing, tinnitus, balance disturbance, and in rare cases deafness, but the risks are small [39].

Conclusion

Ear and hearing problems are common in girls and women with Turner syndrome which is why an otolaryngologist should be connected to all Turner centers. In childhood, recurrent otitis media or otitis media with effusion leading to conductive hearing loss is predominant, while a sensorineural hearing loss in the middle- and/or high-frequency region are most common in adulthood. Mild to moderate hearing loss is common hence the need for hearing rehabilitation with hearing aids or middle ear surgery. Severe hearing loss is rare, but occasionally hearing rehabilitation with a cochlear implant is necessary. Mean hearing in girls and women with Turner syndrome is worse than in women in general throughout life. Due to recurrent ear infections and an anatomical predisposition for Eustachian tube dysfunction, girls and women with Turner syndrome have a higher incidence of chronic otitis and cholesteatoma formation. Surgery is often needed.

References

1. Hultcrantz M. Ear and hearing problems in Turner's syndrome. Acta Otolaryngol. 2003;123(2):253–7.
2. Carel JC, Ecosse E, Bastie-Sigeac I, Cabrol S, Tauber M, Leger J, et al. Quality of life determinants in young women with Turner's syndrome after growth hormone treatment: results of the StaTur population-based cohort study. J Clin Endocrinol Metab. 2005;90(4):1992–7.
3. Verver EJ, Freriks K, Thomeer HG, Huygen PL, Pennings RJ, Alfen-van der Velden AA, et al. Ear and hearing problems in relation to karyotype in children with Turner syndrome. Hear Res. 2011;275(1–2):81–8.
4. Stenberg AE, Nylen O, Windh M, Hultcrantz M. Otological problems in children with Turner's syndrome. Hear Res. 1998;124(1–2):85–90.
5. Sculerati N, Ledesma-Medina J, Finegold DN, Stool SE. Otitis media and hearing loss in Turner syndrome. Arch Otolaryngol Head Neck Surg. 1990;116(6):704–7.
6. Hall JE, Richter GT, Choo DI. Surgical management of otologic disease in pediatric patients with Turner syndrome. Int J Pediatr Otorhinolaryngol. 2009;73(1):57–65.
7. Lim DBN, Gault EJ, Kubba H, Morrissey MSC, Wynne DM, Donaldson MDC. Cholesteatoma has a high prevalence in Turner syndrome, highlighting the need for earlier diagnosis and the potential benefits of otoscopy training for paediatricians. Acta Paediatrica. 2014;103(7):e282–7.
8. Davenport ML, Roush J, Liu C, Zagar AJ, Eugster E, Travers S, et al. Growth hormone treatment does not affect incidences of middle ear disease or hearing loss in infants and toddlers with Turner syndrome. Horm Res Paediatr. 2010;74(1):23–32.
9. Roush J, Davenport ML, Carlson-Smith C. Early-onset sensorineural hearing loss in a child with Turner syndrome. J Am Acad Audiol. 2000;11(8):446–53.
10. Cameron-Pimblett A, La Rosa C, King TFJ, Davies MC, Conway GS. The Turner syndrome life course project: karyotype-phenotype analyses across the lifespan. Clin Endocrinol. 2017;87(5):532–8.
11. Hultcrantz M, Sylven L, Borg E. Ear and hearing problems in 44 middle-aged women with Turner's syndrome. Hear Res. 1994;76(1–2):127–32.
12. King KA, Makishima T, Zalewski CK, Bakalov VK, Griffith AJ, Bondy CA, et al. Analysis of auditory phenotype and karyotype in 200 females with Turner syndrome. Ear Hear. 2007;28(6):831–41.
13. Hederstierna C, Hultcrantz M, Rosenhall U. Estrogen and hearing from a clinical point of view; characteristics of auditory function in women with Turner syndrome. Hear Res. 2009;252(1–2):3–8.
14. Barrenas M, Landin-Wilhelmsen K, Hanson C. Ear and hearing in relation to genotype and growth in Turner syndrome. Hear Res. 2000;144(1–2):21–8.
15. Anderson S, White-Schwoch T, Choi HJ, Kraus N. Training changes processing of speech cues in older adults with hearing loss. Front Syst Neurosci. 2013;7:97.
16. Bonnard A, Hederstierna C, Bark R, Hultcrantz M. Audiometric features in young adults with Turner syndrome. Int J Audiol. 2017;56(9):650–6.
17. Hederstierna C, Hultcrantz M, Collins A, Rosenhall U. Hearing in women at menopause. Prevalence of hearing loss, audiometric configuration and relation to hormone replacement therapy. Acta Otolaryngol. 2007;127(2):149–55.
18. Hederstierna C, Hultcrantz M, Collins A, Rosenhall U. The menopause triggers hearing decline in healthy women. Hear Res. 2010;259(1–2):31–5.
19. Johansson MSK, Arlinger SD. Hearing threshold levels for an otologically unscreened, non-occupationally noise-exposed population in Sweden: umbrales auditivos en una población no estudiada, sin exposición a ruido ocupacional en Suecia. Int J Audiol. 2009;41(3):180–94.
20. Sculerati N, Oddoux C, Clayton CM, Lim JW, Oster H. Hearing loss in turner syndrome. Laryngoscope. 1996;106(8):992–7.
21. Dhooge IJ, De Vel E, Verhoye C, Lemmerling M, Vinck B. Otologic disease in Turner syndrome. Otol Neurotol. 2005;26(2):145–50.

22. Bois E, Nassar M, Zenaty D, Leger J, Van Den Abbeele T, Teissier N. Otologic disorders in Turner syndrome. Eur Ann Otorhinolaryngol Head Neck Dis. 2018;135(1):21–4.
23. Bergamaschi R, Bergonzoni C, Mazzanti L, Scarano E, Mencarelli F, Messina F, et al. Hearing loss in Turner syndrome: results of a multicentric study. J Endocrinol Investig. 2008;31(9):779–83.
24. Hall AJ, Maw R, Midgley E, Golding J, Steer C. Glue ear, hearing loss and IQ: an association moderated by the child's home environment. PLoS One. 2014;9(2):e87021.
25. Morimoto N, Tanaka T, Taiji H, Horikawa R, Naiki Y, Morimoto Y, et al. Hearing loss in Turner syndrome. J Pediatr. 2006;149(5):697–701.
26. Barrenas ML, Nylen O, Hanson C. The influence of karyotype on the auricle, otitis media and hearing in Turner syndrome. Hear Res. 1999;138(1–2):163–70.
27. Hultcrantz M, Sylvén L. Turner's syndrome and hearing disorders in women aged 16–34. Hear Res. 1997;103(1–2):69–74.
28. Anderson H, Filipsson R, Fluur E, Koch B, Lindsten J, Wedenberg E. Hearing impairment in Turner's syndrome. Acta Otolaryngol. 1969;247(Suppl):1–26.
29. Rizell S, Barrenas ML, Andlin-Sobocki A, Stecksen-Blicks C, Kjellberg H. 45,X/46,XX karyotype mitigates the aberrant craniofacial morphology in Turner syndrome. Eur J Orthod. 2013;35(4):467–74.
30. Cook KD, Shpargel KB, Starmer J, Whitfield-Larry F, Conley B, Allard DE, et al. T follicular helper cell-dependent clearance of a persistent virus infection requires T cell expression of the histone demethylase UTX. Immunity. 2015;43(4):703–14.
31. Gravholt CH, Andersen NH, Conway GS, Dekkers OM, Geffner ME, Klein KO, et al. Clinical practice guidelines for the care of girls and women with Turner syndrome: proceedings from the 2016 Cincinnati International Turner Syndrome Meeting. Eur J Endocrinol. 2017;177(3):G1–g70.
32. Simonoska R, Stenberg AE, Duan M, Yakimchuk K, Fridberger A, Sahlin L, et al. Inner ear pathology and loss of hearing in estrogen receptor-beta deficient mice. J Endocrinol. 2009;201(3):397–406.
33. Meltser I, Tahera Y, Simpson E, Hultcrantz M, Charitidi K, Gustafsson JA, et al. Estrogen receptor beta protects against acoustic trauma in mice. J Clin Invest. 2008;118(4):1563–70.
34. Stenberg AE, Wang H, Fish J 3rd, Schrott-Fischer A, Sahlin L, Hultcrantz M. Estrogen receptors in the normal adult and developing human inner ear and in Turner's syndrome. Hear Res. 2001;157(1–2):87–92.
35. Ross J, Roeltgen D, Zinn A. Cognition and the sex chromosomes: studies in Turner syndrome. Horm Res. 2006;65(1):47–56.
36. Monzani D, Galeazzi GM, Genovese E, Marrara A, Martini A. Psychological profile and social behaviour of working adults with mild or moderate hearing loss. Acta Otorhinolaryngol Ital. 2008;28(2):61–6.
37. Gopinath B, Hickson L, Schneider J, McMahon CM, Burlutsky G, Leeder SR, et al. Hearing-impaired adults are at increased risk of experiencing emotional distress and social engagement restrictions five years later. Age Ageing. 2012;41(5):618–23.
38. Laplante-Levesque A, Hickson L, Worrall L. Factors influencing rehabilitation decisions of adults with acquired hearing impairment. Int J Audiol. 2010;49(7):497–507.
39. Phillips JS, Yung MW, Nunney I. Myringoplasty outcomes in the UK. J Laryngol Otol. 2015;129(9):860–4.

Chapter 11
Ocular Features in Turner Syndrome

Erin P. Herlihy and Jolene C. Rudell

The prevalence of ocular disorders is higher in patients with Turner syndrome than in the general population. In a cross-sectional observational study, more than 50% of patients with Turner syndrome were found to have one or more eye disorder. More than 40% of these diagnoses were related to impaired vision [10, 23], with 1/3 of patients diagnosed with more than one ocular condition. It is important that patients with Turner syndrome undergo regular ocular screening, as the eye problems may be associated with visual morbidity and, sometimes, preventable visual impairment.

In 2004 Denniston and Butler published a review summarizing the prevalence of ophthalmic findings in patients with Turner syndrome. Their findings are summarized in Table 11.1.

It is not known with certainty why patients with Turner syndrome have such a high prevalence of eye disorders, though a similar genetic pathway for eye and ovary development may exist. The Usp9x gene on the X chromosome is responsible for gonadal dysgenesis in Turner syndrome. The same gene has been shown to play an important role in development of both the eye and the ovary in the fruit fly *Drosophila* [16]. Similar developmental pathways may overlap and direct gonadal dysgenesis in addition to abnormal eye development.

E. P. Herlihy (✉) · J. C. Rudell
Department of Ophthalmology, University of Washington School of Medicine, Seattle, WA, USA

Division of Pediatric Ophthalmology, Seattle Children's Hospital, Seattle, WA, USA
e-mail: erin.herlihy@seattlechildrens.org

© Springer Nature Switzerland AG 2020
P. Y. Fechner (ed.), *Turner Syndrome*,
https://doi.org/10.1007/978-3-030-34150-3_11

Table 11.1 A review
summarizing the prevalence
of ophthalmic findings in
patients with turner syndrome

	Total	%
Amblyopia	45/156	29%
Strabismus	77/274	33%
Hyperopia	65/242	27%
Myopia	23/177	13%
Nystagmus	12/134	9%
Ptosis	46/219	21%
Red-green deficiency	20/241	8%
Presenile cataract	3/96	3%
Congenital glaucoma	1/96	1%

Refractive Error

One of the most commonly reported vision problems in children with Turner syndrome is refractive error, with nearly half of children affected with hyperopia, myopia, and/or astigmatism [10]. Mild refractive error may not be visually significant for many patients, but high degrees of uncorrected refractive error can significantly limit daily functioning and can lead to long-term visual disability. Significant refractive error is treated with glasses, or sometimes with contact lenses, often affording appreciable improvement in quality of life.

Strabismus

Strabismus (misalignment of the eyes) is another common ocular problem among patients with Turner syndrome. The prevalence of strabismus is approximately 5–10 times higher in patients with Turner syndrome than in the general population, with rates ranging from 21% to 33% in patients with Turner syndrome compared to 2–6% children in the general population [6, 23]. The high incidence of strabismus may be related to the high prevalence of refractive error in this population, as some forms of strabismus are associated with high hyperopia or myopia. Clinically significant strabismus is typically diagnosed after 4 months of age, as infants commonly demonstrate transient strabismus that resolves in the first few months of life.

The treatment of strabismus depends on the type of eye misalignment and sometimes on other factors such as patient age, refractive error, and eye alignment control. Common treatment modalities include glasses for refractive strabismus and surgical correction.

Amblyopia

Uncorrected refractive error and strabismus can also cause amblyopia or decreased vision in one or both eyes. Amblyopia develops when poor visual input leads to abnormal development of the neural pathways involved in vision. Amblyopia can occur secondary to many causes, most commonly uncorrected or unequal refractive error between the eyes and strabismus. Rates of amblyopia are higher in patients with Turner syndrome than the general population, ranging from 16% to 41% [1, 10, 23], versus approximately 4% among nonsyndromic children in the United States [15].

Amblyopia is important to detect early, as treatment is especially effective with occlusive therapy or pharmacologic penalization when a child is young, typically under the age of 7 years [11, 12, 14, 19]. As a child gets older, amblyopia therapy is less efficacious, with resultant unilateral or bilateral visual morbidity that may have been prevented.

Screening for Ocular Disorders

The key to detecting refractive error or amblyopia in children is to screen appropriately, beginning in the primary care physician's office. It is important that the acuity for each eye is tested separately, and an adhesive eye patch to cover one eye is preferable to a plastic occluder which may be easy for the child to peek around. If there is a discrepancy in acuity between the eyes, or if vision is poor in both eyes, prompt referral to an ophthalmologist for further evaluation and treatment is paramount.

Due to the high prevalence of refractive error and strabismus in the Turner syndrome population, a yearly screening examination with an experienced pediatric ophthalmologist, beginning at the age of 12–18 months or at the time of diagnosis, is advisable. This examination should include age-appropriate assessment of visual acuity, cycloplegic refraction, examination of ocular motility and alignment, evaluation of the ocular adnexa including eyelid position and configuration, and anterior and posterior segment examinations.

Ptosis

In addition to other characteristic physical features such as webbed neck, low hairline, retrognathia, and high-arched palate, individuals with Turner syndrome may demonstrate hypertelorism (widely spaced eyes), epicanthal folds (skin folds at the inner corners of the eyes), and ptosis (droopy eyelids). These ocular features are also seen in other genetic syndromes such as Noonan syndrome and are typically not visually significant.

Ptosis in particular, however, may affect normal visual development if the eyelid position blocks visual information from entering the eye or if the weight of the droopy eyelid(s) induces a large degree of astigmatism. Children often develop compensatory mechanisms such as adopting a chin up head position and recruiting the frontalis muscle to assist in raising the eyelids. As long as vision develops normally, surgical repair of ptosis is best delayed until 4–5 years of age or older, when the majority of the growth of the frontoorbital complex is complete. However, if the ophthalmologist determines that ptosis is visually significant for a young child with Turner syndrome, surgical correction may be indicated at a younger age.

Color Vision Deficiency

Red-green color vision deficiency, which is most commonly an X-linked recessive trait, is also reported in patients with Turner syndrome due to the single X chromosome. Reported prevalence in Turner syndrome is 5–10%, higher than the 0.5% prevalence in women without Turner syndrome [6, 23]. Severity can range from mild color vision abnormality to more moderate phenotypes.

A number of studies attempt to ascertain whether patients with color vision deficiency have difficulties with activities of daily living. Many studies conclude that patients with color blindness may have difficulty discriminating visual tasks that rely on color. For example, recognizing street signs and traffic lights may be difficult, and this can lead to increased reaction times while driving [2, 9, 13]. Other studies disagree, arguing that decreased color vision does not necessarily translate into increased incidence of traffic accidents and therefore normal color vision should not be a requirement to drive [4, 5, 7, 13, 17, 18, 22].

Some studies suggest that color vision deficiency can make certain jobs more difficult [3]. For example, healthcare professionals may rely on color cues to identify bleeding or rashes. In certain countries and in several occupations such as aviation, color vision screening tests are administered to applicants. There is increasing evidence that such color vision testing is limiting, however, as color vision screens often do not discriminate the severity of color blindness [8, 20, 21]. Individuals with mild color vision abnormalities can often function well in visually demanding occupations.

Other Ocular Disorders

Several other rare ophthalmologic conditions are also more commonly seen in individuals with Turner syndrome than in unaffected children. Nystagmus (unsteady gaze holding) is reported in up to 9% of cases and can be idiopathic or related to other ocular conditions such as cataract. Congenital or childhood cataracts and glaucoma, although rare in any population, are also more frequent in the setting of Turner syndrome and may require surgical intervention if normal visual development is threatened.

Summary

The prevalence of ocular disorders is higher in individuals with Turner syndrome than in the general population. Significant refractive error and strabismus are common and can lead to irreversible amblyopia if not diagnosed and treated in a timely manner. Ptosis and color vision deficiency are also commonly seen, with varying impact on daily activities and visual development. Regular ophthalmologic examinations beginning in the first 12–18 months of life, or sooner if concerns are identified, are important to ensure timely identification and management of ocular disorders to maximize the visual potential of children with Turner syndrome.

References

1. Adhikary HP. Ocular manifestations of Turner's syndrome. Trans Ophthalmol Soc U K. 1981;101(Pt 4):395–6.
2. Atchison DA, Pedersen CA, Dain SJ, Wood JM. Traffic signal color recognition is a problem for both protan and deutan color-vision deficients. Hum Factors. 2003;45(3):495–503.
3. Birch J, Chisholm CM. Occupational colour vision requirements for police officers. Ophthalmic Physiol Opt. 2008;28(6):524–31.
4. Casson EJ, Racette L. Vision standards for driving in Canada and the United States. A review for the Canadian Ophthalmological Society. Can J Ophthalmol. 2000;35(4):192–203.
5. Charman WN. Vision and driving–a literature review and commentary. Ophthalmic Physiol Opt. 1997;17(5):371–91.
6. Chrousos GA, Ross JL, Chrousos G, Chu FC, Kenigsberg D, Cutler G Jr, Loriaux DL. Ocular findings in Turner syndrome. A prospective study. Ophthalmology. 1984;91(8):926–8.
7. Cumberland P, Rahi JS, Peckham CS. Impact of congenital colour vision deficiency on education and unintentional injuries: findings from the 1958 British birth cohort. BMJ. 2004;329(7474):1074–5.
8. Cumberland P, Rahi JS, Peckham CS. Impact of congenital colour vision defects on occupation. Arch Dis Child. 2005;90(9):906–8.
9. Dain SJ, Wood JM, Atchison DA. Sunglasses, traffic signals, and color vision deficiencies. Optom Vis Sci. 2009;86(4):e296–305.
10. Denniston AK, Butler L. Ophthalmic features of Turner's syndrome. Eye (Lond). 2004;18(7):680–4.
11. Eibschitz-Tsimhoni M, Friedman T, Naor J, Eibschitz N, Friedman Z. Early screening for amblyogenic risk factors lowers the prevalence and severity of amblyopia. J AAPOS. 2000;4(4):194–9.
12. Force, U. S. P. S. T. Vision screening for children 1 to 5 years of age: US Preventive Services Task Force Recommendation statement. Pediatrics. 2011;127(2):340–6.
13. Grassivaro Gallo P, Panza M, Viviani F, Lantieri PB. Congenital dyschromatopsia and school achievement. Percept Mot Skills. 1998;86(2):563–9.
14. Holmes JM, Lazar EL, Melia BM, Astle WF, Dagi LR, Donahue SP, Frazier MG, Hertle RW, Repka MX, Quinn GE, Weise KK, G. Pediatric Eye Disease Investigator. Effect of age on response to amblyopia treatment in children. Arch Ophthalmol. 2011;129(11):1451–7.

15. Kemper A, Harris R, Lieu TA, Homer CJ, Whitener BL. Screening for visual impairment in children younger than age 5 years: a systematic evidence review for the U.S. Preventive Services Task Force. Rockville: Agency for Healthcare Research and Quality (US); 2004.
16. Noma T, Kanai Y, Kanai-Azuma M, Ishii M, Fujisawa M, Kurohmaru M, Kawakami H, Wood SA, Hayashi Y. Stage- and sex-dependent expressions of Usp9x, an X-linked mouse ortholog of Drosophila Fat facets, during gonadal development and oogenesis in mice. Mech Dev. 2002;119(Suppl 1):S91–5.
17. Owsley C, McGwin G Jr. Vision impairment and driving. Surv Ophthalmol. 1999;43(6):535–50.
18. Owsley C, McGwin G Jr. Vision and driving. Vis Res. 2010;50(23):2348–61.
19. Pediatric Eye Disease Investigator, G. A randomized trial of atropine vs. patching for treatment of moderate amblyopia in children. Arch Ophthalmol. 2002;120(3):268–78.
20. Rodriguez-Carmona M, O'Neill-Biba M, Barbur JL. Assessing the severity of color vision loss with implications for aviation and other occupational environments. Aviat Space Environ Med. 2012;83(1):19–29.
21. Siu AW, Yap MK. The performance of color deficient individuals on airfield color tasks. Aviat Space Environ Med. 2003;74(5):546–50.
22. Verriest G, Oskar N, Marion M, Andre U. New investigation concerning the relationship between congenital colour vision defects and road traffic security. Int Ophthalmol. 1980;2:87–99.
23. Wikiera B, Mulak M, Koltowska-Haggstrom M, Noczynska A. The presence of eye defects in patients with Turner syndrome is irrespective of their karyotype. Clin Endocrinol. 2015;83(6):842–8.

Chapter 12
Gastrointestinal and Hepatic Issues in Women with Turner Syndrome

Ghassan T. Wahbeh, Amanda Bradshaw, Lauren White, and Dale Lee

Introduction

The digestive tract is a dynamic area with a constant interplay between the ingested nutrients, the microbiome, endocrine and exocrine systems, nervous system, and immune arsenal. Commonly children, including individuals with Turner syndrome, will present to the general provider or specialist with gastrointestinal symptoms, most likely due to common conditions such as functional constipation, lactose intolerance, excess refined sugar consumption, food malprocessing due to fast eating and poor chewing, gut infections, or allergies (including eosinophilic esophagitis). It is important to consider these more common causes of GI symptoms before assessing for less common ones while being aware that patients with TS are more likely than the general population to have specific GI inflammatory and noninflammatory conditions. Celiac disease and inflammatory bowel disease cause growth failure and delayed puberty, therefore posing a significant diagnostic challenge in TS, where they occur more commonly than in peers. Additionally both conditions may impact the response to hormonal therapy if untreated. Gastrointestinal bleeding and hepatic manifestations are other relevant topics that merit review in this chapter as well.

G. T. Wahbeh (✉)
Pediatrics-Gastroenterology, Inflammatory Bowel Disease Center, Seattle Children's Hospital, University of Washington, Seattle, WA, USA
e-mail: ghassan.wahbeh@seattlechildrens.org

A. Bradshaw · L. White
Gastroenterology, Seattle Children's Hospital, Seattle, WA, USA
e-mail: amanda.bradshaw@seattlechildrens.org; Lauren.White@seattlechildrens.org

D. Lee
Pediatrics-Gastroenterology, Clinical Nutrition & Celiac Program, Seattle Children's Hospital, University of Washington, Seattle, WA, USA
e-mail: Dale.Lee@seattlechildrens.org

© Springer Nature Switzerland AG 2020
P. Y. Fechner (ed.), *Turner Syndrome*,
https://doi.org/10.1007/978-3-030-34150-3_12

Inflammatory Bowel Disease (IBD)

IBD is chronic idiopathic inflammation of the gastrointestinal tract with a spectrum of inflammation either limited to the colonic mucosa (ulcerative colitis (UC)) or the full thickness of the bowel from mouth to anus (Crohn's disease (CD)). Extraintestinal manifestations can occur in around 1 out of 5 children involving the skin, joints, liver, eyes, and beyond. Incidence of IBD has increased over the past several decades, fueling theories about etiology [1]. More than 163 genes have been linked to risk of IBD and the monozygotic twin concordance is under 50% [2]. This leaves the notion of an imbalanced interaction between the immune system, dietary exposures, and microbiome as *the* focus of current research and therapeutic targets.

Incidence

IBD occurs more commonly in TS patients. A study in England estimated the risk ratio of a TS cohort of 2459 individuals of 5.3 for CD (95% CI 3.5–7.8) and 3.9 for UC (95% CI 2.3–6.1) [3]. This increased risk was similar to what was described in the United States [4]. Bakalov et al. showed that women with TS had higher pro-inflammatory (e.g., IL-6) and lower anti-inflammatory (e.g. IL-10) cytokines compared to karyotypically normal women with or without ovarian insufficiency. Interestingly, multiple X-chromosome genes relate to immune regulation including *FOXP3*, deletion of which is associated with IPEX syndrome (immunodysregulation, polyendocrinopathy, and enteropathy X-linked). Further understanding of such genetic regulation may help us understand the reason why IBD is more common in TS, similar to other immune-mediated conditions [5].

Clinical Presentation and Diagnosis

IBD presenting symptoms are often nonspecific: abdominal pain, weight loss, chronic diarrhea, rectal bleeding, and in some perianal pain (abscess). Growth failure and short stature are frequently seen in IBD, leading to a potential delay in referral in children with TS who have growth concerns independently. Similarly short stature can be missed Turner syndrome in IBD and non-IBD patients. Unexplained iron deficiency anemia should also prompt considering IBD as a cause, in addition to celiac disease or vascular malformations, all of which are more often seen in TS patients. Infrequently, perianal fistula and abscess may be the presenting complaint. A thorough history and physical exam with a complete blood count, serum albumin, C-reactive peptide, and/or sedimentation rate should adequately help to differentiate functional from inflammatory bowel disease. Stool inflammatory markers such as lactoferrin and calprotectin can also be helpful screening tools in nonbloody diarrhea as elevation suggests bowel inflammation [6]. Suspicion for IBD should prompt a referral to a gastroenterologist. The differential diagnosis includes gastrointestinal infections (less likely to be chronic), celiac disease, allergic inflammation, polyps, or vascular malformation if bleeding is present.

The gold standard for confirming IBD is esophagogastroduodenoscopy and colonoscopy with biopsies for histologic exam, in addition to imaging studies. Macroscopically, the colon usually shows continuous superficial mucosal ulceration in UC, while microscopically the mucosal architecture is disrupted with abundance of inflammatory cells [7]. The upper GI tract can show reactive inflammation, but without the noncaseating granulomas typically seen in Crohn's disease. Macroscopically, Crohn's inflammation can be patchy with variable superficial and deep ulceration. The characteristic noncaseating granulomas are not seen in all patients. Imaging of the bowel is best done with cross-sectional modalities such as CT and MR, with MR having the advantage of being radiation-free. In Crohn's disease, thickening of the bowel wall indicates inflammation. Strictures, internal and perianal fistulae, and abscesses are also best assessed by imaging.

Management

There is no known medical cure for IBD today. Current therapies focus on nutritional approach, immunomodulators, and biologic therapies (including anti-TNF and anti-adhesion therapies) all with the goals of inducing remission of symptoms, restoring growth, improving bone health, and supporting psychosocial well-being. Avoiding prolonged or repeat use of corticosteroids is an important goal. Among the many corticosteroid adverse events, growth suppression and osteopenia are particularly concerning for patients with TS. Surgery is necessary in medically intractable UC after which patients could have restorative ileal pouch in continuity with the anus. In Crohn's disease, symptomatic strictures and internal fistulae are best managed with local resection. Little is known in the medical literature about the course of IBD specifically for patients with TS. When treated, children and adolescent with both TS and IBD should continue to receive routine care and health maintenance, including follow-up on bone density and growth [8]. Many therapies with immune-suppressive effects preclude the use of live vaccines. Frequent use of NSAIDs is also discouraged [9]. When in remission, there are no specific restrictions on activities. Care for a patient with IBD and TS is best provided by a multidisciplinary team including expert gastroenterologist, endocrinologist, nurse, dietician, and psychologist.

Celiac Disease

Gluten-sensitive enteropathy or celiac disease is a permanent condition where exposure to dietary gluten causes an immune-mediated inflammatory response within the small intestine in genetically predisposed individuals. Gluten is a protein made up of glutenin and gliadin molecules which collectively provide the dough elasticity and strength, allowing the use of wheat in so many cooked varieties. Gluten is also present in rye and barley. These proteins are resistant to digestion by proteases. A key step in the pathophysiology of celiac disease is the ability of the gluten epitopes to traverse the gut lumen into the submucosa and lamina propria, where enzymatic modification and subsequent immune response generate the histologic manifestations of villous blunting and intraepithelial lymphocytosis. These changes can cause malabsorption of nutrients, due to the atrophy of the villi, in addition to extraintestinal manifestations (e.g., arthritis), pathophysiology of which remains incompletely understood. Intriguingly, some individuals may be asymptomatic despite having advanced histologic celiac changes, only to be diagnosed after serology screening. Symptoms in celiac disease are nonspecific, including: failure to thrive, diarrhea, constipation, abdominal distention, vomiting, short stature, iron deficiency anemia, dermatitis herpetiformis, pubertal delay, aphthous stomatitis, dental enamel defects, and osteoporosis/osteopenia. Celiac confers a higher risk of malignancy. Known risk factors for celiac disease include first-degree relatives of celiac disease patients, autoimmune thyroiditis, Williams syndrome, insulin-dependent diabetes, IgA deficiency, trisomy 21, and Turner syndrome [10–12].

Incidence and Prevalence

The prevalence of the disease within the general population is estimated to be 0.5–1% [13]. The incidence of celiac disease varies geographically, being highest within Western European countries [14]. Compared with the general population, individuals with TS are three times as likely to develop celiac disease [15]. The estimated prevalence of celiac disease in TS is 4.1–8.1% [13], with an apparent geographic variation. In a study of 256 subjects with Turner syndrome in the UK, 4.7% individuals had biopsy-confirmed celiac disease [16]. Prevalence in Italy, British Columbia, and Brazil was estimated as 6.4%, 2.2%, and 3.6%, respectively [17–19]. A Swedish study of 7548 patients with celiac disease found that 20 of the female subjects also had confirmed Turner syndrome (0.26%), compared to 34,492 subjects from the general population, where only 21 (0.06%) had Turner syndrome [15]. The cause for the increased risk of celiac disease within the Turner syndrome population is not entirely understood. Similar to what is theorized about the cause of higher incidence of IBD in TS, women with Turner syndrome exhibit higher levels of pro-inflammatory cytokines (e.g., IL6, TGF β2) and decreased levels of anti-inflammatory cytokines (e.g., IL 10,TGF β1) [4]. Similarly, the prevalence of autoantibodies is higher than in healthy peers [20].

Clinical Presentation

A major concern for patients with both Turner syndrome and celiac disease (and similarly inflammatory bowel disease) is poor physical thriving. The facts that both condition affect growth and that celiac disease can be asymptomatic or cause non-specific symptoms can make the diagnosis of celiac disease within this population quite challenging. A delay in making the diagnosis can cause delays which are detrimental to restituting appropriate growth and thriving [21]. The median age at diagnosis of celiac disease was 1 year later for Turner syndrome patients compared to the general population [15]. In a study of TS celiac patients, it was observed that 4% were below the third percentile for the Turner syndrome growth curve. Additionally, one quarter of the subjects were asymptomatic at the time of their celiac disease diagnosis. Of those that were symptomatic, 28% exhibited delayed growth and anorexia. Other exhibited symptoms included: abdominal distention, chronic diarrhea, vomiting, constipation, low hemoglobin, elevated aminotransferases, and low serum iron levels [17]. This illustrates the importance of early screening regardless whether symptoms of celiac disease are present or not [14]. Untreated celiac may well interfere with growth hormone therapy and compromise growth potential despite treatment [20, 22]. Therefore hormone therapy, if appropriate, is best instituted *after* appropriate screening for celiac disease to mitigate the concern that celiac disease might thwart improvement [17].

The North American Society for Pediatric Gastroenterology, Hepatology, and Nutrition (NASPGHAN) recommends considering celiac screening in individuals with persistent suggestive symptoms, or those with known risk factors, but not the general population at this time (Fig. 12.1). Initial serologic screening should be done with IgA antibody to recombinant transglutaminase (TTG). When elevated, it is recommended that a referral is made to a pediatric gastroenterologist to confirm the diagnosis with the possible use of duodenal biopsy. Upon confirmation of diagnosis, the recommendation for treatment is strict lifelong adherence to a gluten-free diet [13].

Certainly, celiac testing should be considered whenever gastrointestinal symptoms are present. An important question is when and how to screen for celiac disease in the setting of Turner syndrome without gastrointestinal symptoms. The optimal time and frequency of screening must account for two issues: gluten exposure is necessary to develop celiac, and the exact age at which celiac disease actually develops is not well defined. One case-control study showed that females with Turner syndrome were at *twofold* risk of developing celiac disease in the first 2 years of life and *fivefold* risk in the first 5 years of life [15]. Screening is recommended by the Turner Consensus Study Group starting at 2–3 years of age [23]. Screening is recommended with the tissue transglutaminase IgA ELISA testing [17]. HLA

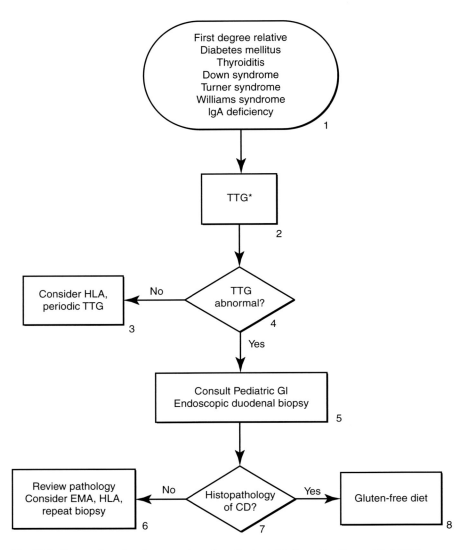

Fig. 12.1 Proposed workup for asymptomatic patients at risk for celiac disease (Ref. [13])

genotyping can identify whether an individual has HLA DQ8 and/or DQ2, which makes up the vast majority of genes concerning for celiac disease. However, both HLA DQ8 and DQ2 are also present in the general healthy population and cannot predict whether an individual with one of these genes may develop celiac disease. HLA testing may be more valuable in certain instances for its negative predictive value as absence of both markers dramatically reduces the chance of developing celiac disease [24]. It should be noted that in a one study of 256 women with TS, eight had positive endomysial antibody tests (a high specificity, lower sensitivity, higher cost test than tTG IgA). Seven of the eight individuals had biopsy-confirmed celiac disease on, yet one patient was found to be HLA DQ2/8 negative [13]. This raises concern for false negativity if HLA testing is used as a screening method [16], reiterating the message that screening should be with the tissue transglutaminase IgA. A duodenal biopsy while on gluten-containing diet remains the gold standard for confirming celiac disease. Nevertheless, there is ongoing debate whether a very high positive titer in a patient with symptoms and/or risk factors is enough to establish a diagnosis of celiac, in a patient who is willing to commit to a lifelong gluten-free diet [25].

Management and Follow-Up

Early diagnosis of celiac disease can help mitigate the related symptoms and reduce short- and long-term complication risk. If initial screening appears negative, and patient appears to be asymptomatic, screening should be considered periodically going forward, with a suggested interval of 2–5 years [23]. Progress on gluten-free should be monitored. After initial diagnosis, symptoms, growth, and nutritional indices are routinely followed along with tissue transglutaminase IgA level (TTG IgA) which should be retested after 6 months of initiating a strict gluten-free diet, in order to assess recovery. A decreasing TTG IgA level indicates adherence to the diet and correlated with intestinal healing. For patients with persistent or recurrent symptoms, a careful reexamination of the diet is usually done, and other common conditions (e.g., lactose intolerance) should be considered. If the TTG IgA level remains high, a redo endoscopic exam is usually offered. Once normal, the tTG IgA monitoring is done yearly [13]. One should not underestimate the additional psychosocial stress that patients and families face with the burden of a strict dietary elimination. Resources including access to an experienced dietician, support group, and mental health specialists should be made available. These recommendations illustrate the need for patients with celiac disease diagnosis to have regular thoughtful follow-up with their healthcare provider.

Gastrointestinal Bleeding

It has been recognized since 1947 that individuals with Turner syndrome have a higher risk of vascular gut bleeding [26]. The incidence is thought to approach 7% [27]. Eroglu et al. published an extensive review on gut bleeding in TS [28]. Clinical presentation is variable: occult indolent bleeding with iron deficiency anemia may cause few if any symptom due to the body's compensatory mechanism. In contrast, overt acute or recurrent upper or lower gastrointestinal bleeding may be life-threatening and require blood transfusion. When overt, the presenting symptoms may be hematemesis (indicating bleeding proximal to the ligament of Treitz), melanotic stools (dark, tarry, sticky, liquid stools indicating bleeding proximal to the ileocecal valve), or hematochezia (bright red blood indicating usually distal colonic source).

Etiology

In children, the most common sources of upper intestinal bleeding, proximal to the ligament of Treitz, are esophageal trauma (such as a Mallory Weiss lesion), gastric bruising due to retching or vomiting, *Helicobacter pylori*-associated gastroduodenitis with or without an ulcer, and NSAID intake. Ingested blood from the mouth or nasal passages can be mistaken for digestive tract source blood. On the other hand, lower gastrointestinal bleeding is most commonly caused by a polyp, anal fissure, stool trauma, benign lymphonodular hyperplasia (infants and toddlers), or infectious and noninfectious colitis [29]. The above sources should be considered in all patients with TS with suspected blood loss.

Bleeding from vascular lesions of the gastrointestinal tract is rare, yet more likely to be seen in TS. Examples of vascular lesion malformation forms in TS are telangiectasias (dilated arteriovenous structures), hemangiomas (essentially endothelial cell tumors), and venous ectasias (dilated venous structures). The first episode of GI bleeding in TS tends to happen in the first two decades of life [30]. Lesions may regress with age [31, 32].

Management

The primary step in managing children with acute gastrointestinal bleeding is urgent/emergent evaluation and stabilization: assessment of vital signs, serial hematocrit/hemoglobin measurements, hydration, and transfusion if necessary. Once stabilized, the next step is to identify the source of bleeding (Fig. 12.2). A physical exam can reveal a source of usually insignificant bleeding such as nasal cavity or perianal hemorrhoids or fissures. The gold standard for detecting the bleeding source is esophagogastroduodenoscopy, then prepped colonoscopy (must weigh safety of waiting and colonic cleanout with laxatives vs need to intervene). Endoscopic intervention allows for use of heat coagulation, bleeding site clipping, or vasoconstrictor injection. Subsequent investigation if no source is found in a clinically stable patient is capsule endoscopy (Fig. 12.3) which has a high yield for identifying small bowel bleed where standard endoscopy cannot reach [33, 34]. When available, a lesion identified on capsule endoscopy can be addressed with small bowel enteroscopy or laparoscopy. When not feasible (e.g., lack of expertise or patient's small size) intraoperative endoscopy may be needed [35]. For active clinically significant bleeding, angiography and tagged RBC scans should be considered, with the former allowing for intervention at the same time. Cross-

Fig. 12.2 Overview of bleeding investigations

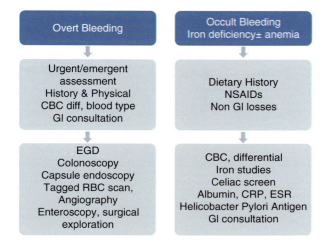

Overt Bleeding	Occult Bleeding Iron deficiency± anemia
Urgent/emergent assessment History & Physical CBC diff, blood type GI consultation	Dietary History NSAIDs Non GI losses
EGD Colonoscopy Capsule endoscopy Tagged RBC scan, Angiography Enteroscopy, surgical exploration	CBC, differential Iron studies Celiac screen Albumin, CRP, ESR Helicobacter Pylori Antigen GI consultation

Fig. 12.3 Large jejunal angiectasia seen with capsule endoscopy (Ref. [34])

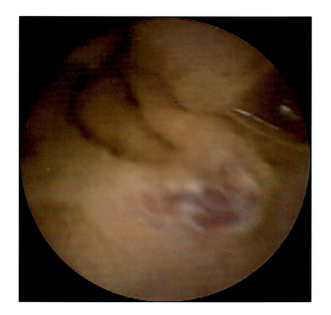

sectional imaging such as magnetic resonance or computed tomography may have a limited role in demonstrating vascular lesions, especially when not associated with a mass. Some vascular lesions may best be detected on laparoscopy if prominent on the serosal bowel surface (Fig. 12.4) [28].

Endoscopic or radiologic interventions may not always be feasible, especially if the bleeding lesion is not readily reachable or too diffuse. Surgical resection may also be unfavorable when the vascular lesions are extensive. Estrogen supplementation (with or without progesterone) in addition to iron supplementation has been shown

Fig. 12.4 Diffuse abnormal venous structures seen on small intestine on laparoscopy (Ref. [49])

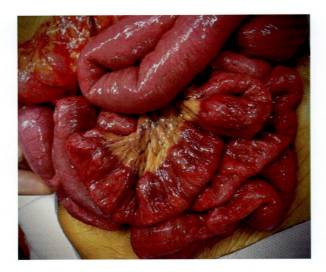

to decrease the bleeding frequency and intensity in TS patient and others with vascular malformations [36–38]. Estrogen's proposed mechanism of action may include its procoagulation effect, enhance microcirculation stasis, induce trophic effects on the intestinal mucosa, or directly stabilize the endothelium of the abnormal vessels [28]. Long-acting somatostatin analogues (which are thought to increase platelet aggregation and vascular bed resistance, reduce splanchnic blood flow, and downregulate vascular endothelial growth factor) have been shown to reduce rebleeding and transfusion requirements in patients with refractory small bowel angiodysplasia [39], although not specifically in TS. It should be noted that no randomized clinical trials have been performed to better define the role of medical therapy in vascular bleeding in TS.

Hepatic Manifestations

Hepatic abnormalities in Turner syndrome patients have been recognized in the medical literature since 1959 when Bridwell first described a case study of a Turner syndrome patient with portal fibrosis [40]. Since that time, a small but growing number of publications have shed light on the prevalence and etiology of hepatic abnormalities in TS.

Elevated liver enzymes are common, seen in 20–80% of TS patients [41]. Several studies suggest that such elevations are benign and remain static over time without clinical or histologic progression [42–44]. However, this may not be the case for all, similarly to the general population, making follow-up and referral to a hepatologist necessary. Mild elevations of the liver enzymes can be followed for a trend and if symptomatic, persistent, or severely elevated, prompt further evaluation with serology and imaging and consultation are needed. The published guidelines on care for individuals with TS suggest screening labs to assess liver function starting in the school-aged years [23].

The differential diagnosis for elevated liver enzymes in the general population is quite extensive and includes conditions such as viral, autoimmune, or alcoholic hepatitis, Wilson's disease, alpha-1 antitrypsin deficiency, celiac disease, biliary structural or obstructive lesions, pancreatitis, muscle diseases, nonalcoholic fatty liver disease (NAFLD), drug reactions or drug overdoses, malignancy, hemochromatosis, adrenal insufficiency, and thyroid disease. Further testing with serology and imaging for these causes is tailored depending on the clinical picture. However, there are certain hepatic conditions that have been historically more prevalent in TS: nonalcoholic steatohepatitis (NASH), liver architectural changes, and biliary lesions. Celiac disease is discussed earlier in this chapter.

Nonalcoholic Steatohepatitis

NASH, a type of nonalcoholic fatty liver disease, has been widely reported as a cause of elevated liver enzymes in the general population as well as TS. In NASH, the excess fat accumulation in the liver can disrupt the normal liver function and lead to inflammation, tissue damage, and cirrhosis. NASH is most often correlated with overweight status, which is a known concern in TS where BMIs of over 25 are frequently reported [41]. As rates of obesity have risen, increased frequency of NASH has been observed worldwide. The treatment approach to NASH has long focused on lifestyle changes such as improved diet and increased activity level. However, because NASH patients are at risk for development of cirrhosis and long-term cardiovascular and metabolic diseases, they should be regularly followed by a trained gastroenterologist or hepatologist.

The exact dynamic of overweight, NASH, and elevated liver enzymes in TS remains to be defined. While several studies linked overweight and NASH with transaminitis in TS [41–43], a more recent study by Calcaterra in 2014 found no significant association between abnormal liver enzymes and metabolic syndrome, obesity, or hepatic steatosis [45]. These contrasting findings suggest that further research is needed in order to elucidate the relationship between NASH, obesity, and abnormal liver enzymes in Turner syndrome patients. Similar to the recommendation in general pediatric and adult medicine diet, exercise and weight management should be optimized to address NASH and for general health.

Hepatic Architectural Changes

It has been suggested that TS patients are at risk of liver architectural changes since the first case report of an architectural abnormality was described by Bridwell in 1959, when a patient presenting with melena was found to have portal fibrosis on liver biopsy [40]. Histologic changes seen in TS may include: cirrhosis, hepatic adenoids, nodular regenerative hyperplasia (NRH), and focal nodular hyperplasia (FNH) [41, 44]. Of these, cirrhosis is perhaps the most concerning, as the irreversible scar tissue that progressively replaces healthy liver tissue in cirrhosis can eventually significantly impair normal liver function. Hepatic adenomas, NRH, and FNH are all considered to be different types of benign liver tumors (Fig. 12.5) – hepatic adenomas are usually well-defined solitary lesions that are most often associated with the long-term use of OCPs or pregnancy, and FNH typically also presents as a well-circumscribed, nonneoplastic lesion that develops in response to a disruption in blood supply to the liver. NRH is somewhat distinct from these other types of benign tumors, as it occurs when normal hepatic tissue transforms into small regenerative nodules in the liver [46]. This process typically occurs as a response to a vascular injury. While largely benign, these hepatic tumors have potential to result in complications such as bleeding, hemorrhage, or portal hypertension.

In Roulot et al.'s investigation of vascular liver involvement in Turner syndrome patients, 1/3 of subjects showed signs of major architectural changes on liver biopsy: NRH, FNH, or cirrhosis [47]. It was further noted that major medical complications occurred in three out of the ten patients affected. These medical complications included uncontrolled refractory ascites leading to pleural effusion and cardiac failure, as well as uncontrolled or recurrent variceal bleeding. Another study by Gravholt of almost 600 women with TS in Denmark demonstrated a five- to sixfold increase in the relative risk of cirrhosis in TS [48].

It has been postulated that there is a link between the hepatic architectural change, diverse vascular abnormalities, and the underlying genetic change in TS. Building on this, in 2013 Lee noted evidenced to suggest that the increased risk of cirrhosis may be attributable to higher rates of coarctation of the aorta causing secondary hepatic ischemia and hypoperfusion. One case report describes congenital absence of the portal vein in a patient with TS and GI bleed [49]. Taken together, these findings suggest that it is important to monitor Turner syndrome patients for potential liver abnormalities via routine screening of liver function tests. With persistent blood work abnormalities, subspecialty evaluation by a hepatologist is indicated.

Lee et al. and Roulot et al. further noted that Turner syndrome patients may be at risk of biliary lesions such as small duct sclerosing cholangitis, bile duct paucity, and biliary atresia [41, 42]. Sclerosing cholangitis is inflammation of the bile ducts either inside or outside the liver with subsequent damage and scarring. Lee noted that TS patients with concurrent IBD seemed to be at highest risk for developing this issue, but Roulot's 2004 study noted that none of the TS patients with ductal fibrosis in her study had concurrent IBD. As opposed to primary sclerosing cholangitis, which primarily affects extrahepatic ducts, TS patients most often experience sclerosing cholangitis that affects the intrahepatic ducts. Roulot postulated that this issue could potentially be due to altered blood supply from arterial damage. Apart from sclerosing cholangitis, Lee additionally noted a case of biliary atresia reported in a neonate with TS. In this case, it was postulated that a vascular malformation triggered bile duct paucity and the subsequent biliary atresia.

Fig. 12.5 Liver
architectural changes and
vascular lesions in patients
with Turner's syndrome.
(**a**) Multiple focal nodular
hyperplasia; (*inset*) fibrotic
area containing abnormal
vessels; (**b**) nodular
regenerative hyperplasia;
(**c**) numerous vessels
within fibrosis (Ref. [41])

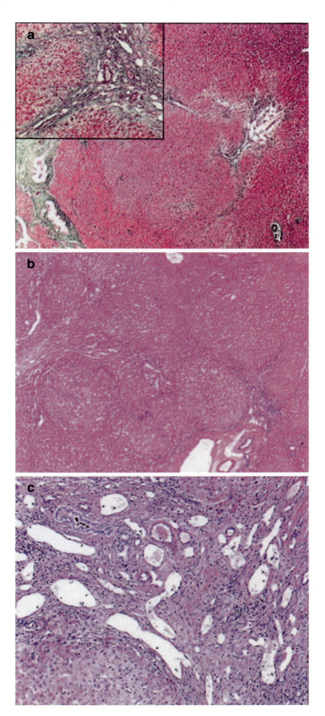

The Role of Hormone Replacement Therapy

Over the past few decades, several studies have looked at the connection between elevated liver enzyme levels in Turner syndrome patients and hormone replacement therapy, as estrogen and growth hormone replacement therapies specifically are commonly prescribed to address the gonadal failure, lack of pubertal development, and growth failure in TS. While the exact relationship between hormone replacement therapy and elevated liver enzymes remains unclear, there is more evidence to suggest that use of hormone replacement therapy does *not* contribute to the development of hepatic complications. In 2004, Roulot noted that there was no evidence of liver toxicity from estrogen replacement therapy, and in 2007 Bondy noted that estrogen therapy was not associated with adverse effects on the liver [23, 47]. Indeed, several studies have suggested that hormone replacement therapy may actually have a hepatoprotective effect. Specifically, in 2001 Elsheikh noted that hormone replacement therapy actually resulted in a decline in liver enzymes in his study population, and Koulouri et al. noted in their 2008 study that increasing doses of hormone replacement therapy actually led to an improvement in several hepatic markers such as GGT, ALT, bilirubin, and albumin [44, 50]. While these results are promising, the overall body of literature addressing the link between hormone replacement therapy and abnormal liver indices is relatively small and further research is needed in order to elucidate the potential risks or benefits of prescribing hormone replacement therapy in TS.

References

1. Benchimol EI, Fortinsky KJ, Gozdyra P, Van den Heuvel M, Van Limbergen J, Griffiths AM. Epidemiology of pediatric inflammatory bowel disease: a systematic review of international trends. Inflamm Bowel Dis. 2011;17:423–39.
2. Loddo I, Romano C. Inflammatory bowel disease: genetics, epigenetics, and pathogenesis. Front Immunol. 2015;6:551.
3. Goldacre MJ, Seminog OO. Turner syndrome and autoimmune diseases: record-linkage study. Arch Dis Child. 2014;99:71–3.
4. Bakalov VK, Gutin L, Cheng CM, Zhou J, Sheth P, Shah K, Arepalli S, Vanderhoof V, Nelson LM, Bondy CA. Autoimmune disorders in women with Turner syndrome and women with karyotypically normal primary ovarian insufficiency. J Autoimmun. 2012;38:315–21.
5. Pessach IM, Notarangelo LD. X-linked primary immunodeficiencies as a bridge to better understanding X-chromosome related autoimmunity. J Autoimmun. 2009;33:17–24.
6. Holtman GA, Lisman-van Leeuwen Y, Reitsma JB, Berger MY. Noninvasive tests for inflammatory bowel disease: a meta-analysis. Pediatrics. 2016;137:e20152126.
7. Bousvaros A, Antonioli DA, Colletti RB, Dubinsky MC, Glickman JN, Gold BD, Griffiths AM, Jevon GP, Higuchi LM, Hyams JS, Kirschner BS, Kugathasan S, Baldassano RN, Russo PA. Differentiating ulcerative colitis from Crohn disease in children and young adults: report of a working group of the North American Society for Pediatric Gastroenterology, Hepatology, and Nutrition and the Crohn's and Colitis Foundation of America. J Pediatr Gastroenterol Nutr. 2007;44:653–74.

8. Rufo PA, Denson LA, Sylvester FA, Szigethy E, Sathya P, Lu Y, Wahbeh GT, Sena LM, Faubion WA. Health supervision in the management of children and adolescents with IBD: NASPGHAN recommendations. J Pediatr Gastroenterol Nutr. 2012;55:93–108.
9. Long MD, Kappelman MD, Martin CF, Chen W, Anton K, Sandler RS. Role of nonsteroidal anti-inflammatory drugs in exacerbations of inflammatory bowel disease. J Clin Gastroenterol. 2016;50:152–6.
10. Crone J, Rami B, Huber WD, Granditsch G, Schober E. RBHWDGGSE: prevalence of celiac disease and follow-up of EMA in childrend and adolescents with type 1 diabetes mellitus. J Pediatr Gastroenterol Nutr. 2003;37:67.
11. Giannotti A, Tiberio G, Castro M, Virgilii F, Colistro F, Ferretti F, Digilio MC, Gambarara M, Dallapiccola B. Coeliac disease in Williams syndrome. J Med Genet. 2001;38:767.
12. Fasano A, Berti I, Gerarduzzi T, Not T, Colletti RB, Drago S, Elitsur Y, Green PH, Guandalini S, Hill ID, Pietzak M, Ventura A, Thorpe M, Kryszak D, Fornaroli F, Wasserman SS, Murray JA, Horvath K. Prevalence of celiac disease in at-risk and not-at-risk groups in the United States: a large multicenter study. Arch Internal Med. 2003;163:286.
13. Hill ID, Dirks MH, Liptak GS, Colletti RB, Fasano A, Guandalini S, Hoffenberg EJ, Horvath K, Murray JA, Pivor M, Seidman EG. Guidelines for diagnosis and treatment of celiac disease in children: recommendations of the North American Society of Pediatric Gastroenterology, Hepatology and Nutrition. J Pediatr Gastroenterol Nutr. 2005;40:1–19.
14. Moayeri HB. Prevalence of celiac disease in patients with Turner's syndrome. Acta Med Iran. 2005;43:287–90.
15. Mårild K, Størdal K, Hagman A, Ludvigsson JF. Turner syndrome and celiac disease: a case-control study. Pediatrics. 2016;137:e20152232.
16. Frost AR, Band MM, Conway GS. Serologically screening for coeliac disease in adults with Turner's syndrome: prevalence andc linical significance of endomysium antibody positivity. Eur J Endocrinol. 2009;160:877–81.
17. Bonamico M, Pasquino AM, Mariani P, Danesi HM, Culasso F, Mazzanti L, et al. Prevalence and clinical picture of celiac disease in Turner syndrome. J Clin Endocrinol Metab. 2002;87:5495–8.
18. Gillett PM, Gillett HR, Israel DM, Metzger DL, Stewart L, Chanoine JP, et al. Increased prevalence of celiac disease in girls with Turner syndrome detected using antibodies to endomysium and tissue transglutaminase. Can J Gastroenterol. 2000;14:915.
19. Dias M, Castro L, Gandolfi L, Almeida R, Corboda M, Pratesi R. Screening for celiac disease among patients with Turner syndrome in Brasilia, DF, Midwest region of Brazil. Arg Gastroenterol. 2010;47:246–9.
20. Bettendorf M, Doerr HG, Hauffa BP, Lindberg A, Mehls O, Partsch CJ, et al. Prevalence of autoantibodies associated with thyroid and celiac disease in Ullrich-Turner syndrome in relation to adult height after growth hormone treatment. J Pediatric Endocrinol. 2006;19:149–54.
21. Mortensen KH, Cleemann L, Hjerrild BE, Nexo E, Locht H, Jeppesen EM, Gravholt CH. Increased prevalence of autoimmunity in Turner syndrome-influence of age. Clin Exp Immunol. 2009;156:205–10.
22. Arslan D, Kuyucu T, Kendirci M, Kurtoglu S. Celiac disease and Turner's syndrome: patient report. J Pediatr Endocrinol. 2000;13:1629–31.
23. Gravholt CH, Andersen NH, Conway GS, et al. Clinical practice guidelines for the care of girls and women with Turner syndrome: proceedings from the 2016 Cincinnati International Turner Syndrome Meeting. Eur J Endocrinol. 2017;177(3):G1–G70.
24. Sollid LM, Lie BA. Celiac disease genetics: current concepts and practical applications. Clin Gastroenterol Hepatol. 2005;3:843–51.
25. Mills JR, Murray JA. Contemporary celiac disease diagnosis: is a biopsy avoidable? Curr Opin Gastroenterol. 2016;32:80–5.
26. Lisser H, Curtis LE, et al. The syndrome of congenitally aplastic ovaries with sexual infantilism, high urinary gonadotropins, short stature and other congenital abnormalities; tabular presentation of 25 previously unpublished cases. J Clin Endocrinol Metab. 1947;7:665–87.

27. Haddad HM, Wilkins L. Congenital anomalies associated with gonadal aplasia; review of 55 cases. Pediatrics. 1959;23:885–902.
28. Eroglu Y, Emerick KM, Chou PM, Reynolds M. Gastrointestinal bleeding in Turner's syndrome: a case report and literature review. J Pediatr Gastroenterol Nutr. 2002;35:84–7.
29. Boyle JT. Gastrointestinal bleeding in infants and children. Pediatr Rev. 2008;29:39–52.
30. Schultz LS, Assimacopoulos CA, Lillehei RC. Turner's syndrome with associated gastrointestinal hemorrhage: a case report. Surgery. 1970;68:485–8.
31. Scott T. Turner's syndrome and vermiform phlebectasia of the bowel. Trans Am Clin Climatol Assoc. 1968;79:45–50.
32. Frame B, Rao DS, Ohorodnik JM, Kwa DM. Gastrointestinal hemorrhage in Turner syndrome. Long-term follow-up with postmortem examination. Arch Intern Med. 1977;137:691–2.
33. Qureshi MA, Mouzaki M, Le T. Diagnosis of small bowel telangiectasia in Turner's syndrome using capsule endoscopy. J Pediatr Endocrinol Metab. 2009;22:759–62.
34. Nudell J, Brady P. A case of GI hemorrhage in a patient with Turner's syndrome: diagnosis by capsule endoscopy. Gastrointest Endosc. 2006;63:514–6.
35. Jolley C, Langham MR Jr, Dillard R, Novak D. Intraoperative endoscopy in a child with Turner's syndrome and gastrointestinal hemorrhage: a case report. J Pediatr Surg. 2001;36:951–2.
36. O'Hare JP, Hamilton M, Davies JD, Corrall RJ, Mountford R. Oestrogen deficiency and bleeding from large bowel telangiectasia in Turner's syndrome. J R Soc Med. 1986;79:746–7.
37. Van Cutsem E. Georges Brohee Prize. Oestrogen-progesterone, a new therapy of bleeding gastrointestinal vascular malformations. Acta Gastroenterol Belg. 1993;56:2–10.
38. Vase P. Estrogen treatment of hereditary hemorrhagic telangiectasia. A double-blind controlled clinical trial. Acta Med Scand. 1981;209:393–6.
39. Holleran G, Hall B, Breslin N, McNamara D. Long-acting somatostatin analogues provide significant beneficial effect in patients with refractory small bowel angiodysplasia: results from a proof of concept open label mono-centre trial. United European Gastroenterol J. 2016;4:70–6.
40. Bridwell T. Gonadal dysgenesis (Turner's syndrome) with associated liver disease and bleeding esophageal varices. Henry Ford Hosp Med Bull. 1959;7:156–60.
41. Roulot D. Liver involvement in Turner syndrome. Liver Int. 2013;33:24–30.
42. Lee MC, Conway GS. Liver dysfunction in Turner syndrome and its relationship to = exogenous oestrogen. Eur J Gastroenterol Hepatol. 2013;25:1141–5.
43. Larizza D, Locatelli M, Vitali L, Vigano C, Calcaterra V, Tinelli C, Sommaruga MG, Bozzini A, Campani R, Severi F. Serum liver enzymes in Turner syndrome. Eur J Pediatr. 2000;159:143–8.
44. Koulouri O, Ostberg J, Conway GS. Liver dysfunction in Turner's syndrome: prevalence, natural history = and effect of exogenous oestrogen. Clin Endocrinol. 2008;69:306–10.
45. Calcaterra V, Brambilla P, Maffe GC, Klersy C, Albertini R, Introzzi F, Bozzola E, Bozzola M, Larizza D. Metabolic syndrome in Turner syndrome and relation between body = composition and clinical, genetic, and ultrasonographic characteristics. Metab Syndr Relat Disord. 2014;12:159–64.
46. Chiche L, Adam JP. Diagnosis and management of benign liver tumors. Semin Liver Dis. 2013;33:236–47.
47. Roulot D, Degott C, Chazouilleres O, Oberti F, Cales P, Carbonell N, Benferhat S, Bresson-Hadni S, Valla D. Vascular involvement of the liver in Turner's syndrome. Hepatology. 2004;39:239–47.
48. Gravholt CH, Naeraa RW, Nyholm B, Gerdes LU, Christiansen E, Schmitz O, Christiansen JS. Glucose metabolism, lipid metabolism, and cardiovascular risk factors in adult Turner's syndrome. The impact of sex hormone replacement. Diabetes Care. 1998;21:1062–70.
49. Cheah E, La Hei E, O'Loughlin E. Melena and hyperammonemic seizures in a Turner syndrome patient. Gastroenterology. 2015;148:302–3.
50. Elsheikh M, Hodgson HJ, Wass JA, Conway GS. Hormone replacement therapy may improve hepatic function in women with Turner's syndrome. Clin Endocrinol. 2001;55:227–31.

Chapter 13
Dermatologic Conditions in Turner Syndrome

Alessandra Haskin and Eve Lowenstein

Abbreviations

TS   Turner syndrome
hGH   Human growth hormone
CVG   Cutis verticis gyrata
CDP   Complete decongestive physiotherapy

Introduction

Turner syndrome (TS) is a multisystem disorder with many dermatologic manifestations. As it is not always diagnosed in the neonatal period, it is important that clinicians are aware of the diverse clinical stigmata that may provide clues for diagnosis [1]. Dermatologic cues may also predict specific TS karyotypes and, in some cases, may even predict severity of organ involvement. Some of the common and less frequently reported cutaneous findings observed in TS patients are outlined in Table 13.1. The unique dermatologic sequelae of TS also provide important clinical implications that must be considered when managing these patients. The objective of this chapter is to provide an overview of the dermatologic issues prevalent in patients with TS.

A. Haskin · E. Lowenstein (✉)
Department of Dermatology, SUNY Health Science Center at Brooklyn, Brooklyn, NY, USA

© Springer Nature Switzerland AG 2020   221
P. Y. Fechner (ed.), *Turner Syndrome*,
https://doi.org/10.1007/978-3-030-34150-3_13

Table 13.1 Approximate
frequencies of cutaneous
abnormalities in turner
syndrome [1, 13]

Very frequent (>50% of individuals)
Congenital lymphedema
Low posterior hairline
Hyperconvex nails
Unusual shape/rotation of ears
Prominent inner canthal folds
Micrognathia
Broad shield chest with widely spaced nipples
Hypoplastic/inverted nipples
Frequent (<50% of individuals)
Webbed neck
Increased numbers of pigmented nevi
Altered dermatoglyphics
Low/undetermined frequency
Alopecia areata
Keloid/hypertrophic scar tendency
Psoriasis
Persistent lymphedema
Vitiligo
Pilomatricomas
Pigmentary mosaicism
Cutis verticis gyrate
Café au lait macules
Premature skin aging

Lymphatic Abnormalities

Lymphatic abnormalities are frequently observed in TS patients and are thought to contribute to the pathogenesis of many of the associated phenotypic features [2]. Embryonic lymphatic obstruction is believed to be due to hypoplasia or agenesis of the lymphatic ducts [1, 3, 4]. These malformations result in subcutaneous accumulation of lymph fluid and clinical lymphedema [4].

Lymphedema is more common in TS patients with the 45,X karyotypes than in those with mosaic or other karyotypes and is linked to a higher incidence of cardiac and renal anomalies [5]. Vascular endothelial growth factor-D (VEGF-D), mapped to Xp22, is the locus implicated in the lymphedema phenotype in TS [6, 7]. Mutations in VEGF receptor-3 have been associated with Milroy disease, a familial primary lymphedema [6, 8, 9]. Furthermore, a recent study using a zebra fish model has also suggested a potential link between VEGFD and mutations in the transcription factor gene SOX18, which is associated with hypotrichosis-lymphedema-telangiectasia syndrome [8, 10]. Further research is needed to determine whether specific genes or gene loci are responsible for the high prevalence of lymphedema in TS patients. Lymphatic abnormalities are important to recognize as presenting manifestations of TS; however these changes may not be clinically evident at birth.

Any infant presenting with congenital lymphedema of the extremities or neck should undergo karyotype analysis [1].

Congenital Acral Lymphedema

Congenital lymphedema of the dorsal hands and feet is thought to be present in more than 60% of infants with TS and facilitates early diagnosis in approximately one third of patients [2, 11]. The lymphedema seen at birth rarely persists and typically resolves spontaneously by 2 years of age [1]. Infrequently, unilateral or bilateral lymphedema of the lower extremities may recur in late childhood and has been associated with the initiation of salt-retaining therapies such as human growth hormone (hGH) or estrogen replacement therapy [1, 2, 12]. In cases where lymphedema recurs or persists beyond childhood, it tends to run a benign course, with the typical complications (cellulitis, thrombosis, elephantiasis nostras verrucosa, etc.) not previously reported in TS patients [1].

Treatments such as the use of low-stretch support garments or stockings, elevation of affected extremities, and exercise may be effective [2, 13]. Diuretics are of limited use [12]. Complete decongestive physiotherapy (CDP), which uses manual lymphatic drainage, may be considered in severe or refractory cases [2, 13].

Cystic Hygroma

Cystic hygromas, which appear as single or multiloculated fluid-filled cavities in the nuchal region, are one of the most common manifestations of lymphatic malformations in TS [3]. This abnormality may be observed as increased nuchal translucency on ultrasound scanning at 10–14 weeks gestation [4, 14]. Cystic hygromas are a result of jugular lymphatic obstruction during embryogenesis, which is thought to be due to developmental delay in the formation of connections between lymphatic and venous structures [1, 3, 4]. The impeded drainage of interstitial fluid results in congestion of large diameter vessels at the junction of the dermis and subcutis in nuchal skin and the formation of hygromas [3, 4]. Cystic hygromas typically resolve before birth with the development of accessory pathways for lymphatic drainage, leaving redundant nuchal folds, webbed neck (pterygium coli), and low-set hairline over the nape of the neck [1, 2]. In utero facial edema may also cause the formation of epicanthal folds [11]. While still controversial, several studies have demonstrated a possible association between webbed neck and flow-related heart defects, with an incidence of congenital heart disease estimated to be 150-fold higher than in the general population [1, 15–18]. A pathogenic relationship has been implicated with increased hydrostatic pressure resulting in distention of cardiac lymphatics, compression of the aorta, and a subsequent increase in resistance to left-sided heart blood flow [15].

Although webbed neck and hairline abnormalities rarely cause functional limitations, they often present aesthetic concerns [19]. Surgical correction of these anomalies has been described using a variety of different techniques. The use of lateral approach methods such as Z-plasties or modified Z-plasties, which access the lateral portions of the neck, have been most frequently reported in TS patients [19–21]. While these techniques provide good fold reduction, some of the disadvantages include visible scars on the lateral surfaces of the neck and abnormal hairline displacement [19, 22]. Posterior approach techniques have also been reported to provide good fold reduction; however sutures are often applied with increased tension, which can favor the formation of keloids and hypertrophic scarring or even reoccurrence of webbing [1, 22]. Tissue expanders have been used to address this issue, with reports indicating successful results [23, 24]. Some physicians favor the use of posterior approach techniques due to the ability to restore the neck outline and provide a more natural posterior hairline [21, 22]. Patients should consult experienced surgeons to determine the most appropriate surgical technique, based on their presentation.

Dermatoglyphics

Congenital acral edema has also been implicated in the development of unusual dermatoglyphics, which can be described as the dermal ridge configurations on the digits, palms, and soles [25, 26]. Edema in the developing digits results in an increased surface area, requiring an increased number of finger ridges [26, 27]. TS is also associated with an increased angle of the axial triradius and triradii at the bases of the index and fifth fingers, which has been linked to an elevated risk of congenital heart disease (Fig. 13.1: dermatoglyphics) [1, 26].

Nails

Alterations in nail anatomy have also been observed in patients with TS. While the exact underlying mechanism remains unknown, they are believed to be due to the effects of lymphedema on the distal phalanges [28]. Hyperconvex or concave nails with an increased Lovibond's angle (angle of nail insertion), giving the nails an upturned appearance, are common findings (Fig. 13.2: upturned toenails) [2, 28]. The toenails are more frequently affected than the fingernails [2]. These abnormalities may result in recurrent paronychia or pain when wearing shoes; therefore frequent clipping of the nails may be recommended [2].

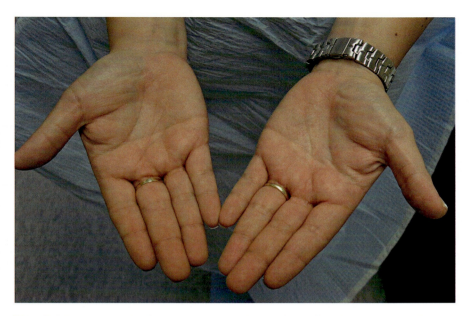

Fig. 13.1 Dermatoglyphics showing an increased angle of the axial triradius and triradii at the bases of the index and fifth fingers

Fig. 13.2 Upturned nails in a TS patient with acral lymphedema

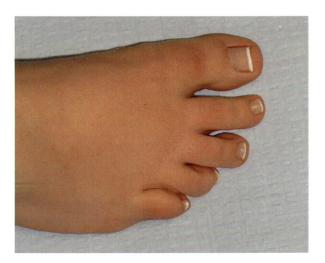

Neonatal Cutis Verticis Gyrata

Neonatal cutis verticis gyrata (CVG) is a rare condition clinically defined as redundant skin folds of the scalp that mimic the gyral pattern of the cerebral cortex [5, 29, 30]. It has been postulated that this condition may result from resolved intrauterine scalp lymphedema [31]. Of the reported cases of CVG in TS patients, these lesions appear to persist unchanged into childhood and adolescence [5], with one report of regression at 2 years of age [29]. In many cases, these lesions are excised within the first few years of life, after closure of the fontanelles, and have not been associated with abnormalities in psychomotor development [5, 32]. In addition to TS, CVG has also been frequently associated with other chromosomal anomalies such as Noonan syndrome, Klinefelter syndrome, and fragile X syndrome [30].

Melanocytic Nevi

An increased number of benign melanocytic nevi have been reported in TS patients, with prevalence of 25–70% [1, 27, 33–36]. In one study, the average number of nevi was 115, which is significantly higher than the reported average of 20–40 in the general population [33, 37]. There has been no evidence to indicate a relationship between this increase in nevi count and specific TS karyotypes [18]. Nevi in TS are usually acquired in late childhood and are commonly localized to the face, back, and extremities (Fig. 13.3, benign melanocytic nevus on the forearm, and Fig. 13.4, multiple nevi on the back) [18, 33]. These nevi are typically small with an average size of 1–5 mm in diameter and benign in appearance and do not exhibit increased dysplastic features on histology (Fig. 13.5: benign vulvar nevus under dermoscopy) [33, 38, 39]. Similar to the general population, the number of nevi appears to increase with age and in individuals with fair skin [40]. Interestingly, an increased prevalence of halo nevi, clinically defined as melanocytic nevi encircled by an acquired halo of depigmentation, has been reported in TS patients [41].

Although increased number of nevi is a strong risk factor for melanoma [42, 43], the reported incidence of melanoma in TS patients is strikingly reduced [40]. A small number of cutaneous melanomas have been reported in TS patients, including melanoma in a patient with a concurrent meningioma, melanoma in situ, melanoma in situ in a patient with concurrent glioblastoma in situ [44], lentigo maligna in a

Fig. 13.3 An atypical appearing benign melanocytic nevus on the forearm

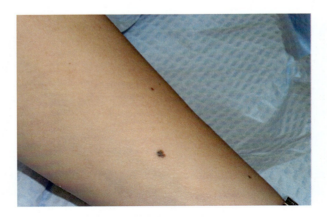

Fig. 13.4 Alopecia totalis in a patient with TS. This photo also shows an increased number of melanocytic nevi on the back

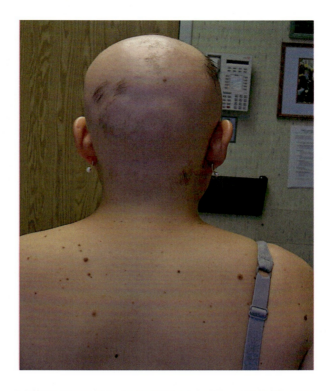

Fig. 13.5 Benign vulvar melanocytic nevus on dermoscopy

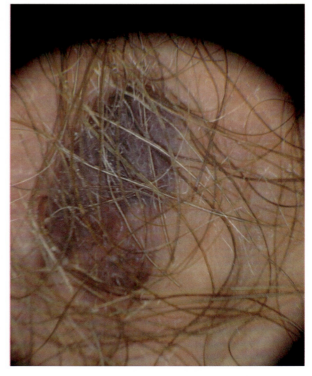

patient with over 200 nevi [33], and two cases of advanced metastatic melanoma [36, 45]. Additionally, two cases of rare non-cutaneous melanomas (anorectal malignant melanoma and ocular choroidal melanoma) have also been reported [40, 46].

The unexpectedly low incidence of melanoma in TS has given rise to speculation as to its cause. The presence of a protective tumor suppressive factor has been posited [40]. Alternatively, the deficiency of circulating sex hormones in young girls with TS may suppress the development of cutaneous melanomas [40]. This is supported by studies associating the onset of menopause in the general female population with a decline in the incidence of cutaneous melanoma, an observation not noted in the male population [40]. However the exact mechanism behind this relationship is not fully understood. Another theory posits that chromosomal deletion syndromes may offer some unknown protection against carcinogenesis, based on the significantly reduced cutaneous tumor incidence observed in syndromes such as fragile X syndrome and Down syndrome [47].

The role of hGH on nevogenesis in TS patients has also been examined. The use of hGH for the treatment of short stature has been implicated in dysplastic changes in nevocyte morphology, such as anisokaryosis (excessive variation in nuclei size) and HMB-45 staining positivity; however there is a lack of proven biologic significance of these changes [39]. One study reported an increase in growth rate and size of nevi in children treated with hGH [38]; however this has been refuted in additional studies, which have shown no pathologic impact of hGH on the number or density of melanocytic nevi [36, 48–50]. Additionally, although hGH receptors are expressed on both melanoma and benign melanocytes [51], hGH treatment has not been shown to stimulate melanoma tumor growth in vitro [52]. Studies on the use of oral contraceptives or hormone replacement for ovarian failure in TS have also failed to demonstrate an effect on melanoma risk [53]. Despite the low incidence of melanoma in TS patients, there is a lack of long-term data on this association; therefore in patients who have many nevi, periodic skin examinations and photoprotection education are recommended [1].

Autoimmune Cutaneous Conditions

Individuals affected by chromosomal abnormalities have a predisposition for autoimmune disease [54, 55]. All main karyotypes of TS have been correlated with a two- to threefold increase in the risk of developing an autoimmune pathology [56]. It has been suggested that this increased risk may in part be due to the haploinsufficiency of genes on the X chromosome [57]. Pro-inflammatory cytokines, such as interleukin-6, interleukin-8, and tumor necrosis factor α, appear to be upregulated in women with TS [58]. These findings are also corroborated by the increased frequency of certain histocompatibility alleles implicated in autoimmunity (HLA-A31, B38, DR-7, DQ2, and DQ9) found in TS patients [59]. Despite the increased prevalence of autoimmune disorders in TS, autoimmune antibodies in most cases are not associated with overt disease [59]. TS has been associated with a variety of autoimmune disorders such as Hashimoto thyroiditis, vitiligo, psoriasis, psoriatic arthritis, alopecia areata, and celiac disease [1, 60]. It is important to note that many of these cutaneous autoimmune conditions are correlated with increased psychiatric or psychological disturbances; therefore multidisciplinary management including psychological and behavioral therapies should be included if necessary [61].

Alopecia Areata

Alopecia areata, presenting as recurrent patches of non-scarring hair loss, has been reported to be three times more frequent in TS patients compared to the general population (Fig. 13.4: alopecia totalis) [59–63]. This increased frequency may be related to HLA-DR and DQ loci in TS [59, 62, 64]. Similar to alopecia areata seen in association with Down syndrome and autoimmune thyroid disease, this condition may be slow to respond to traditional therapies in TS patients [1].

Vitiligo

Vitiligo, an acquired autoimmune skin depigmentation disorder, has been reported as one of the cutaneous findings of TS [35, 41]. However, one study indicated that the slight increase in prevalence of vitiligo in TS patients may not be significant and may merely reflect increased physician awareness [41, 65]. Interestingly, the association between vitiligo and halo nevi has been studied in TS patients [41, 54]. When coincident, halo nevi tend to antedate the onset of generalized vitiligo [41, 54].

Psoriasis

Although infrequently reported, psoriasis has been associated with TS and typically presents as sharply demarcated erythematous scaly plaques most commonly localized to extensor surfaces (elbows and knees), scalp, hands, and trunk (including the intergluteal fold) [54, 55, 60, 61, 66–70]. In particular, several reports have implicated an increased prevalence of pustular psoriasis, which can present as sterile pustules on generalized desquamative erythema (generalized pustular psoriasis), at the edge of existing psoriatic plaques or localized to the palms and soles (pustulosis of the palms and soles) [54, 66, 67, 69]. One study indicated that the prevalence of psoriasis was significantly higher in TS patients (17%) compared to controls (1.6%) [60]. While no susceptibility loci for psoriasis have been detected on the X chromosome, it has been postulated that a protein encoded on the X chromosome may indirectly influence the development of psoriasis in TS [54].

Interestingly, several of the reported cases of psoriasis in TS patients developed after the initiation of hGH therapy [55, 61, 70]. Psoriasis induced by hGH treatment has also been reported in two children with normal chromosomal karyotypes [71, 72]. In both cases the psoriatic lesions improved after withdrawal or dose reduction of hGH therapy [71, 72]. It has been suggested that transient eruptions of psoriasis can occur during hGH therapy, and it is not necessary to cease treatment [70, 72]. hGH affects almost every organ in the body and hGH receptors are found in all skin layers, except the stratum corneum [70]. Many of the metabolic actions of hGH are mediated by local or circulating insulin-like growth factor I (IGF-I), which is believed to influence the effects of hGH on keratinocyte differentiation and stratification [70]. While the exact mechanism behind the association between hGH therapy and psoriasis has yet to be determined, it has been suggested that the genetic predisposition to psoriasis in TS patients may surface with the initiation of hGH therapy [70]. Therefore it is recommended that TS patients be monitored closely for skin eruptions, especially during hGH replacement therapy [70]. In most cases psoriatic lesions were successfully managed with topical measures [55, 61, 70–72].

Mild to moderate cases can usually be managed with topical corticosteroids and/or vitamin D analogues (calcipotriene/calcipotriol) [55, 61, 70]. Coal tar shampoos are particularly useful for scalp psoriasis [61]. More severe or widespread involvement may require systemic therapies such as phototherapy, methotrexate, cyclosporine, systemic retinoids, or biologic therapies [54, 66].

Hypertrophic Scarring and Keloid Formation

An increased propensity for hypertrophic scarring and keloid formation has long been thought to be intrinsic to TS [27, 34]. This association was examined in a study of more than 400 patients, of which 92 underwent 103 operations [5]. Of these patients only three developed keloids at cardiac or nuchal repair sites (high-risk areas for keloid formation) and two developed hypertrophic scars [5]. These findings have raised questions as to whether this association truly reflects inherent differences in the tissue response to injury in TS patients or whether this perceived increased risk is due to the increased prevalence of procedures in locations with a propensity for keloiding (e.g., the neck and upper chest) [5]. Until this possible association is better understood, the risk of scarring should be discussed with patients before any surgeries are undertaken, especially cosmetic or elective procedures [1, 2].

Acne

An apparent decrease in the prevalence of acne in TS patients has been reported [1, 73]. Androgens and their active metabolites have been implicated in the pathogenesis of acne, by inducing increased sebum production [74, 75]. It has been proposed that the decreased prevalence of acne in TS is due to a relative decrease in androgen exposure with gonadal failure [1]. In a recent study of 22 patients affected by TS, a significant decrease in sebum secretion was found in all facial regions, compared to controls [76]. Studies have also demonstrated lower serum androgen levels in TS patients compared to age-matched controls [77, 78]. Specifically, there was a reduction in circulating androstenedione, testosterone, free testosterone, and dihydrotestosterone in patients with TS [78]. The role played by low androgens in the decreased prevalence of acne in TS was further confirmed in a study that found a significant decrease in acne in TS patients without spontaneous menarche, but an increase in acne in TS patients with spontaneous menarche who had complete pubertal development [73]. Further research into this association is needed to elucidate the exact mechanism of peripheral androgen production in TS patients and its effects on acne production.

Other Related Dermatologic Conditions

Variations in Hair Growth

Hair growth variations have been observed in TS patients, with unusual patches of short and long hair having been described [79]. Luxuriant arm and leg hair has also been observed in a small number of cases; however axillary and pubic hair is often scanty [1, 35]. Interestingly, the axillary hair is implanted more distally along the inner surface of the arm, as seen in men, instead of high in the axillary fossa [35]. Hypertrichosis and facial hirsutism can also present in patients with TS [1, 2].

Pigmentary Mosaicism

Pigmentary mosaicism (cutaneous hyper- or hypopigmentation along Blaschko's lines) associated with TS has only been reported in individuals with the mosaic phenotype, with patients often presenting with hyper- or hypopigmented macules, streaks, or broad bands following Blaschko's lines [80–87]. TS patients with extensive pigmentary mosaicism have been reported to exhibit extracutaneous abnormalities affecting the musculoskeletal, ocular, and central nervous systems [88]. It is therefore important that patients with pigmentary mosaicism be referred for genetic counseling to facilitate early diagnosis and management of potentially severe complications.

Pilomatricomas

Pilomatricoma is an uncommon benign cutaneous adnexal tumor thought to arise from cells of the hair follicle matrix [89, 90]. Although the prevalence of this neoplasm among the general population is unknown, one study found a relatively high prevalence of pilomatricomas (2.6%) in patients with TS [89]. In the majority of cases, patients present with enlarging papules or mobile subcutaneous nodules that develop as single or multiple lesions on the face, trunk, or extremities [89–92]. No association with prior hGH treatment has been identified [89]. These lesions can be excised and histology confirmed [93].

Conclusion

There are still many unanswered questions regarding the pathogenesis of many of the cutaneous conditions associated with TS. Further research on TS is needed to better elucidate the genetic mechanisms responsible for the observed phenotypic changes and how they contribute to the clinical manifestations of this disorder. Specifically, studies on the role of the X chromosome in autoimmune disease, lymphatic abnormalities, and the risk of melanoma could yield important information that may influence the development of improved preventative and management strategies. In general, patients should be advised to adopt basic sun safety practices, which include the use of a broad-spectrum (UVA/UVB) sunscreen with an SPF of 30 or higher daily. When caring for patients with TS, clinicians should closely monitor for cutaneous changes or abnormalities and refer patients to dermatology for further diagnosis and management.

References

1. Lowenstein EJ, Kim KH, Glick SA. Turner's syndrome in dermatology. J Am Acad Dermatol. 2004;50(5):767–76.
2. Gunther DF, Sybert VP. Lymphatic, tooth and skin manifestations in Turner syndrome. Int Congr Ser. 2006;1298:58–62.
3. Chervenak FA, Isaacson G, Blakemore KJ, Breg WR, Hobbins JC, Berkowitz RL, et al. Fetal cystic hygroma. Cause and natural history. N Engl J Med. 1983;309(14):822–5.
4. von Kaisenberg CS, Nicolaides KH, Brand-Saberi B. Lymphatic vessel hypoplasia in fetuses with Turner syndrome. Hum Reprod. 1999;14(3):823–6.
5. Larralde M, Gardner SS, Torrado MV, Fernhoff PM, Santos Munoz AE, Spraker MK, et al. Lymphedema as a postulated cause of cutis verticis gyrata in Turner syndrome. Pediatr Dermatol. 1998;15(1):18–22.
6. Boucher CA, Sargent CA, Ogata T, Affara NA. Breakpoint analysis of Turner patients with partial Xp deletions: implications for the lymphoedema gene location. J Med Genet. 2001;38(9):591–8.
7. Ogata T, Muroya K, Matsuo N, Shinohara O, Yorifuji T, Nishi Y, et al. Turner syndrome and Xp deletions: clinical and molecular studies in 47 patients. J Clin Endocrinol Metab. 2001;86(11):5498–508.
8. Irrthum A, Devriendt K, Chitayat D, Matthijs G, Glade C, Steijlen PM, et al. Mutations in the transcription factor gene SOX18 underlie recessive and dominant forms of hypotrichosis-lymphedema-telangiectasia. Am J Hum Genet. 2003;72(6):1470–8.

9. Karkkainen MJ, Ferrell RE, Lawrence EC, Kimak MA, Levinson KL, McTigue MA, et al. Missense mutations interfere with VEGFR-3 signalling in primary lymphoedema. Nat Genet. 2000;25(2):153–9.
10. Duong T, Koltowska K, Pichol-Thievend C, Le Guen L, Fontaine F, Smith KA, et al. VEGFD regulates blood vascular development by modulating SOX18 activity. Blood. 2014;123(7):1102–12.
11. Atton G, Gordon K, Brice G, Keeley V, Riches K, Ostergaard P, et al. The lymphatic phenotype in Turner syndrome: an evaluation of nineteen patients and literature review. Eur J Hum Genet. 2015;23(12):1634–9.
12. Bondy CA, Turner Syndrome Study G. Care of girls and women with Turner syndrome: a guideline of the Turner Syndrome Study Group. J Clin Endocrinol Metab. 2007;92(1):10–25.
13. Frias JL, Davenport ML, Committee on G, Section on E. Health supervision for children with Turner syndrome. Pediatrics. 2003;111(3):692–702.
14. Rizell S. Dentofacial morphology in Turner syndrome karyotypes. Swed Dent J Suppl. 2012;225:7–98.
15. Berdahl LD, Wenstrom KD, Hanson JW. Web neck anomaly and its association with congenital heart disease. Am J Med Genet. 1995;56(3):304–7.
16. Brady AF, Patton MA. Web-neck anomaly and its association with congenital heart disease. Am J Med Genet. 1996;64(4):605–6.
17. Ferencz C, Rubin JD, McCarter RJ, Brenner JI, Neill CA, Perry LW, et al. Congenital heart disease: prevalence at livebirth. The Baltimore-Washington Infant Study. Am J Epidemiol. 1985;121(1):31–6.
18. Sybert VP. Turner syndrome. In: Cassidy S, Allanson J, editors. Management of genetic syndromes. New York: Wiley and Sons; 2001. p. 459–84.
19. Zielinski T, Lorenc-Podgorska K, Antoszewski B. Surgical correction of a webbed-neck deformity in Turner's syndrome. Pol Przegl Chir. 2015;87(3):134–8.
20. Hikade KR, Bitar GJ, Edgerton MT, Morgan RF. Modified Z-plasty repair of webbed neck deformity seen in Turner and Klippel-Feil syndrome. Cleft Palate Craniofac J. 2002;39(3):261–6.
21. Leandris M, Ricbourg B. Surgical treatment of pterygium colli. A case report and review of the literature. Ann Chir Plast Esthet. 1997;42(6):615–22.
22. Chaput B, Chavoin JP, Lopez R, Meresse T, Nadon F, Herlin C, et al. The "posterior cervical lift": a new approach to pterygium colli management. Plast Reconstr Surg Glob Open. 2013;1(6):e46.
23. Miller LB, Kanter M, Wolfort F. Treatment of webbed neck in Turner's syndrome with tissue expansion. Ann Plast Surg. 1990;24(5):447–50.
24. Niranjan NS. Webbing of the neck: correction by tissue expansion. Plast Reconstr Surg. 1989;84(6):985–8.
25. Preus M, Fraser FC. Dermatoglyphics and syndromes. Amer J Dis Child. 1972;124:933–43.
26. Verbov J. Clinical significance and genetics of epidermal ridges–a review of dermatoglyphics. J Invest Dermatol. 1970;54(4):261–71.
27. Hall JG, Gilchrist DM. Turner syndrome and its variants. Pediatr Clin N Am. 1990;37(6):1421–40.
28. Kaplowitz PB, Chernausek SD, Horn JA. Fingernail angle in girls with Ullrich-Turner syndrome. Am J Med Genet. 1993;46(5):570–3.
29. Auada MP, Cintra ML, Puzzi MB, Viana D, Cavalcanti DP. Scalp lesions in Turner syndrome: a result of lymphoedema? Clin Dysmorphol. 2004;13(3):165–8.
30. Debeer A, Steenkiste E, Devriendt K, Morren M. Scalp skin lesion in Turner syndrome: more than lymphoedema? Clin Dysmorphol. 2005;14(3):149–50.
31. Shepard TH, Wener MH, Myhre SA, Hickok DE. Lowered plasma albumin concentration in fetal Turner syndrome. J Pediatr. 1986;108(1):114–6.
32. Snyder MC, Johnson PJ, Hollins RR. Congenital primary cutis verticis gyrata. Plast Reconstr Surg. 2002;110(3):818–21.

33. Becker B, Jospe N, Goldsmith LA. Melanocytic nevi in Turner syndrome. Pediatr Dermatol. 1994;11(2):120–4.
34. Lemli L, Smith DW. The XO syndrome. A study of the differentiated phenotype in 25 patients. J Pediatr. 1963;63:577–88.
35. Polani PE. Turner's syndrome and allied conditions. Clinical features and chromosome abnormalities. Br Med Bull. 1961;17:200–5.
36. Zvulunov A, Wyatt DT, Laud PW, Esterly NB. Influence of genetic and environmental factors on melanocytic naevi: a lesson from Turner's syndrome. Br J Dermatol. 1998;138(6):993–7.
37. Bataille V, Snieder H, MacGregor AJ, Sasieni P, Spector TD. Genetics of risk factors for melanoma: an adult twin study of nevi and freckles. J Natl Cancer Inst. 2000;92(6):457–63.
38. Bourguignon JP, Pierard GE, Ernould C, Heinrichs C, Craen M, Rochiccioli P, et al. Effects of human growth hormone therapy on melanocytic naevi. Lancet. 1993;341(8859):1505–6.
39. Pierard GE, Pierard-Franchimont C, Nikkels A, Nikkels-Tassoudji N, Arrese JE, Bourguignon JP. Naevocyte triggering by recombinant human growth hormone. J Pathol. 1996;180(1):74–9.
40. Gibbs P, Brady BM, Gonzalez R, Robinson WA. Nevi and melanoma: lessons from Turner's syndrome. Dermatology. 2001;202(1):1–3.
41. Brazzelli V, Larizza D, Martinetti M, Martinoli S, Calcaterra V, De Silvestri A, et al. Halo nevus, rather than vitiligo, is a typical dermatologic finding of Turner's syndrome: clinical, genetic, and immunogenetic study in 72 patients. J Am Acad Dermatol. 2004;51(3):354–8.
42. Bauer J, Garbe C. Acquired melanocytic nevi as risk factor for melanoma development. A comprehensive review of epidemiological data. Pigment Cell Res. 2003;16(3):297–306.
43. Grob JJ, Gouvernet J, Aymar D, Mostaque A, Romano MH, Collet AM, et al. Count of benign melanocytic nevi as a major indicator of risk for nonfamilial nodular and superficial spreading melanoma. Cancer. 1990;66(2):387–95.
44. Larizza D, Albanesi M, De Silvestri A, Accordino G, Brazzelli V, Maffe GC, et al. Neoplasia in Turner syndrome. The importance of clinical and screening practices during follow-up. Eur J Med Genet. 2016;59(5):269–73.
45. Gare M, Ilan Y, Sherman Y, Ben-Chetrit E. Malignant melanoma in Turner's syndrome. Int J Dermatol. 1993;32(10):743–4.
46. Buckley CA, Cheng H. Intraocular melanoma, diabetes, and Turner's syndrome: presentation with proptosis. Br J Ophthalmol. 1981;65(7):460–3.
47. Schultz-Pedersen S, Hasle H, Olsen JH, Friedrich U. Evidence of decreased risk of cancer in individuals with fragile X. Am J Med Genet. 2001;103(3):226–30.
48. Zvulunov A, Wyatt DT, Rabinowitz LG, Esterly NB. Effect of growth hormone therapy on melanocytic nevi in survivors of childhood neoplasia. Arch Dermatol. 1997;133(6):795–6.
49. Zvulunov A, Wyatt DT, Laud PW, Esterly NB. Lack of effect of growth hormone therapy on the count and density of melanocytic naevi in children. Br J Dermatol. 1997;137(4):545–8.
50. Wyatt D. Melanocytic nevi in children treated with growth hormone. Pediatrics. 1999;104(4 Pt 2):1045–50.
51. Ginarte M, Garcia-Caballero T, Fernandez-Redondo V, Beiras A, Toribio J. Expression of growth hormone receptor in benign and malignant cutaneous proliferative entities. J Cutan Pathol. 2000;27(6):276–82.
52. Fiebig HH, Dengler W, Hendriks HR. No evidence of tumor growth stimulation in human tumors in vitro following treatment with recombinant human growth hormone. Anti-Cancer Drugs. 2000;11(8):659–64.
53. English JS, Swerdlow AJ, MacKie RM, O'Doherty CJ, Hunter JA, Clark J, et al. Relation between phenotype and banal melanocytic naevi. Br Med J (Clin Res Ed). 1987;294(6565):152–4.
54. Oiso N, Ota T, Kawara S, Kawada A. Pustular psoriasis and vitiligo in a patient with Turner syndrome. J Dermatol. 2007;34(10):727–9.
55. Watabe H, Kawakami T, Kimura S, Fujimoto M, Ono T, Mizoguchi M, et al. Childhood psoriasis associated with Turner syndrome. J Dermatol. 2006;33(12):896–8.
56. Jorgensen KT, Rostgaard K, Bache I, Biggar RJ, Nielsen NM, Tommerup N, et al. Autoimmune diseases in women with Turner's syndrome. Arthritis Rheum. 2010;62(3):658–66.

57. Invernizzi P, Miozzo M, Selmi C, Persani L, Battezzati PM, Zuin M, et al. X chromosome monosomy: a common mechanism for autoimmune diseases. J Immunol. 2005;175(1):575–8.
58. Gravholt CH, Hjerrild BE, Mosekilde L, Hansen TK, Rasmussen LM, Frystyk J, et al. Body composition is distinctly altered in Turner syndrome: relations to glucose metabolism, circulating adipokines, and endothelial adhesion molecules. Eur J Endocrinol. 2006;155(4):583–92.
59. Larizza D, Martinetti Bianchi M, Lorini R, Maghnie M, Dugoujon JM, Cuccia Belvedere M, et al. Autoimmunity, HLA, Gm and Km polymorphisms in Turner's syndrome. Autoimmunity. 1989;4(1–2):69–78.
60. Dacou-Voutetakis C, Kakourou T. Psoriasis and blue sclerae in girls with Turner syndrome. J Am Acad Dermatol. 1996;35(6):1002–4.
61. Rosina P, Segalla G, Magnanini M, Chieregato C, Barba A. Turner's syndrome associated with psoriasis and alopecia areata. J Eur Acad Dermatol Venereol. 2003;17(1):50–2.
62. Tebbe B, Gollnick H, Muller R, Reupke HJ, Orfanos CE. Alopecia areata and diffuse hypotrichosis associated with Ullrich-Turner syndrome. Presentation of 4 patients. Hautarzt. 1993;44(10):647–52.
63. Lee WS, Yoo MS. Alopecia areata in a patient with Turner's syndrome. Br J Dermatol. 1996;135(6):1013.
64. de Andrade M, Jackow CM, Dahm N, Hordinsky M, Reveille JD, Duvic M. Alopecia areata in families: association with the HLA locus. J Investig Dermatol Symp Proc. 1999;4(3):220–3.
65. Lleo A, Moroni L, Caliari L, Invernizzi P. Autoimmunity and Turner's syndrome. Autoimmun Rev. 2012;11(6–7):A538–43.
66. Kawakami Y, Oyama N, Kishimoto K, Yamazaki K, Nishibu A, Nakamura K, et al. A case of generalized pustular psoriasis associated with Turner syndrome. J Dermatol. 2004;31(1):16–20.
67. Ito M, Maejima Y, Okazaki S, Isobe M, Saeki H. Generalized pustular psoriasis associated with Turner syndrome and dilated cardiomyopathy. J Dermatol. 2016;43(7):829–30.
68. Dogruk Kacar S, Ozuguz P, Polat S. Coexistence of psoriasis, and alopecia areata with trachyonychia in a pediatric patient with Turner syndrome. Arch Argent Pediatr. 2014;112(5):e209–12.
69. Asahina A, Uno K, Fujita H. Pustular psoriasis in a patient with Turner syndrome: profile of serum cytokine levels. Int J Dermatol. 2014;53(1):e29–32.
70. Acikgoz G, Ozmen I, Tunca M, Akar A, Arca E, Saifurrahman S. Psoriasis induced by growth hormone therapy in a patient with Turner's syndrome. Int J Dermatol. 2015;54(5):e132–5.
71. Maghnie M, Borroni G, Larizza D, Lorini R, Girani MA, Rabbiosi G, et al. Relapsing eruptive psoriasis and immunological changes triggered by growth hormone therapy in a growth hormone-deficient girl. Dermatologica. 1990;181(2):139–41.
72. Pirgon O, Atabek ME, Sert A. Psoriasis following growth hormone therapy in a child. Ann Pharmacother. 2007;41(1):157–60.
73. Brazzelli V, Larizza D, Muzio F, Calcaterra V, Fornara L, Klersy C, et al. Low frequency of acne vulgaris in adolescent girls and women with Turner's syndrome: a clinical, genetic and hormonal study of 65 patients. Br J Dermatol. 2008;159(5):1209–11.
74. Deplewski D, Rosenfield RL. Role of hormones in pilosebaceous unit development. Endocr Rev. 2000;21(4):363–92.
75. Thiboutot D. Hormones and acne: pathophysiology, clinical evaluation, and therapies. Semin Cutan Med Surg. 2001;20(3):144–53.
76. Brazzelli V, Calcaterra V, Muzio F, Klersy C, Larizza D, Borroni G. Reduced sebum production in Turner syndrome: a study of twenty-two patients. Int J Immunopathol Pharmacol. 2011;24(3):789–92.
77. Apter D, Lenko HL, Perheentupa J, Soderholm A, Vihko R. Subnormal pubertal increases of serum androgens in Turner's syndrome. Horm Res. 1982;16(3):164–73.
78. Gravholt CH, Svenstrup B, Bennett P, Sandahl Christiansen J. Reduced androgen levels in adult Turner syndrome: influence of female sex steroids and growth hormone status. Clin Endocrinol. 1999;50(6):791–800.
79. Smith DW, Hanson JW. Letter: asynchronous growth of scalp hair in XO Turner syndrome. J Pediatr. 1975;87(4):659–60.

80. Capaldi L, Gray J, Abuelo D, Torrelo A, Nieto J, Lapidus C, et al. Pigmentary mosaicism and mosaic Turner syndrome. J Am Acad Dermatol. 2005;52(5):918–9.
81. Moss C, Larkins S, Stacey M, Blight A, Farndon PA, Davison EV. Epidermal mosaicism and Blaschko's lines. J Med Genet. 1993;30(9):752–5.
82. Nehal KS, PeBenito R, Orlow SJ. Analysis of 54 cases of hypopigmentation and hyperpigmentation along the lines of Blaschko. Arch Dermatol. 1996;132(10):1167–70.
83. Niessen RC, Jonkman MF, Muis N, Hordijk R, van Essen AJ. Pigmentary mosaicism following the lines of Blaschko in a girl with a double aneuploidy mosaicism: (47,XX,+7/45,X). Am J Med Genet A. 2005;137A(3):313–22.
84. Ruiz-Maldonado R, Toussaint S, Tamayo L, Laterza A, del Castillo V. Hypomelanosis of Ito: diagnostic criteria and report of 41 cases. Pediatr Dermatol. 1992;9(1):1–10.
85. Sybert VP, Pagon RA, Donlan M, Bradley CM. Pigmentary abnormalities and mosaicism for chromosomal aberration: association with clinical features similar to hypomelanosis of Ito. J Pediatr. 1990;116(4):581–6.
86. Thomas IT, Frias JL, Cantu ES, Lafer CZ, Flannery DB, Graham JG Jr. Association of pigmentary anomalies with chromosomal and genetic mosaicism and chimerism. Am J Hum Genet. 1989;45(2):193–205.
87. Flannery DB, Byrd JR, Freeman WE, Perlman SA. Hypomelanosis of Ito: a cutaneous marker of chromosomal mosaicism. Am J Hum Genet. 1985;37:A93.
88. Deza G, Lopez Aventin D, Salido M, Espinet B, Gilaberte M, Pujol RM. Hyperpigmentation following the Blaschko's lines: a subtle cutaneous manifestation of Turner syndrome with complex mosaicism. Br J Dermatol. 2016;175:1379.
89. Handler MZ, Derrick KM, Lutz RE, Morrell DS, Davenport ML, Armstrong AW. Prevalence of pilomatricoma in Turner syndrome: findings from a multicenter study. JAMA Dermatol. 2013;149(5):559–64.
90. Maeda D, Kubo T, Miwa H, Kitamura N, Onoda M, Ohgo M, et al. Multiple pilomatricomas in a patient with Turner syndrome. J Dermatol. 2014;41(6):563–4.
91. Bengtzen AR, Grossniklaus HE, Bernardino CR. Multiple pilomatrixoma in Turner syndrome. Ophthal Plast Reconstr Surg. 2009;25(3):229–30.
92. Noguchi H, Kayashima K, Nishiyama S, Ono T. Two cases of pilomatrixoma in Turner's syndrome. Dermatology. 1999;199(4):338–40.
93. Wood S, Nguyen D, Hutton K, Dickson W. Pilomatricomas in Turner syndrome. Pediatr Dermatol. 2008;25(4):449–51.

Chapter 14
Orthopedic Manifestations in Turner Syndrome

Anna M. Acosta, Suzanne E. Steinman, and Klane K. White

Introduction

Skeletal deformity in Turner syndrome has been extensively described in the literature [32]. It has been associated with short stature, angular deformities of both upper and lower extremities, coronal and sagittal deformities of the spine, altered bone growth, and early-onset osteoporosis. In the past, these skeletal differences were hypothesized to be related to the gonadal dysgenesis found in patients with Turner syndrome. However, more recently, research into the genetic changes in patients with Turner syndrome has revealed a deficiency in the short stature homeobox (SHOX)-containing gene within the bone regulatory center for longitudinal growth.

In this chapter, we will address the orthopedic issues that arise in patients with Turner syndrome. We will review the literature published regarding these orthopedic concerns. And we will discuss the current recommendations for treatment of the common and uncommon skeletal deformities found in patients with Turner syndrome.

A. M. Acosta
Memorial Care and Miller Children's and Women's Hospital, Long Beach, CA, USA

S. E. Steinman · K. K. White (✉)
Department of Orthopedics and Sports Medicine, Seattle Children's Hospital, Seattle, WA, USA

Department of Orthopaedics and Sports Medicine, University of Washington, Seattle, WA, USA
e-mail: suzanne.steinman@seattlechildrens.org; klane.white@seattlechildrens.org

© Springer Nature Switzerland AG 2020
P. Y. Fechner (ed.), *Turner Syndrome*,
https://doi.org/10.1007/978-3-030-34150-3_14

SHOX Gene

In utero, the SHOX gene is initially expressed in the cells of mesenchymal tissue. At sixth gestational week, the cells begin to differentiate and transform into chondrocytes to form a skeletal model where ossification eventually begins (endochondral ossification) [7]. SHOX expression condenses in the perichondrial layer along the diaphysis of long bones [7] and is most strongly expressed within the mesomelic region of the limbs. Dosage insufficiency of this gene can lead to bowing and shortening in these regions, specifically in the forearms and lower legs. Clinically, this may cause shortened limbs, cubitus varus, and genu valgum.

It has been proposed that the SHOX gene may influence the timing of growth plate fusion and skeletal maturation [9]. Skeletal tissues with a haploinsufficient SHOX gene appear to be more susceptible to premature growth plate fusion with exposure to estrogens. Studies of individuals/families with SHOX mutations (without Turner syndrome) show similar skeletal features to Turner syndrome patients. However, radiographic differences in non-Turner syndrome individuals with SHOX deficiency (Leri-Weill dyschondrosteosis, LWD) appeared more severe than in patients with Turner syndrome. It is hypothesized that this results from the effects of endogenous estrogen production in pubertal girls with non-Turner SHOX deficiency, which is absent in females with Turner syndrome [6, 17].

Short Stature

Short stature is the single most common skeletal anomaly found in patients with Turner syndrome. The incidence of short stature in these patients ranges from 88% to 100% [29]. All other skeletal anomalies common in Turner syndrome such as short metacarpals, cubitus valgus, high-arched palate, micrognathia, and short neck only occur with an incidence of 35–60% [17]. Short stature in patients with Turner syndrome is thought to result from growth retardation throughout development. Most patients show mild growth impairment in utero and are delivered short for age. Infancy (up to 24 months) appears to be the period most affected by slow growth. Davenport et al. reviewed the growth charts of 62 children with Turner syndrome at the University of North Carolina from 1992 to 1998. They found that the mean height in girls with Turner syndrome fell from −0.5 SDS at birth to −1.5 SDS at age 1 year and −1.8 SDS by 1.5 years [8]. Patients also show delayed onset and slow growth during childhood, as well as failure to undergo a normal pubertal growth spurt [8]. Turner syndrome is an important diagnosis for providers to consider when evaluating young infants less than 2 years of age who have fallen off the height growth curve.

Short stature may be the first physical abnormality found in an undiagnosed patient with Turner syndrome. By age 4–8 years old, the mean height of girls with Turner syndrome is −2.3 SDS from the norm [8]. On average, individuals with

Turner syndrome, not treated with growth hormone, are 20 cm shorter than the average female adult of corresponding ethnic population [8, 29]. The final height for most adults with Turner syndrome ranges from 54 to 60 inches tall [2].

Mesomelic Growth

Mesomelic growth is a disorder of bone growth in which the middle parts of the limbs (forearm and leg) are disproportionately short. Mild mesomelic growth of both the upper and lower limbs in patients with Turner syndrome has been described in the literature [2]. However, more extreme mesomelia may be seen in patients who carry a diagnosis of LWD. LWD is a skeletal dysplasia on the severe end of the spectrum for SHOX gene disorders. It can result from either a complete SHOX deletion or a SHOX single-nucleotide variant [3]. Clinically, LWD is defined by symmetric shortening of the forearms and lower legs and the typical presence of a Madelung deformity in the forearm [4].

Delayed Skeletal Maturation

Multiple authors have noted a delay in skeletal maturation when evaluating patients with Turner syndrome. It has been reported that bone age wrist X-rays often appear normal for age in Turner syndrome patients less than 11 years. However, bone age wrist X-rays will progressively become more delayed as the patient ages. A maximum of 2-year bone age delay can be seen by the age of 16 years in patients with Turner syndrome. This is believed to be due to a failure in growth plate closure, possibly secondary to SHOX haploinsufficiency and the absence of pubertal hormone onset [6, 17].

Upper Extremity

The upper extremity can be involved to varying degrees in Turner syndrome with classic findings of cubitus valgus, brachymetacarpia of the fourth digit, and Madelung deformity. The most cited cause for these findings is SHOX haploinsufficiency [4, 27, 28, 32]. The SHOX gene expression is greatest in the ulna, radius, and elbow in the upper extremity which is felt to contribute to the phenotypes identified in the syndrome [7].

Cubitus valgus is an increase in the carrying angle of the elbow (Fig. 14.1) and affects roughly 45% of patients with Turner syndrome [9, 28]. This can also be accompanied by bowing and shortening of the forearms. This is most commonly asymptomatic and requires no treatment other than observation.

Fig. 14.1 Cubitus valgus

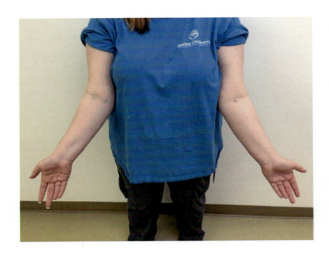

Brachymetacarpia, or shortening of the fourth metacarpal, can be identified in 37% of patients with Turner syndrome [9]. This is rarely symptomatic and is often only noted as the fourth metacarpophalangeal being shorter than the others clinically or the incidental finding of a short metacarpal on X-ray (Fig. 14.2). Treatment, as with cubitus valgus, is observation.

The most discussed upper extremity difference but least common is Madelung deformity (Fig. 14.3a, b). Madelung deformity is a classic finding of abnormal growth of the volar-ulnar aspect of the distal radius resulting in increased radial inclination and volar tilt, proximal migration of the carpus, and the appearance of volar subluxation of the wrist on the forearm. This is sometimes accompanied by the finding of Vickers ligament, an abnormally thickened radial-carpal ligament that tethers the volar-ulnar distal radial physis and the lunate (Fig. 14.4) [33]. Although routinely discussed as a finding in Turner syndrome, it is identified in only 2–7% of patients [9, 32]. A more common finding, although still found in a limited number of patients, is an increased distal radio-ulnar physeal disparity where the ulnar physis lies more proximally than the radial physis (ulnar negative variance). This is the opposite finding to Madelung deformity where there is commonly an ulnar positive variance [32]. Initial treatment of Madelung deformity is observation if asymptomatic and not progressing on surveillance posterior to anterior and lateral radiographs of the forearm. If pain does develop, then the first treatment is activity modification. If symptoms continue or progression is noted and the patient is still skeletally immature, then an epiphysiolysis and interposition fat graft of the region of growth disturbance at the volar-ulnar aspect of the distal radius physis with or without release of Vickers ligament can restore growth. There is, however, risk of further injury to the physis and possible greater growth disturbance [33]. If the patient is approaching skeletal maturity and is symptomatic, then a dome osteotomy to correct the multiplanar deformity with or without an ulnar shortening osteotomy is recommended [15]. Wrist arthrodesis is recommended as a salvage procedure for severe pain in the skeletally mature.

Fig. 14.2 Brachymetacarpia of the fourth digit

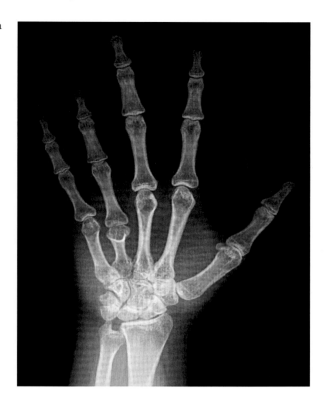

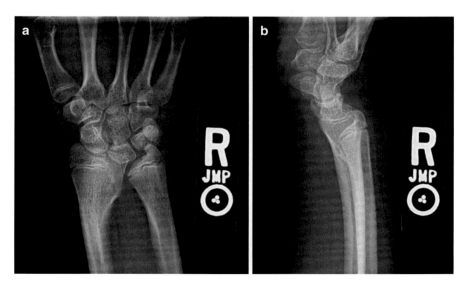

Fig. 14.3 (a) PA X-ray of a wrist with Madelung deformity. (b) Lateral X-rays of a wrist with Madelung deformity

Fig. 14.4 MRI
demonstrating Vickers
ligament of the volar wrist

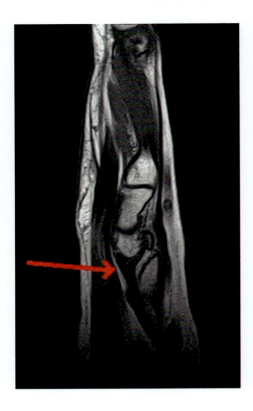

Spinal Deformity

SHOX gene expression has been demonstrated in vertebral body growth plates, with upregulation having been demonstrated in cases of idiopathic and congenital scoliosis [9]. There has long been known the presence of irregular vertebral epiphyseal growth rings and anterior vertebral wedging in Turner syndrome [19, 22, 23]. Spinal deformity, both in the frontal plane and sagittal plane, appears to occur more frequently in patients with Turner syndrome when compared to the general population. Historically, the incidence of scoliosis in Turner syndrome has been estimated to be approximately 10%. However, more recent literature raises this figure to as high as 59% [25]. Kyphotic deformity has been estimated to be as high as 48%. The presence of these deformities appears to be later in onset compared to the general population, and therefore the prevalence increases with age, well into the second decade of life. As a result, general screening by physical exam and selective radiography has been recommended up to 20 years of age.

Scoliosis in Turner syndrome is clinically and radiographically similar to idiopathic scoliosis. However, a small percentage has been associated with vertebral body malformations (congenital scoliosis) [9, 16]. The mean age at presentation for scoliosis in larger studies is typically between 12 and 13 years of age [9, 25], with onset described as young as 3 years of age and as old as 18 years. The deformities observed are usually mild (Cobb angles < 20°). Ricotti et al. reported 29 of 29 patients with deformities between 10 and 20° [25], while Day et al. reported 8 of 13 patients with curves < 20° and the remaining five with curves up to 55° [9]. This study did not report on brace or surgical therapies. Kim et al. reported an incidence of 5 out of 43 patients with scoliosis (11.6%), of which two were braced and three underwent surgical treatment [16].

The anterior vertebral wedging and irregular vertebral epiphyseal growth rings result in "Scheuermann-like disease" in Turner syndrome [10]. The incidence of hyperkyphosis has been reported at 35–48%, with an increasing prevalence with age, suggesting late-onset presentation (40% of hyperkyphosis presenting after age 14 years) [25]. Elder et al. specifically studied the incidence of hyperkyphosis in Turner syndrome. In their survey, 40% (10/25) had excessive kyphosis, defined as an anterior to posterior curvature exceeding 40°. The majority of these patients demonstrated vertebral body wedging, suggesting that these two entities go hand in hand [10].

The association between growth hormone therapy and the incidence of scoliosis is controversial. Previous reports have suggested that the use of human growth hormone (HGH) supplementation may accelerate preexisting scoliosis [1, 5, 34]. Looking at the effect of HGH on the development of scoliosis in Australian patients with short stature, Day et al. reported that scoliosis progression occurred in 5 of 13 subjects during HGH therapy [9]. HGH treatment was not stopped in any patient because of scoliosis progression. Two patients (2/13) had curves that progressed to 45°, while a third (1/13) progressed to 55° and was treated surgically. These authors did remark on their increased incidence of scoliosis at 29%, which was higher than previous reports at about 10%. This suggested that either scoliosis was more common in Turner syndrome than previously believed or that HGH may lead to an increased prevalence of scoliosis. Ricotti et al. reported that patients with scoliosis tended to be taller than those without scoliosis and that patients were more likely to be on HGH at baseline [25]. In this study, all cases of scoliosis were felt to be minor in degree. Three of the 29 subjects with scoliosis at baseline demonstrated progression of their deformity; however, this was not quantified. Furthermore, less than half of the patients (9/20) without scoliosis at baseline developed scoliosis, and in all of these cases, the severity of the deformity was not felt to be consequential.

Lower Extremity

The lower extremity can also be involved to varying degrees in Turner syndrome, the most commonly reported finding being genu valgum and less commonly tarsal coalitions and brachymetatarsia. These phenotypic differences have been traced back to the SHOX gene haploinsufficiency as discussed earlier. The strongest expression of SHOX in the lower extremity is in the tibia and fibula, most specifically around the knee [7].

Genu Valgum

Genu valgum, commonly referred to as "knocked knees," is an increased femoral-tibial angle at the knee. This can be a normal physiologic finding in adolescents between ages 3 and 4 years with an average angle of 2–20° [21]. Most adolescents in the general population correct this femoral-tibial angle to less than 12° by the age of 7 years. The increased expression of SHOX in the perichondrium around the knee in patients with Turner syndrome can cause growth impairment and lead to the development of genu valgum that does not correct [7]. Mild or moderate genu valgum is most commonly asymptomatic and requires no treatment other than observation. However, if patients have severe genu valgum (mechanical axis of the lower extremity passing through beyond the lateral cortex of the tibial plateau) or moderate genu valgum with pain (mechanical axis passing through the lateral half of the lateral femoral condyle), treatment may need to include surgical correction. For the skeletally immature with 1–2 years of growth remaining, this consists of guided growth techniques [30]. In the skeletally mature patients with less than 1–2 years of growth remaining, a varus-producing osteotomy may be more appropriate [21].

In 1973, Beals reported that 7 of 11 patients (63%) in his series of Turner syndrome had knee abnormalities. The increased expression of SHOX in the perichondrium around the knee in patients with Turner syndrome may cause growth impairment, leading to early or partial closure of growth plate and adaptive changes in the epiphysis resulting in deformity [2]. The proximal tibia is a common site of physeal/epiphyseal changes found in patients with Turner syndrome. Patients have been observed to have medial projections from the metaphysis, depression of the medial plateau, or superior or inferior beaking of the medial border overlying the epiphysis. The overlying medial femoral condyle becomes enlarged, which can result in a lateral shift of the tibia [2], thus creating an almost "Blount-type deformity" without genu varum [18].

Brachymetatarsia

Brachymetatarsia, or a shortened metatarsal, most commonly in the fourth digit, has been suggested as a rare finding in patients with Turner syndrome [12]. Early closure of the distal physis, likely related to SHOX deficiency, may lead to a shortened metatarsal in the foot. This skeletal difference is rarely symptomatic and is most often only found incidentally on foot X-ray. The treatment, as with brachymetacarpia, is observation.

Coalitions

Bony coalitions can be fairly common findings in patients with Turner syndrome. Sternal coalitions are the most common. Phalanx coalitions, carpal coalitions, tarsal coalitions, and vertebral coalitions have also been described [2]. Most of the coalitions are incidental findings and are rarely symptomatic. Vertebral coalitions, however, may result in significant scoliosis and should be referred to an orthopedic spine surgeon for evaluation and long-term follow-up. Tarsal coalitions that cause pain and are unrelieved by conservative measures should be referred to an orthopedic surgeon for evaluation of surgical management.

Other General Orthopedic Concerns

Hip Dysplasia

It has been proposed that infants with Turner syndrome may have an increased risk of dislocation of the hip (about 5% of patients) [29, 31]. However, there has been little research to support this. Orthopedic recommendations for hip evaluation in infants with Turner syndrome remain equal to the general population. Evaluation of the hips using Ortolani and Barlow examinations, Galeazzi sign, and hip range of motion is recommended at all well-baby checks by the primary care practitioner. Breech presentation, family history of hip disease, and instability by examination at birth are indications for a screening ultrasound [26].

Bone Mineral Density

Multiple studies have reviewed data on osteoporosis in patients with Turner syndrome. Although still a very controversial topic, bone mineral density (BMD) and bone fragility continue to be considered a major lifelong comorbidity in patients with Turner syndrome [11]. Early studies showed a high correlation of low BMD and Turner syndrome based on DXA evaluation. However, these DXA studies were completed using a comparison to the average population based on age and were limited secondary to the body size of the typical Turner syndrome patient. With new, more precise tools for bone imaging such as peripheral quantitative computer tomography (pQCT) or volumetric transformation of DXA data, a more detailed description of BMD in Turner syndrome has become available.

At a young age, patients with Turner syndrome have been found to have a lower cortical bone density but normal trabecular bone density when compared to age-matched norms [11]. It has been hypothesized that these differences are due to a combination of estrogen deficiency and X chromosome abnormality (SHOX haploinsufficiency) in patients with Turner syndrome [13]. A decreased bone cortical density, along with differences in bone geometry (size, shape, and microarchitecture secondary to continuous remodeling), may predispose Turner syndrome patients to fragility fractures [11, 13]. Gravholt et al. published a study reviewing the medical morbidities of 594 females with Turner syndrome over 10 years in the Danish National Registry. They reported 2.66 times the relative risk (1.37–4.64, 95% CI) of "potential osteoporotic fractures" (fractures of the spine, femoral neck, and radius/

ulna) in patients with Turner syndrome when compared to age-matched norms [14]. When taking into consideration the other common comorbidities in Turner syndrome such as obesity, decreased physical activity, hearing impairment, and low vitamin D, these patients may be at even higher risk for fragility fractures. More recent studies have focused on the evaluation of the elevated risk of fragility fractures in patients with Turner syndrome. An increased risk of fracture was seen only in those greater than 45 years of age. However, all younger study subjects had previously been treated, since childhood, with hormone replacement therapy compared to the older subjects who had not. Hormone factors were seen to be of great importance in the development of peak bone mass and the maintenance of BMD in these patients [20]. Thus, it could be that growth-promoting treatments during childhood and adolescence in Turner syndrome could be of lifelong benefit for bone health [24].

Growth Hormone Replacement and SCFE

Treatment with growth hormone may increase risk of slipped capital femoral epiphysis (SCFE) in children. Young patients with Turner syndrome may also be predisposed to obesity and hypothyroidism which further increases their risk for SCFE. Any child/adolescent with Turner syndrome complaining of prolonged hip or knee pain should be evaluated radiographically with orthogonal views of the hip. Surgical stabilization is recommended in cases of SCFE, particularly in the presence of an endocrine disorder (use of growth hormone or hypothyroidism).

Summary

The skeletal manifestations of Turner syndrome have been extensively reviewed, but several topics still remain controversial. Current literature has shown the SHOX gene to be the major cause of skeletal deformity in Turner syndrome. The combination of SHOX haploinsufficiency and estrogen deficiency likely leads to the short stature and delayed skeletal maturation seen in these patients. Hormone replacement therapies used in the treatment of young patients with Turner syndrome are hypothesized to be beneficial for future bone health. Practitioners should be aware of the lower BMDs and increased risk of fragility fractures at a younger age in patients with Turner syndrome that have not been treated with hormone replacement therapy. Patients with Turner syndrome have a higher incidence of scoliosis and kyphosis and should be followed by an orthopedic surgeon for curves > 20°. The upper and lower extremity abnormalities found in Turner syndrome may be evident on clinical examination but rarely require surgical treatments unless symptomatic.

The goal of this chapter was to address the skeletal issues that arise in patients with Turner syndrome, to discuss the natural history of these anomalies, and to review current treatment recommendations. Although there are several skeletal abnormalities found in patients with Turner syndrome, it remains a rare diagnosis to be seen in the orthopedic clinic. While the majority of these skeletal manifestations remain nonoperative, it is important for the primary practitioner to be knowledgeable about the natural history of these abnormalities and the current standards of treatment so that they may refer to specialty care provider when needed.

References

1. Ahn UM, Ahn NU, Nallamshetty L, Buchowski JM, Rose PS, Miller NH, Kostuik JP, Sponseller PD. The etiology of adolescent idiopathic scoliosis. Am J Orthop. 2002;31:387–95.
2. Beals RK. Orthopedic aspects of the XO (Turner's) syndrome. Clin Orthop Relat Res. 1973;97:19–30.
3. Binder G, Rappold GA. SHOX deficiency disorders. GeneReviews. 2015. https://www.ncbi.nlm.nih.gov/books/NBK1215/.
4. Blaschke RJ, Rappold GA. SHOX: growth, Leri-Weill and Turner syndromes. Trends Endocrinol Metab. 2000;11(6):227–30.
5. Burwell RG. Aetiology of idiopathic scoliosis: current concepts. Pediatr Rehabil. 2003;6:137–70.
6. Child CJ, Kalifa G, Jones C, Ross JL, Rappold GA, Quigley CA, Zimmermann AG, Garding G, Cutler GB Jr, Blum WF. Radiological features in patients with short stature homeobox-containing (SHOX) gene deficiency and turner syndrome before and after 2 years of GH treatment. Horm Res Paediatr. 2015;84:14–25.
7. Clement-Jones M, et al. The short stature homeobox gene SHOX is involved in skeletal abnormalities in turner syndrome. Hum Mole Genet. 2000;9(5):695–702.
8. Davenport ML, Punyasavatsut N, Gunther D, Savendahl L, Stewart PW. Turner syndrome: a pattern of early growth failure. Acta Paediatr Suppl. 1999;433:118–21.
9. Day G, Szvetki A, Griffiths L, McPhee IB, Tuffley J, LaBrom R, Askin G, Woodland P, McClosky E, Torode I, Tomlinson F. SHOX gene is expressed in vertebral body growth plates in idiopathic and congenital scoliosis: implications for the etiology of scoliosis in turner syndrome. J Orthop Res. 2009;27:807–13.
10. Elder DA, Roper MG, Henderson RC, Davenport ML. Kyphosis in a turner syndrome population. Pediatrics. 2002;109(6):1–5.
11. Faienza MF, Ventura A, Colucci S, Cavallo L, Grano M, Brunetti G. Bone fragility in turner syndrome: mechanisms and prevention strategies. Front Endocrinol. 2016;7(34):1–8.
12. Formosa N, Buttigieg M, Torpiano J. Congenital brachymetatarsia and Turner syndrome. Arch Dis Child. 2016;101:332.
13. Gravholt CH, Lauridsen AL, Brixen K, Mosekilde L, Heickendorff L, Christiansen JS. Marked disproportionality in bone size and mineral, and distinct abnormalities in bone markers and calcitropic hormones in adult turner syndrome: a cross-sectional study. J Clin Endocrinol Metab. 2002;87(6):2798–808.
14. Gravholt CH, Juul S, Naeraa RW, Hansen J. Morbidity in turner syndrome. J Clin Epidemiol. 1998;51(2):147–58.
15. Harley BJ, Brown C, Cummings K, Carter PR, Ezaki M. Volar ligament release and distal radial dome osteotomy for the correction of Madelung deformity. J Hand Surg Am. 2006;31(9):1499–506.
16. Kim JY, Rosenfeld SR, Keyak JH. Increased prevalence of scoliosis in turner syndrome. J Pediatr Orthop. 2001;21:765–6.
17. Kosho T, Muroya K, Nagai T, Fujimoto M, Yokoya S, Sakamoto H, Hirano T, Terasaki H, Ohashi H, Nishimura G, Sato S, Matsuo N, Ogata T. Skeletal features and growth patterns in 14 patients with haploinsufficiency of SHOX: implications for the development of turner syndrome. J Clin Endocrinol Metab. 1999;84(12):4613–21.

18. Kosowicz J. Changes in the medial tibial condyle – a common finding in Turner's syndrome. Acta Endocrinol. 1959;31:321–3.
19. Kosowicz J. Skeletal changes in Turner's syndrome and their significance in differential diagnosis. Polish Med Hist Sci Bull. 1959;2:23–6.
20. Landin-Wilhelmsen K, Bryman I, Windh M, Wilhelmsen L. Osteoporosis and fractures in turner syndrome – importance of growth promoting and oestrogen therapy. Clin Endocrinol. 1999;51:497–502.
21. Morrissy RT, Weinstein SL. Lovell and Winter's pediatric orthopaedics. 6th ed: Lippincott, Williams and Wilkins: Philadelphia, PA; 2006. p. 1184–9. (The lower extremity: knock-knees and genu valgum).
22. Muller G, Gschwend N. Endocrine disorders and Scheuermann's disease. Arch Orthop Unfallchir. 1969;65:357–62.
23. Preger L, Steinbach HL, Moskowitz P, Scully AL, Goldberg MB. Roentgenographic abnormalities in phenotypic females with gonadal dysgenesis. AJR Am J Roentgenol. 1968;104:899–910.
24. Ranke MB, Saenger P. Turner's syndrome. Lancet. 2001;358:309–14.
25. Ricotti S, Petrucci L, Carenzio G, Klersy C, Calaterra V, Larizza D, Toffola FD. Prevalence and incidence of scoliosis in Turner syndrome: a study in 49 girls followed-up for 4 years. Eur J Phys Rehabil Med. 2011;47:447–53.
26. Roof AC, Jinguji TM, White KK. Musculoskeletal screening: developmental dysplasia of the hip. Pediatr Ann. 2013;42:229–35.
27. Ross J, Scott C, Marttila P, Kowal K, Nass A, Papenhausen P, Abboudi J, Osterman L, Kushner H, Carter P, Ezaki M, Elder F, Wei F, Chen H, Zinn A. Phenotypes associated with SHOX deficiency. J Clin Endocrinol Metab. 2001;86(12):5674–80.
28. Ross J, Kowal K, Quigley C, Blum W, Cutler G, Crowe B, Hovanes K, Elder F, Zinn A. The phenotype of short stature homeobox gene (SHOX) deficiency in childhood: contrasting children with Leri-Weill dyschondrosteosis and Turner syndrome. J Pediatr. 2005;147(4):499–507.
29. Saenger P, Albertsson Wikland K, Conway GS, et al. Recommendations for the diagnosis and management of Turner syndrome. J Clin Endocrinol Metab. 2001;86:3061–9.
30. Stevens PM, Klatt JB. Guided growth for pathological physes: radiographic improvement during realignment. J Pediatr Orthop. 2008;28:632–9.
31. Sybert VP, McCauley E. Turner's syndrome. N Engl J Med. 2004;351:1227–38.
32. Tauber M, Lounis N, Coulet J, Baunin C, Cahuzac JP, Rochiccioli P. Wrist anomalies in turner syndrome compared with Leri-Weill dyschondrosteosis: a new feature in Turner syndrome. Eur J Pediatr. 2004;163:475–81.
33. Vickers D, Nielsen G. Madelung deformity: surgical prophylaxis (physiolysis) during the late growth period by restriction of the dyschondrosteosis lesion. J Hand Surg Br. 1992;17(4):410–07.
34. Wang ED, Drummond DS, Dormans JP, Moshang T, Davidson RS, Gruccio D. Scoliosis in patients treated with growth hormone. J Pediatr Orthop. 1997;17:708–11.

Chapter 15
Oral Manifestations in Turner Syndrome

Carolina Di Blasi and Harlyn Susarla

Dental abnormalities described in Turner syndrome (TS) include (1) variations in eruption patterns; (2) changes in crown size such as small mesiodistal dimensions of teeth, small primary and permanent teeth, thinner enamel, and abnormal dentin; (3) variations in root morphology, including bifurcated roots of mandibular first and second premolars and reduced root length with an increased risk of root resorption and early tooth loss; (4) recessed and small mandible; (5) an abnormal palate; (6) malocclusion, particularly an anterior and posterior open bite; and (7) periodontal issues, for example, increased tooth mobility and periodontal pockets. Occasionally, these patients also report having a cleft lip and palate.

TS is a genetic disorder caused by numerical and/or structural aberrations of the X chromosome, with a prevalence of 1/2000 female live births. X-chromosome monosomy (45,X) is the most frequent karyotype. TS is an anomaly that dentists are likely to encounter; in fact, the dental and oral findings may give the first clue leading to the diagnosis at an early age.

Studies of chromosome aberrations have shown that both the X and the Y chromosomes promote dental growth; therefore, sex chromosomes contain genes involved in tooth development [1].

Patients with TS may present with different oral and craniofacial manifestations. The facial features of TS include a heart-shaped face, depressed corners of the mouth, prominent low-set ears, and multiple ocular findings including ptosis, cataracts, strabismus, epicanthus, color blindness, blue sclera, and corneal nebula.

Paradoxically, the prevalence of caries in this population is lower despite the findings of poorer oral hygiene when compared with controls [2].

The first extensive dental examination of Turner patients was performed by Filipsson et al. [3], who reported a tendency for the early eruption of teeth, which was later verified by other authors. In the study by Midtbo et al. [4], patients with

C. Di Blasi (✉) · H. Susarla
Seattle Childrens Hospital, University of Washington, Seattle, WA, USA
e-mail: Carolina.DiBlasi@seattlechildrens.org

© Springer Nature Switzerland AG 2020
P. Y. Fechner (ed.), *Turner Syndrome*,
https://doi.org/10.1007/978-3-030-34150-3_15

249

TS demonstrated delayed skeletal development, advanced dental development, and normal to moderately advanced dental eruption. However, tooth formation and eruption are essentially different processes, which are influenced differently by genetic, environmental, and hormonal factors. The relationship of various factors for skeletal, dental, and sexual maturity has been investigated in normal populations. Generally, there is a low correlation between dental maturity and skeletal/sexual maturity [5–8]. In contrast, the correlation between skeletal and sexual maturity is high [6–9]. This indicates that the variables of height, skeletal, and sexual maturity are regulated by the same factors, unlike dental development.

Delayed skeletal maturity is more pronounced in girls of older age groups, which is likely caused by hormonal factors. Dental development appears unrelated to other developmental systems. Dental development is subject to less variation when compared to chronologic age and appears to be controlled independently [6]. The correlation between dental and skeletal maturity has been shown to be lower in girls with TS than in normal karyotype girls. In fact, in girls with TS, the skeletal maturity was retarded, while the dental maturity was advanced and the teeth eruption was close to normal. In investigations by Midtbo et al., dental maturity was advanced by 1 year [4], which was in accordance with other authors. According to Ogiuchi et al. [10], this may be explained by the fact that shorter roots are found in those with TS. Because the roots are shorter in length, root formation is completed sooner in these patients, thus leading to advanced dental maturity.

Midtbo et al. observed several local eruption disturbances in the lateral segments of the maxilla. Dental maturity appears unaffected or even accelerated by the shortage of estrogen, which has the opposite effect on skeletal maturation. There is a significant disparity between delayed linear growth, an absent or delayed pubertal growth spurt, and delayed skeletal age, with the paradoxically advanced dental age.

Evaluation of these factors is crucial to formulate a dental treatment plan for females with TS as they often present with dental and skeletal malocclusions that should be treated according to skeletal age and maturity [11, 12]. Knowledge of the disparity between dental age versus skeletal age and pubertal development is crucial to formulate the correct dental treatment plan.

It has been found that TS patients have reduced tooth crown size and altered tooth morphology [2, 13, 14]. In fact, reduced crown height is the most predominant finding in TS. Since growth and its regulatory mechanism appear to be influenced by genes on the X chromosome, these genes also seem to influence tooth size. The mechanism whereby partial and total X monosomy results in abnormalities is still unknown. Tooth development involves many complex biological processes, which include epithelial-mesenchymal relationships, morphogenesis, fibrillogenesis and mineralization. The dental anomalies observed in TS indicate that several of those processes are influenced by the X-chromosome deficiency [15].

Patients with TS have a greater reduction of the mesiodistal crown dimension compared to the labiolingual dimension [3]. This difference may relate to the fact that the enamel thickness contributes more to the mesiodistal crown than to the labiolingual diameter [13]. Radiographic analysis of the thickness of dental hard tissues showed that the X chromosome mainly influences enamel deposition and has little or no effect on dentin growth [16]. The human enamel protein gene amelogenin is expressed from both the X and Y chromosomes; it is postulated that chromosomal aneuploidy can directly influence enamel formation and crown size.

There are multiple underlying causes of decreased tooth size in TS. The tooth size is dependent on the number of X chromosomes: the more X chromosomes present, the larger the tooth size, mainly due to an increase in enamel layer [15], while the dentin is affected only to a minor degree. X-chromosome mapping allows the location of the genes involved in the odontogenesis on the short arm, Xp22.3-p22.1. Amelogenin coding gene, AMELX, is the gene encoding an enamel organic matrix protein produced by the ameloblasts, which regulates the formation of crystallites during the secretory stage of enamel formation [17]. The majority of the genes on either the maternal or the paternal X chromosomes are silenced as a result of X-chromosome inactivation, but about 15% of the genes escape silencing and another 10% show a variable inactivation pattern [18]. Most of the escaping genes are located in the pseudoautosomal regions (PAR1 and PAR2) on the X chromosome, but there is also a lower proportion of genes that escape inactivation in the X-added region (XAR), where AMELX is located. It is therefore feasible that the enamel volume is reduced as the loss of one AMELX gene will reduce the amount of its gene product amelogenin [19]. In the study by Rizell et al., patients with TS with an isochromosome exhibited the smallest dental crown width, indicating some consideration to the number of intact X-chromosome p-arm on crown width.

Dental elements in patients with TS often cause defects in enamel: reduced crown size and enamel hypoplasia. This highlights the need for early preventive measures, such as fluoride exposure and use, proper oral hygiene practices, good systemic health with periodic checkups, and dietary recommendations, including reduced sugar consumption [20, 21].

Reduced root length of incisors, canines, and premolars was also found in patients with TS [15]. In the Turner patients, there was a high prevalence of supernumerary roots of mandibular molars. The tendency for increased root division in mandibular molars was associated with all karyotypes of the syndrome.

Growth of the dental arches may be influenced by the number of sex chromosomes [22, 23]. It is suggested that several TS features map to the short arm of the X chromosome [24]. Widths and lengths of the maxillary and mandibular alveolar arches in patients with TS were determined by Laine and Alvesalo. The mandibular arch was broader and shorter, whereas the maxillary alveolar arch was narrower but of normal length, reflecting the imbalanced facial growth in subjects with TS. The finding of decreased anteroposterior dimensions of the mandible in 45,X females seems to be uniform in different studies. As the narrow maxillary and broad mandibular alveolar arches found result in a bilateral posterior crossbite, the prevalence of bilateral posterior crossbites is high [25].

A high palatal arch is regarded as a significant clinical feature of TS. There are reports of lateral palatal ridges, which together with the narrower maxillary arch might give the palate vault a false appearance of being higher [26]. The position of the tongue is thought to be of importance for development of the lateral palatal ridges, which constitutes bulges of fibrous tissue appearing between the palatal midline and the alveolar processes. It has been suggested to use the denomination "narrow palatal vault" instead of using the term "high palatal vault" for the typical TS feature [27].

The craniofacial morphology of TS patients also shows some specific alterations. The cranial base is flattened, the jaws are more posteriorly positioned, and a retrognathic face type is common [28].

The shape of the craniofacial complex in children with TS was described by Rongen et al. [29]. The main abnormalities in the skull of patients with TS are located in the posterior cranial base and the mandible. The presence of cranial abnormalities in young children indicates that the origin of these abnormalities must occur very early in infancy or even prenatally. A cartilage growth disorder has been suggested. It is further suggested that the narrow retropharyngeal space found in patients with TS plays a role in the frequently occurring upper airway infections of these girls. During childhood, the depth of the retropharyngeal space increases gradually, while the incidence of infections decreases simultaneously. This finding was also supported by Dumancic et al. [30].

As growth hormone therapy is widely used in children with TS, its effects on craniofacial growth has been studied. It has been shown that growth hormone has an important role in growth of the craniofacial skeleton.

It is believed that the growth disorder in TS is not caused by growth hormone deficiency [31]. A previous study indicated that in TS both interstitial and appositional cartilage growth are affected, suggesting that the growth disorder is likely the result of chondrodysplasia and not growth hormone deficiency [29].

The dose of growth hormone use in TS is higher than the substitution doses. Furthermore, because patients with TS have disproportionate craniofacial morphology, growth hormone treatment might stimulate growth differently in the less versus more affected bone segments, resulting in an undesirable increase in the disproportions and risks for acromegalic effects in the craniofacial region, including enlargement of the chin and nose. In the study performed by Rongen-Westerlaken et al., patients with TS treated with growth hormone for 2 years demonstrated a significant increase (normalization) in the length of the ramus of the mandible. Growth hormone affects the condylar cartilage but not the cartilage of the spheno-occipital synchondrosis, which is responsible for growth of the cranial base. The following factors might contribute to these different responses: cells of the condylar cartilage are derived from non-cartilage precursors, whereas the cartilage cells of the spheno-occipital synchondrosis are derived from other cartilage cells by division. It has been reported that the mature condyle can be reactivated by hypersecretion of growth hormone. In the cited study, there were no indications during the 2 years of growth hormone intervention that the more affected structures, the mandible and the posterior cranial base, grew less than the remaining structures. On the contrary, the initially short ramus of the mandible normalized during treatment, and the mandible rotated forward toward normal position [32]. Juloski et al. concluded that long-term growth hormone therapy has a positive influence on craniofacial development in TS patients, with the greatest impact being on the posterior facial height and the mandibular ramus. However, although there are positive effects, growth hormone therapy does not regulate the craniofacial characteristics related to TS [33]. Although no signs of acromegalic growth were noted in previous studies, additional long-term studies are needed to confirm that long-term growth hormone does not result in relative mandibular overgrowth and a prognathic mandible [34].

Short stature in those with TS is the result of short lower limbs with a normal trunk length [35]. Reduced circulating nocturnal levels of growth hormone were initially thought to cause a delay and reduction of growth. However, the selective growth reduction of only certain body structures suggested that TS may involve a growth plate abnormality. Of all craniofacial structures, the posterior cranial base and mandible are primarily affected in TS, supporting a possible alteration in endochondral growth [32, 36], but the absolute cause of the abnormal growth and the morphologic characteristics of the craniofacial structures associated with TS are unclear. Growth hormone treatment has been shown to increase the annual growth rate of patients with TS and may also influence craniofacial growth. Because of the effects on growth, orthodontic treatment should be delayed until growth hormone treatment has been completed, growth has ceased, and the craniofacial relationship has stabilized. Dental morphology should be reviewed, as the variations from normal may require treatment modifications to achieve optimal results [12].

Orthodontic anomalies of patients with TS were reported at an increased frequency. Occlusion problems are common in this population. The most common anomaly is protrusion, crossbite, and open bite [2]. A dental/orthodontic evaluation is recommended at diagnosis if no previous care was established. The differences in crown and root morphology in these patients and their increased risk for root absorption increase the risk of tooth loss during orthodontic treatment.

Considerations during orthodontic treatment may include (1) antibiotic prophylaxis, if required for their cardiac defect; (2) modifications in occlusion due to anomalous dental morphology; (3) adjustments in timing of treatment due to differences in growth, as well as biologic and dental age; and (4) growth hormone therapy [12].

In summary, females with TS have a variety of dental problems. Dental abnormalities described include variation in eruption patterns, changes in crown and root morphology with an increased risk of tooth resorption and early tooth loss, a recessed and small mandible, an increased cranial base and abnormal palate, an anterior and lateral open bite, small primary and permanent teeth, thinner enamel and abnormal dentin, and occasionally cleft palate. The oral manifestations described can be used by dentists to ascertain undiagnosed TS.

Knowledge of the disparity between dental age versus skeletal age and pubertal development is crucial to formulate the correct dental treatment plan. The childhood growth period is longer for patients with TS, and the normal pubertal growth spurt is often absent. Distinctions among early dental eruption, dental age, chronological age, delayed skeletal age, and craniofacial growth rate must be made to correctly plan treatment for patients with TS.

Growth hormone has an important role in the growth of the craniofacial skeleton, although its positive effects do not overcome the craniofacial characteristics of

TS. Therefore, the importance of continual monitoring of craniofacial growth, especially in patients undergoing long-term growth hormone intervention, is warranted.

Multiple reports suggest that for patients with TS, greater emphasis should be placed on early diagnosis and treatment of dental problems.

A comprehensive assessment should involve a pediatrician or endocrinologist, a cardiologist, and, if indicated, a cleft palate team because of the risk of hypernasal speech and velopharyngeal insufficiency, as well as a pediatric dentist and prosthodontist for comprehensive dental care. It is recommended that dental/orthodontic evaluation is completed at diagnosis if not done previously. Future management should utilize the standard of dental/orthodontic care, individual clinical findings, and patient needs.

References

1. Alvesalo L, Osborne RH, Kari M. The 47,XYY male, Y chromosome, and tooth size. Am J Hum Genet. 1975;27(1):53–61.
2. Szilágyi A, Keszthelyi G, Nagy G, Madléna M. Oral manifestations of patients with Turner syndrome. Oral Surg Oral Med Oral Pathol Oral Radiol Endod. 2000;89(5):577–84.
3. Filipsson R, Lindsten J, Almqvist S. Time of eruption of the permanent teeth, cephalometric and tooth measurement and sulphation factor activity in 45 patients with Turner's syndrome with different types of X chromosome aberrations. Acta Endocrinol. 1965;48:91–113.
4. Midtbo M, Halse A. Skeletal maturity, dental maturity, and eruption in young patients with Turner syndrome. Acta Odontol Scand. 1992;50(5):303–12.
5. Filipsson R, Hall K. Correlation between dental maturity, height development and sexual maturation in normal girls. Ann Hum Biol. 1976;3(3):205–10.
6. Demirjian A, Buschang PH, Tanguay R, Patterson DK. Interrelationships among measures of somatic, skeletal, dental, and sexual maturity. Am J Orthod. 1985;88(5):433–8.
7. Hagg U, Taranger J. Dental emergence stages and the pubertal growth spurt. Acta Odontol Scand. 1981;39(5):295–306.
8. Hagg U, Taranger J. Maturation indicators and the pubertal growth spurt. Am J Orthod. 1982;82(4):299–309.
9. Hagg U, Taranger J. Skeletal stages of the hand and wrist as indicators of the pubertal growth spurt. Acta Odontol Scand. 1980;38(3):187–200.
10. Ogiuchi H, Takano K, Tanaka M, Hizuka N, Takagi S, Sangu Y, et al. Oro-maxillofacial development in patients with Turner's syndrome. Endocrinol Jpn. 1985;32(6):881–90.
11. Gravholt CH, Andersen NH, Conway GS, Dekkers OM, Geffner ME, Klein KO, et al. Clinical practice guidelines for the care of girls and women with Turner syndrome: proceedings from the 2016 Cincinnati International Turner Syndrome Meeting. Eur J Endocrinol. 2017;177(3):G1–G70.
12. Russell KA. Orthodontic treatment for patients with Turner syndrome. Am J Orthod Dentofac Orthop. 2001;120(3):314–22.
13. Townsend G, Jensen BL, Alvesalo L. Reduced tooth size in 45,X (Turner syndrome) females. Am J Phys Anthropol. 1984;65(4):367–71.
14. Varrela J, Townsend G, Alvesalo L. Tooth crown size in human females with 45,X/46,XX chromosomes. Arch Oral Biol. 1988;33(5):291–4.
15. Midtbo M, Halse A. Root length, crown height, and root morphology in Turner syndrome. Acta Odontol Scand. 1994;52(5):303–14.

16. Alvesalo L, Tammisalo E. Enamel thickness of 45,X females' permanent teeth. Am J Hum Genet. 1981;33(3):464–9.
17. Salido EC, Yen PH, Koprivnikar K, Yu LC, Shapiro LJ. The human enamel protein gene amelogenin is expressed from both the X and the Y chromosomes. Am J Hum Genet. 1992;50(2):303–16.
18. Carrel L, Willard HF. X-inactivation profile reveals extensive variability in X-linked gene expression in females. Nature. 2005;434(7031):400–4.
19. Rizell S, Barrenas ML, Andlin-Sobocki A, Stecksen-Blicks C, Kjellberg H. Turner syndrome isochromosome karyotype correlates with decreased dental crown width. Eur J Orthod. 2012;34(2):213–8.
20. American Academy on Pediatric Dentistry. Policy on dietary recommendations for infants, children, and adolescents. Pediatr Dent. 2012;37(6):56–8.
21. Faggella A, Guadagni MG, Cocchi S, Tagariello T, Piana G. Dental features in patients with Turner syndrome. Eur J Paediatr Dent. 2006;7(4):165–8.
22. Laine T, Alvesalo L. Palatal and alveolar arch dimensions in 47,XXY (Klinefelter syndrome) men. Hum Biol. 1993;65(1):131–8.
23. Laine T, Alvesalo L. Palatal and mandibular arch morphology in 47,XYY men and in other sex-chromosome anomalies. Arch Oral Biol. 1993;38(2):101–5.
24. Ogata T, Matsuo N. Turner syndrome and female sex chromosome aberrations: deduction of the principal factors involved in the development of clinical features. Hum Genet. 1995;95(6):607–29.
25. Laine T, Alvesalo L, Savolainen A, Lammi S. Occlusal morphology in 45,X females. J Craniofac Genet Dev Biol. 1986;6(4):351–5.
26. Perkiomaki MR, Alvesalo L. Palatine ridges and tongue position in Turner syndrome subjects. Eur J Orthod. 2008;30(2):163–8.
27. Rizell S, Barrenas ML, Andlin-Sobocki A, Stecksen-Blicks C, Kjellberg H. Palatal height and dental arch dimensions in Turner syndrome karyotypes. Eur J Orthod. 2013;35(6):841–7.
28. Laine T, Alvesalo L. Size of the alveolar arch of the mandible in relation to that of the maxilla in 45,X females. J Dent Res. 1986;65(12):1432–4.
29. Rongen-Westerlaken C, vd Born E, Prahl-Andersen B, Rikken B, Teunenbroek V, Kamminga N, et al. Shape of the craniofacial complex in children with Turner syndrome. J Biol Buccale. 1992;20(4):185–90.
30. Dumancic J, Kaic Z, Varga ML, Lauc T, Dumic M, Milosevic SA, et al. Characteristics of the craniofacial complex in Turner syndrome. Arch Oral Biol. 2010;55(1):81–8.
31. Wit JM, Massarano AA, Kamp GA, Hindmarsh PC, van Es A, Brook CG, et al. Growth hormone secretion in patients with Turner's syndrome as determined by time series analysis. Acta Endocrinol. 1992;127(1):7–12.
32. Rongen-Westerlaken C, vd Born E, Prahl-Andersen B, von Teunenbroek A, Manesse P, Otten BJ, et al. Effect of growth hormone treatment on craniofacial growth in Turner's syndrome. Acta Paediatr. 1993;82(4):364–8.
33. Juloski J, Dumancic J, Scepan I, Lauc T, Milasin J, Kaic Z, et al. Growth hormone positive effects on craniofacial complex in Turner syndrome. Arch Oral Biol. 2016;71:10–5.
34. Simmons KE. Growth hormone and craniofacial changes: preliminary data from studies in Turner's syndrome. Pediatrics. 1999;104(4 Pt 2):1021–4.
35. Rongen-Westerlaken C, Rikken B, Vastrick P, Jeuken AH, de Lange MY, Wit JM, et al. Body proportions in individuals with Turner syndrome. The Dutch Growth Hormone Working Group. Eur J Pediatr. 1993;152(10):813–7.
36. Babic M, Scepan I, Micic M. Comparative cephalometric analysis in patients with X-chromosome aneuploidy. Arch Oral Biol. 1993;38(2):179–83.

Chapter 16
The Turner Syndrome Resource Center: An Interdisciplinary Approach to the Care of Girls and Women with Turner Syndrome

Philippe Backeljauw and Sarah Corathers

Introduction

Turner syndrome (TS) affects approximately 1 in 2000 live-born phenotypic females [1, 2]. This makes TS one of the most common chromosomal abnormalities. There are at least an estimated 75,000 girls and women living in the United States with TS. As the previous chapters in this book have illustrated, an individual with TS may have to deal with a wide variety of comorbidities throughout life. In many instances, living with TS may have a profound effect on the quality of life. Because of the rather complex nature of this syndrome, the increased frequency of prenatal detection of TS, and the development of sophisticated diagnostic tools and therapeutic interventions to address the TS health issues, there is an ever-increasing need for an integrated approach to the management of TS individuals' healthcare across the life span. Primary care providers (pediatricians, family practitioners, internists) remain an essential part of the healthcare team for TS individuals (provision of standard health maintenance, childhood immunizations, etc.), and most primary care physicians will be somewhat familiar with the typical clinical features characteristic of TS, so that they can have an important impact on the long-term care of TS patients. Nevertheless, it becomes quickly evident that the primary care physician will need to collaborate with a team of other healthcare providers to address the multifaceted and time-intensive care issues specific to TS individuals. There are several reasons why the care of girls and women with TS should be coordinated through a team of specialists, under the supervision of a central coordinator, which is in most cases a pediatric endocrinologist. Table 16.1 lists the reasons for such inter- or multidisciplinary approach to the healthcare management of TS individuals.

P. Backeljauw (✉) · S. Corathers
The Cincinnati Center for Pediatric and Adult Turner Syndrome Care, Cincinnati Children's Hospital Medical Center, University of Cincinnati College of Medicine, Cincinnati, OH, USA
e-mail: philippe.backeljauw@cchmc.org; sarah.corathers@cchmc.org

© Springer Nature Switzerland AG 2020
P. Y. Fechner (ed.), *Turner Syndrome*,
https://doi.org/10.1007/978-3-030-34150-3_16

Table 16.1 Reasons why chronic healthcare management for TS individuals should be done by a team of specialists under supervision from a care coordinator

(a) Primary care providers may have limited exposure to TS patients and therefore are less familiar with the many comorbidities of TS
(b) Coordinating the clinical care of TS patients is time-intensive
(c) Centralization of testing and specialty consults reduces burden and promotes completion of indicated services
(d) Ability to centralize TS care promotes the development of expertise
(e) Support systems are more likely to be available in a larger center than in private practice
(f) Availability of research resources/support
(g) Navigating fragmented systems of care is difficult for many families

This chapter provides an overview of the different care models available to provide inter- or multidisciplinary care to girls and women with TS. Part of this chapter further discusses the development of a TS resource center, a unit to provide different areas of specialty care for TS patients. In addition to the delineation of the different roles that care providers have within a TS resource center, the value of peer support systems, advocacy groups, and social networking is also addressed. In another part of this chapter, the issues related to transition from pediatric to adult TS care will also be discussed.

Models Providing Interdisciplinary Clinical Care to Girls and Women with Turner Syndrome

Girls and women with TS currently face a number of major health and well-being issues [3]. These include, but are not limited to, a lack of knowledge about TS comorbidities (especially in the adult TS population), suboptimal access to appropriate developmental evaluation, and inadequate insurance coverage for their medical care, diagnostic test, and recommended treatments. In addition to these major health issues, several barriers to better healthcare provision are often encountered: identification of knowledgeable providers, lack of collaboration between specialists who evaluate TS patients, lack of care coordination, and lack of uniformly described criteria for care. Considering all these major issues facing patients with TS, several clinical care models have been proposed to improve medical care for these patients, with several of them involving an interdisciplinary (or multidisciplinary) approach. These teams can provide more knowledge and experience than each of the different medical disciplines operating in isolation.

Providing healthcare through an interdisciplinary team approach implies that the team also will have to deal with the complexities of the clinical setting's internal and external environments. Any type of team approach will need to address the practical needs and demands of the organization which houses the team and any team needs to be able to adapt quickly to the rapidly changing organizational environment – if unable to do so, the team will be unable to function or survive long term. Any successful interdisciplinary team also should carefully embrace all the internal relationships and external factors that can affect the team dynamics. A well-organized TS care team will allow for the effects of any environmental influence, experienced either as positive or negative stress, without jeopardizing its functionality.

There are several approaches to arrive at having a well-functioning TS care team; two are worth discussing here. One approach may be called the "one-stop approach." In such a model, the interdisciplinary care team is providing healthcare services in one physical location with all subspecialty consultations occurring as part of a single appointment on a single day [4]. The different TS providers and specialists will come together either in one clinic setting or in clinic settings close to one another. The approach could be focused or generalized. In the focused approach model, a patient will have one set of issues addressed in greater detail during one clinic visit (e.g., problems related to the cardiovascular system) and another set of health issues addressed on the next visit (e.g., developmental or behavioral problems). The other comorbidities do not get neglected but may only be addressed superficially until the next clinic visit. Because of this, the patient may not always see all specialists within the team at each encounter. In the generalized approach, all systems are given similar attention, and all providers will see the patients. The duration of these clinics can be quite long; some run almost an entire day. The different subspecialties that are available usually include pediatric endocrinology, cardiology, audiology, otolaryngology, developmental pediatrics, and genetics. Visits with these providers, which may be considered as first-tier specialists within the TS care team, are preplanned by a TS center coordinator. In the focused approach, the specialists could be alternating quarterly with second- and third-tier specialists, which include, respectively, nutrition, psychology, gynecology, and reproductive endocrinology and (third-tier) dentistry, orthodontics, ophthalmology, dermatology, and gastroenterology.

The second model could be called the "interfacing approach." For this type of interdisciplinary approach, the main TS provider and the TS coordinator will network with a number of previously identified subspecialty consultants. The key aspect of this model is excellent communication through the presence of the TS care coordinator. The main medical provider is usually a pediatric endocrinologist (pediatric endocrinologists have traditionally coordinated the clinical care for TS patients during the last three to four decades). This interdisciplinary approach works best in a large medical center or university healthcare system. The key specialty services available for interaction include cardiology, audiology, developmental pediatrics, psychology, gynecology, and nutrition. Specific medical providers in the second- and third-tier specialties are also identified, to whom the TS patients can then be referred on an as-needed basis. This also requires that the main physician has developed a significant knowledge base regarding TS diagnosis and treatment. The fact that pediatric endocrinologists have assumed the role of TS care coordinator from a medical perspective is a consequence of the many developments in hormonal therapy, which have greatly improved the potential for growth, development of secondary sexual characteristics, and general well-being in girls and women with TS.

Both interdisciplinary team approaches described have clear advantages over the fragmented care that has been provided in so many settings where the coordination of care was lacking, and individual providers were unable to link with one another to optimize patient management. For example, these models allow very nicely for patient involvement and a patient-centered care approach. It is easier for the team members to meet, instead of having to arrange for case conferences to discuss the patient's complex care. In addition, the described setup allows for a stimulating work environment where some of the assessments and interventions can be applied in a shared fashion (e.g., a social worker can assist in screening for behavioral or neurocognitive problems). With a well-run team, the efficiency of providing care can be facilitated, with both time and cost savings as a result.

Transition to Adult Care

By design and practicality, pediatric care models engage both child and family, whereas adult care models are more often oriented toward patients as individuals. Pediatric care tends to be centralized around a medical home or academic health center, whereas adult care may be more dispersed across providers and institutions. The process of transition between child- and adult-oriented health systems therefore requires purposeful planning to be successful and may vary in length based on complexity of medical needs, personal characteristics, preferences, and local community resources [5, 6]. Transition between health systems usually transpires concurrent with the broader developmental context of moving from adolescence to adulthood, which can include exploration of education, social and professional opportunities, living outside of the family home for the first time, and potentially financial autonomy [7]. General models and tools for transition readiness provide a useful initial framework for navigation between pediatric and adult health systems. Valuable resources include the Got Transition website (www.gottransition.org) and the Transition Readiness Assessment Questionnaire, TRAQ [8].

Among girls and women with TS, the developmental transition to greater independence includes increasing responsibility for chronic medical and mental health needs. Skill development, essential for successful medical transition, includes "cognitive and social skills to communicate and articulate health needs and preferences" [9]. As communication skills and general health literacy among TS girls and women is relatively high, nonverbal learning challenges or other gaps in health knowledge or transition readiness skills may be missed by general assessments. Therefore, there is increasing consensus that condition-specific transition readiness assessments that address the medical, psychological, and cognitive needs of a unique population, such as TS, are indicated [10]. Resources for TS-specific transition readiness including a TS passport [11] and the TS Pediatric to Adult Care Transition Toolkit (http://www.endocrinetransitions.org/turner-syndrome/) are available. Individualized assessment of TS-specific content of personal health history and ongoing adult health recommendations is recommended as part of transition planning.

During adolescence, the frequency of medical visits for girls with TS often decreases as the need for intensive interventions with growth hormone and puberty induction is completed. However, women with TS will have lifelong medical needs. It is well documented that many young adult women with TS are too often lost to follow-up in the transition between pediatric and adult care, which can result in under-recognition and treatment of common comorbidities with suboptimal outcomes [12–14]. Knowledge of personal medical history, understanding of future health risks and impact of self-care behaviors, health navigation, and health literacy skills are all important aspects of transition readiness to assure TS adolescents and young adults are equipped to advocate if necessary and maintain ongoing engagement with appropriate healthcare services.

The Turner Syndrome Resource Center

In the ideal TS resource center, the patient or family is at the center of the care model. Medical care is coordinated by a designated TS care coordinator (often a nurse). The role of the TS care coordinator is to help the TS individual navigate the complexities of the healthcare system, improve the interactions with the TS team, engage with community resources, and facilitate a patient-centered approach. The care coordinator works closely together with the director of the TS clinic, which could be a pediatric endocrinologist or geneticist – both specialists that should have been adequately trained in care provision of TS individuals. Depending on local resources, the TS resource center may continue to provide care across the life span with adult providers. At all ages, partnership with primary care providers is essential. For additional specialty consultation, the different subspecialists required have greater or lesser importance based on the prevalence of the comorbidities encountered in the TS population. The way subspecialists are needed in the TS resource center may vary based on the patient's age. For example, a cardiologist and a pediatric endocrinologist are often more involved with younger patients, but in young adulthood, a psychiatrist or reproductive endocrinologist may become more important to the patient. The TS resource centers will vary in size. For some institutions, smaller clinics following an interfacing approach may be feasible and more realistic than trying to get the different subspecialists come together in a one-stop approach clinic (see above). Larger TS resource centers may be able to follow TS individuals according to either model previously described. The author's preference goes to the interfacing approach rather than the one-stop approach, provided that specific subspecialists can be identified and collaborated with to facilitate consultation for the respective specialties. For example, if a same audiologist always gets the TS patients referred to, that person will be more aware of the specific audiological healthcare needs, compared to referring a patient to one of a set of audiologists available in that

Table 16.2 Important elements of a TS resource center	(a) Comprehensive (regional) centers versus smaller peripheral clinics
	(b) Integrated clinical care (interfacing interdisciplinary versus multidisciplinary)
	(c) Multiple standard-size clinics versus larger one-day clinics operating less frequently
	(d) Educational component
	(e) Group meetings with advocacy representation
	(f) Easier access to behavioral health assessment/screening

department. Larger clinics may have additional resources such as a designated nutritionist or social worker to help screen patients for nutritional issues or psycho-emotional needs. In an interdisciplinary interfacing clinic model, patients can be seen either through smaller clinics offered multiple times per month or through larger clinics that operate less frequently but with more patients coming in for the day. Such larger clinics can then also offer educational and collaborative efforts through an available TS support group. Table 16.2 summarizes the important elements of a TS resource center.

Role of the Turner Syndrome Clinic Coordinator

The TS clinic coordinator or TS health navigator is an individual, usually a nurse, with understanding of the medical and psychosocial needs of TS patients and families. A primary responsibility of the coordinator in the TS resource center is pre-visit planning. For newly diagnosed families, a phone call in advance of the initial clinic visit provides an opportunity to inform families of the purpose of the clinic and review expectations. Families are encouraged to share the story of how their daughter was diagnosed with TS, and an educational packet of materials can be mailed to families in advance that includes a guide for families and clinic and local support group information. For established patients, the coordinator may review the schedule several weeks in advance to determine if labs or other tests are indicated and to identify needs to meet with the dietician or social worker at the upcoming visit. Completion of test prior to the visit allows for face-to-face discussion of results and any indicated intervention at the time of the encounter. Coordination in advance of the visit eliminates the need for follow-up calls from the provider of nurse after the appointment to discuss results and can improve the efficiency of the TS resource center (Table 16.3).

During the clinic visit, the TS coordinator can provide educational materials ranging from TS diagnosis to nonverbal learning disabilities. A nurse coordinator is able to educate families about proper administration of medications such as growth hormone, estrogen, and thyroid hormone. The coordinator may be responsible for pursuing required prior authorization for growth hormone and guiding families

Table 16.3 Roles of Turner syndrome clinic coordinator

(a) Pre-visit planning
(b) Education on administration of medications such as growth hormone and estrogen
(c) Provide resources for educational materials about TS diagnosis, common comorbidities, and treatment options
(d) Coordination of referral services
(e) Integration of clinical team with local support groups
(f) Research recruitment

through this process. The nurse coordinator is an important contact to provide instructions and help address questions that arise in between visits.

Involvement in support group activities outside the clinic setting complements the coordinator's ability to effectively serve the TS population. Annual parent and patient education and social events provide an opportunity to interact with girls and women affected by TS in a nonclinical setting. The TS coordinator may also be a resource for connecting local families to national support programs (e.g., www.turnersyndrome.org and www.turnersyndromefoundation.org).

Adult Care in a Turner Syndrome Resource Center

Adult care in a TS resource center may follow a more consultative model, usually by an adult endocrinologist or internist with experience in TS. Adult women with TS can be evaluated annually to maintain a comprehensive approach to screening and prevention services for common comorbidities. The goal of the annual assessment is to monitor blood pressure; to oversee ordering and interpretation of appropriate labs, tests (e.g., electrocardiography, bone densitometry, etc., as indicated), and referral services; and also to provide select treatment interventions. Adult endocrinologists in a TS resource center can help identify adult specialists with expertise in TS care. The adult endocrinologist may prescribe estrogen replacement and manage hypertension and hyperlipidemia or may coordinate this care with primary care, gynecology, or cardiology, respectively. Frequency of visits for adult endocrinology care will depend on required interventions but is recommended at least annually to avoid loss to follow-up.

The resources that will be required to efficiently run a TS clinic or center are significant. To circumnavigate some of the barriers to quality TS care previously mentioned, administrative support will be crucial. Each center will need support from their institution to enforce clinical activities dedicated to TS patient care. Therefore, the providers attending to these clinics will need divisional support. These medical providers will need to be protected from being overwhelmed by other clinical duties during these clinics so that they can spend the time needed to provide comprehensive TS care. The presence of a TS coordinator is essential, as will be interaction with local advocacy groups. Extramural funding for the long-term survival of these clinics and for educational efforts will be a necessity.

Peer Support, Advocacy Groups, and Social Networking

The value of peer support for children and adolescents, or for adults, with chronic conditions is well established. There are many studies that have demonstrated the effectiveness of peer support [15]. For example, peer support interventions in individuals with chronic illness lead to improvement in behavioral and emotional well-being. Therefore, also for TS individuals, peer support can be valuable adjunct to the medical care they already receive. For example, for adults with TS, such peer support may lead to better outcomes with respect to education or employment, quality of life, and self-esteem. Peer support may further help to foster medication adherence. Peer support may come from interactions in the TS clinic setting itself but may also come through social networking platforms. These provide opportunities for virtual conversations and sharing of experiences, as well as exchange of information regarding available medical care providers. Because of this, it is important to link patients and families with one another.

Another important contributor to the success of a TS resource center is through its interaction with local advocacy groups. TS advocacy groups by history have taken the lead in providing educational and networking forums for patients, families, children, adolescents, and young adults with TS. These advocacy efforts continue to lead important advances in research and improve the care for girls and women with TS. Encouraging TS resource centers to be involved with TS advocacy groups will contribute toward self-empowerment of the TS individuals and their families. TS resource centers should interact closely with patient/advocacy TS groups that offer activities, both locally and regionally, geared toward children, adolescents, and adults to improve their developmental and individual autonomy.

The authors would like to acknowledge the valuable contribution from Lori Casnellie, RN, who is the TS clinic coordinator at the Cincinnati Center for Pediatric and Adult Turner Syndrome Care.

References

1. Gravholt CH, Andersen NH, Conway GS, et al. Clinical practice guidelines for the care of girls and women with Turner syndrome: proceedings from the 2016 Cincinnati International Turner Syndrome Meeting. Eur J Endocrinol. 2017;177(3):G1–G70.
2. Sybert VP, McCauley E. Turner's syndrome. N Engl J Med. 2004;351(12):1227–38.
3. Backeljauw PF, et al. Proceedings from the Turner Resource Network symposium: the crossroads of health care research and health care delivery. Am J Med Genet A. 2015;167A(9):1962–71.
4. Jessup RL. Interdisciplinary versus multidisciplinary care teams: do we understand the difference? Aust Health Rev. 2007;31(3):330–1.
5. Blum RW, et al. Transition from child-centered to adult health-care systems for adolescents with chronic conditions. A position paper of the Society for Adolescent Medicine. J Adolesc Health. 1993;14(7):570–6.
6. American Academy of Pediatrics, et al. Supporting the health care transition from adolescence to adulthood in the medical home. Pediatrics. 2011;128(1):182–200.

7. Arnett JJ. Emerging adulthood. A theory of development from the late teens through the twenties. Am Psychol. 2000;55(5):469–80.
8. Wood DL, et al. The Transition Readiness Assessment Questionnaire (TRAQ): its factor structure, reliability, and validity. Acad Pediatr. 2014;14(4):415–22.
9. Massey PM, et al. Contextualizing an expanded definition of health literacy among adolescents in the health care setting. Health Educ Res. 2012;27(6):961–74.
10. Beal SJ, et al. The associations of chronic condition type and individual characteristics with transition readiness. Acad Pediatr. 2016;16(7):660–7.
11. Rubin K. Transitioning the patient with Turner's syndrome from pediatric to adult care. J Pediatr Endocrinol Metab. 2003;16(Suppl 3):651–9.
12. Devernay M, et al. Determinants of medical care for young women with Turner syndrome. J Clin Endocrinol Metab. 2009;94(9):3408–13.
13. Freriks K, et al. Standardized multidisciplinary evaluation yields significant previously undiagnosed morbidity in adult women with Turner syndrome. J Clin Endocrinol Metab. 2011;96(9):E1517–26.
14. Gawlik A, Malecka-Tendera E. Transitions in endocrinology: treatment of Turner's syndrome during transition. Eur J Endocrinol. 2014;170(2):R57–74.
15. Kohut S, Stinson J, van Wyk M, Giosa L, Luca S. Systematic review of peer support interventions for adolescents with chronic illness. Int J Child Adolesc Health. 2014;7:183–97.

Chapter 17
Future Directions

Patricia Y. Fechner

One of the primary challenges in the care of girls with Turner syndrome (TS) is late diagnosis. A study in Denmark showed that only 50% of individuals with TS are identified as having TS and the average age of diagnosis was 15 years [1]. Thus, 50% of females with TS are not receiving the medical care that they need, and many of those diagnosed are diagnosed late. Another study found that girls are on average 7.7 years when the diagnosis of TS is made [2]. Therefore, a goal in the care of girls with TS is to make the diagnosis in more girls and at an earlier age. Primary care providers need to consider the diagnosis of TS not just in girls who have the classic TS phenotype but also in girls who are short or who have two or more subtle features of TS. The recent availability of guidelines for the care of girls and women with TS provides the opportunity to meet the needs of those diagnosed with TS [3]. As non-invasive prenatal testing (NIPT) becomes more prevalent, more girls with TS will be identified in utero. NIPT though also brings about false positives in the diagnosis of monosomy X as it is a screening tool looking at placental DNA and not fetal DNA. In utero diagnosis of true cases of TS will broaden the phenotypic spectrum of TS since currently 50% of women with TS are undiagnosed and will likely shift the TS phenotype spectrum to a milder phenotype than what is traditionally thought of as TS. Studies of girls identified solely by NIPT will need to be performed in order to provide better prenatal counseling.

Growth hormone is efficacious in increasing adult height in girls with TS, but it needs to be administered while girls still have the potential to grow. An earlier diagnosis of TS allows for earlier initiation of growth hormone therapy if indicated. This will result in improved height during childhood as well as adulthood because there are more years for catch-up growth. This will also allow for a more physiologic onset of puberty if initiation with exogenous estrogen is required. Trials of

P. Y. Fechner (✉)

Division of Endocrinology, Seattle Children's Hospital, University of Washington, Seattle, WA, USA

e-mail: Patricia.Fechner@seattlechildrens.org

© Springer Nature Switzerland AG 2020

P. Y. Fechner (ed.), *Turner Syndrome*,

https://doi.org/10.1007/978-3-030-34150-3_17

long-acting growth hormone, given only once a week or every 2 weeks, are in progress for children with growth hormone deficiency. If these new formulations of growth hormone are FDA approved for children with growth hormone deficiency, then studies in girls with TS will be necessary to see if they too can have improved growth with less frequent injections and perhaps better adherence.

Most girls with TS require exogenous estrogen therapy to induce puberty. Protocols have been developed to adapt the higher dose transdermal estrogen patches to the low doses of estradiol needed to induce and advance puberty in a physiologic manner. Unfortunately, many insurance policies fail to cover transdermal patches for girls with TS. Hopefully with the recent TS guidelines [3] which endorse the use of transdermal estrogen over oral estrogen for induction of puberty, insurance companies will provide better coverage of the transdermal patch which is more physiologic than oral estrogen therapy and can be given in lower doses. Studies are required to determine the optimal duration of increasing estradiol levels for linear growth as many girls are not having a pubertal growth spurt and for optimal uterine growth. Another question is: How is the shape of the breast affected by estradiol and progesterone dosing protocols? Long-term studies looking at bone health outcomes are also important given the increased risk of osteoporosis seen in women with TS.

There needs to be better discussion of options for motherhood whether it be adoption (domestic or international) or pregnancy (spontaneous, oocyte donation, or gestational surrogacy with oocyte donation). A recent study reported that only 67% of families received fertility counseling [4]. Assisted reproductive technology continues to advance, and with these advances women with TS can benefit. However, women with TS have significantly higher mortality associated with pregnancy which needs to be known to the woman with TS as well as to her physician. Prior to becoming pregnant, women with TS need to have a complete multidisciplinary evaluation to determine increased risk. They also require close monitoring due to the higher cardiovascular disease and risk for obstetrical complications while pregnant. Girls with TS experience premature loss of oocytes with only 2–7% having spontaneous pregnancy. Oocyte preservation after ovarian stimulation is no longer considered experimental and does not require a partner as embryo preservation does. However, girls need to be post-menarchal in order to have mature oocytes for preservation, and many have already lost fertility potential due to premature loss of oocytes. Anti-Müllerian hormone may be useful in determining ovarian reserve. Ovarian tissue cryopreservation is an option for prepubertal girls, but it is experimental and requires a research protocol and consent. Ovarian tissue cryopreservation in the future may be a possibility for the girl with 45,X/46,XY karyotype who has a gonadectomy due to high risk of gonadoblastoma. Any fertility preservation in a girl less than 18 years requires ethical consideration as it is the parents who are providing consent and the girl assent. As more options for fertility become available, the question of how to make pregnancy safer for the woman with TS remains an important area of study.

Preventive cardiovascular care has improved for girls and women with TS. At least one cardiac magnetic resonance imaging study is now standard of care which allows for added information on anatomy. The MRI is usually obtained after the girl no longer requires sedation for the study. As blood pressure monitoring for the general population has become more prevalent, so has 24-h ambulatory BP monitoring in TS. Subtle difference in blood pressure levels may allow for earlier intervention. Cardiovascular morbidity and mortality are high in TS, and outcome research needs to be done to show the effectiveness in increased cardiac MR and 24-h ambulatory BP monitoring. Women with TS who have aortopathies are helping scientists understand better the role of aortopathy in cardiac disease. An exciting discovery is that hemizygousity for TIMP1 (tissue inhibitor of matrix metalloproteinase 1) located on Xp11.3 and a variant in TIMP3, found on chromosome 22, increase the risk of bicuspid aortic valve and aortic aneurysm by 16-fold in women with TS [5]. Will this variant in TIMP3 be useful in identifying which women with TS and bicuspid aortic valve have the highest risk for aortic aneurysm? What about a role in men who all are hemizygous for TIMP1? Are therapies used in the treatment for Marfan aortopathy relevant for women with TS aortopathy?

Girls and women with TS may have increased social and behavioral concerns. The neurocognitive and psychosocial issues can decrease self-esteem and quality of life. Making an earlier diagnosis of TS will allow earlier educational, cognitive-behavioral, and pharmacologic interventions to improve social and behavioral outcomes in the long term. Girls with TS should have routine neuropsychological assessments during childhood and adolescence to identify problems and allow for additional services to support them. Primary care providers should perform annual developmental and behavioral screening so that referrals can be made early. Knowledge gained from the care of children with other conditions such as ADHD (attention deficit hyperactivity disorder) and autism may benefit girls and women with TS. Future research in social issues is a primary concern for those with TS.

Females with TS are well cared for by pediatric subspecialists with the pediatric endocrinologist often taking the lead, and the girls have their parents to provide support and advocacy. However, when they age out of pediatrics and transition, there is no specific provider who can ensure that they are getting the multispecialty care that they require. Young women are now on their own to navigate the health-care system, and some may have decreased executive function which can make it even more difficult for them to coordinate the complexities of multispecialty care. The issues that women with TS face are the same issues that many other women face; unfortunately, they face them at a younger age-premature ovarian failure, metabolic syndrome, early sensorineural hearing loss, risk of osteoporosis, and autoimmune disease, to name a few. Cardiologists who care for adults may not be as familiar with congenital heart disease. But they do have experience with hypertension and aortic dissection. Gynecologists care for women with premature ovarian failure and have experience in hormone replacement therapy. Reproductive endocrinologists deal with infertility, but they need to know the increased risk of pregnancy in a woman with TS. Endocrinologists are familiar with metabolic syndrome, autoimmune disease, and osteoporosis, but they need to know when and how often to screen women with TS. This is where the TS guidelines [3] will play an important role. They give the medical care provider the tools to know how often to screen for the illnesses that women with TS are at increased risk.

An online TS research registry was developed through the TS Society of the United States using "Platform for Engaging Everyone Responsibly" or PEER. This is a registry used by other patient advocacy organizations with the goal of collecting health information from girls and women with TS and then sharing the information with researchers studying TS. It is hoped that by having a critical mass of individuals with TS, new studies can be done and that younger investigators will choose to study women with TS because there is a study population available to them. Research is key to improving the long-term outcomes in women with TS, and it is important to take into account what areas of research are important to women with TS.

References

1. Stochholm K, Juul S, Juel K, Naeraa RW, Gravholt CH. Prevalence, incidence, diagnostic delay, and mortality in Turner syndrome. J Clin Endocrinol Metab. 2006;91:3897–902.
2. Savendahl L, Davenport ML. Delayed diagnoses of Turner's syndrome: proposed guidelines for change. J Pediatr. 2000;137:455–9.
3. Gravholt CH, Andersen NH, Conway GS, et al. Clinical practice guidelines for the care of girls and women with Turner syndrome: proceedings from the 2016 Cincinnati International Turner Syndrome Meeting. Eur J Endocrinol. 2017;177(3):G1–G70.
4. Morgan TL, Kapa HM, Creand CE, Kremen J, Tishelman A, Davis S, Nahata L. Fertility counseling and preservation discussions for females with Turner syndrome in pediatric centers: practice patterns and predictors. Fertil Steril. 2019;112(4):740–8.
5. Corbitt H, Morris SA, Gravholt CH, Mortensen KH, Tippner-Hedges R, Silberbach M, Maslen CL, GenTAC Registry Investigators. TIMP3 and TIMP1 are risk genes for bicuspid aortic valve and aortopathy in Turner syndrome. PLoS Genet. 2018;14:e1007692.

Index

A

Acne, 230, 231
Acromegalic effects, 252
Alopecia areata, 229
Amblyopia, 200, 201
Ambulatory blood pressure monitoring
 (ABPM), 148
American College of Medical Genetics and
 Genomics (ACMG), 24
Analysis of covariance (ANCOVA), 49–51
Anatomic renal anomalies, 140
Anti-Müllerian hormone (AMH), 79, 80
Aortic dissection, 128
 dilation, 128
 dimensions assessment, 128, 129
 medical/operative management, 129, 130
 surveillance, 130, 131
Ascending aortic size index (ascending
 ASI), 129
Auditory brainstem response (ABR), 188
Autism, 18
Autim spectrum disorder (ASD), 18
Autoimmune disease
 alopecia areata, 229
 pro-inflammatory cytokines, 228
 psoriasis, 229, 230
 psychiatric/psychological
 disturbances, 229
 risk of, 228
 vitiligo, 229

B

Bayley Scales, 180
Benton Facial Recognition Test, 176
Bicuspid aortic valve (BAV), 126

Bone anchored hearing aid system
 (BAHS), 193, 194
Bone mineral density (BMD), 113, 166,
 245, 246
Brachymetacarpia, 240, 241

C

Celiac disease
 clinical presentation, 209–211
 follow-up, 211
 immune-mediated inflammatory
 response, 207
 incidence of, 208
 management, 211
 pathophysiology, 208
 prevalence, 208
 screening, 209, 210
 symptoms, 208
Child Behavior Checklist (CBCL), 180
Cholesteatoma formation, 192
Chorionic villus sampling (CVS), 23
Chronic kidney disease, 147
Chronic otitis, 192
Cochlear implants, 195
Cochlear nerve, 187
Coeliac disease, 159
Color vision deficiency, 202
Complete decongestive physiotherapy
 (CDP), 223
Conductive hearing loss, 186, 188
Congenital/childhood cataracts, 202
Congenital heart disease
 aortic arch abnormalities, 126
 assessment, 125
 BAV, 126

© Springer Nature Switzerland AG 2020
P. Y. Fechner (ed.), *Turner Syndrome*,
https://doi.org/10.1007/978-3-030-34150-3